CODE BLUE

Inside America's Medical Industrial Complex

Also by Mike Magee

Basic Science for the Practicing Urologist

CODE BLUE

Inside America's Medical Industrial Complex

Mike Magee, MD

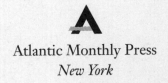

Atlantic Monthly Press
New York

FIRST EDITION

Published simultaneously in Canada
Printed in the United States of America

First Grove Atlantic hardcover edition: May 2019

This book was set in 11-point Janson Text LT by Alpha Design & Composition of Pittsfield, NH.

Library of Congress Cataloging-in-Publication data is available for this title.

ISBN 978-0-8021-2905-5
eISBN 978-0-8021-4687-8

Atlantic Monthly Press
an imprint of Grove Atlantic
154 West 14th Street
New York, NY 10011

Distributed by Publishers Group West

groveatlantic.com

19 20 21 22   10 9 8 7 6 5 4 3 2 1

To my wife, Trish, who encouraged me with these words—
"Write an important book."

CONTENTS

About the Title

"Code Blue" is the phrase customarily announced over hospital public address systems to alert the staff to an urgent medical emergency requiring immediate attention. It is a call to action and a request for specialized personnel and resources to resuscitate and stabilize the victim of some catastrophe, and eventually transport him or her to safety so that full recovery can begin. I chose the phrase as the title of this book to communicate my sense that the American health care system is in critical condition and that it urgently needs to be resuscitated. Ironically, the color blue is also associated with Pfizer and with its most famous product. The Pfizer company color is blue, and Wall Street and competitors often refer to Pfizer as "Big Blue." The Pfizer logo combines two shades of blue, French (#0070BF) and Vivid Cerulean (#00AFF0). Pfizer's most famous product, Viagra, is often called "the little blue pill."

Chapter 1

The Constant Gardener

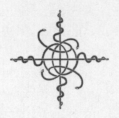

In 2005, my wife, Trish, and I went to see the film of John Le Carré's *The Constant Gardener*, a thriller about a pharmaceutical company's exploitation of Nigerian children in a corrupt clinical trial that leads to murder.[1] As we were walking out of the theater, Trish said, "That's based on Pfizer, isn't it?"

For me, that was a life-changing comment. For eight years I had been the physician-spokesman for Pfizer's most noted product, Viagra. For eight years I had been part of the large, well-financed team wheeling and dealing with the American Medical Association (AMA), the insurance industry, the academic research establishment, state and federal lawmakers, and government regulators all over the world. From the time I'd started there, I'd been astonished by the resources this single company had been able to marshal to launch this single drug—we lobbied the pope, after all. Yet until I turned away in a kind of revulsion at the manipulation and well-financed maneuvering, I was right in there, helping give moral cover and scientific legitimacy to the world's largest drugmaker, which also happens to be an industry leader in penalty fees paid to the government for regulatory infractions—$2.3 billion in 2009 for one settlement alone.[2]

I mention my experience with Viagra and Pfizer not just as a point of access to the much larger story I want to tell, but also because the new model of "corporate affairs on steroids" that Pfizer developed for this one drug has become standard operating procedure throughout the health care industry. And this raw corporate power is only one of the many imbalances and contradictions at the heart of the entire $4 trillion enterprise, an increasingly organized economic syndicate in which, as Saint Augustine said, "plunder is divided according to an agreed convention," and that now represents more than 20 percent of our total gross domestic product (GDP).

When Donald Trump expressed his cluelessness—"Nobody knew that healthcare could be so complicated"[3]—before a meeting of state governors in February 2017, he was referring to our approach to health *insurance*, which has been a political piñata whacked by both left and right for decades. But even when we Americans acknowledge the absurdity of our convoluted system of third-party payers, and the pretzel positions our politicians weave into and out of as they try to justify it, reform it, then unreform it, many still find solace in telling themselves, "Well, we still have the best health care in the world."

In point of fact, we're not even close to having the best health care in the world. As legendary Princeton health economist Uwe Reinhardt said, "At international health care conferences, arguing that a certain proposed policy would drive some country's system closer to the U.S. model usually is the kiss of death."[4] Our system is marked by extreme variability, a nation of health care haves and have-nots. The fortunate receive services from immensely talented and dedicated physicians, nurses, and other caregivers, and they have access to drugs, devices, and facilities that are the envy of the world. All others struggle just to stay healthy without going broke. Americans spend from 50 percent to 100 percent more on health care as a share of GDP than people in other industrialized countries do, and for all our high expenditure we get collective outcomes that are demonstrably worse.[5] In fact, we get outcomes that are, in general, truly dismal.

American women, on average, are three times as likely to die in pregnancy as British or Canadian women, with 28 deaths per 100,000 births versus just 8 in the United Kingdom and 11 in Canada.[6] In Germany and Japan, two countries whose universal health care systems were rebuilt from scratch by the American military as part of the Marshall

Plan following World War II, maternal deaths per 100,000 are 7 and 6, respectively. According to World Bank data, American children are about twice as likely to die in the first five years of life as are British, Canadian, German, or Japanese children.[7] A 2017 study by the Commonwealth Fund comparing the health care performance of 11 nations ranked the United States last in health system performance.[8] This was the same position the US held six years earlier when compared with 15 other industrialized nations. That study revealed that the US rates of premature death (the rate of preventable death amenable to timely and effective care) were 68 percent higher than those of the best-performing nations; this figure translated into 91,000 lives needlessly cut short each year.[9]

As for cost-efficiency, in the 2016 Bloomberg index of health care efficiency rankings of 55 nations, the only nations with lower scores than ours were Jordan, Colombia, Azerbaijan, Brazil, and Russia.[10] We pay on average *twice* as much for our drugs as any other developed nation does and waste $375 billion a year on billing and insurance-related services simply because we rely on a complex multi-payer system of insurers rather than having—like every other advanced economy in the world—a more streamlined and coordinated single-payer/multi-plan approach.[11] All of which contributes to Americans' receiving medical care that has consistently ranked *last* over the past decade among developed nations, not just in terms of efficiency and equity, but also in terms of overall quality, with the death rate from treatable diseases nearly 70 percent higher than the rates in Australia, France, and Sweden.[12]

Although health insurance is only one part of this sorry state of affairs, our approach to it underscores the core problem of our health care overall, a truth so fundamental and so blindingly obvious that we often overlook it. The simple fact is that nothing about our system was ever envisioned as a holistic way to logically and efficiently provide for the overall health and well-being of our nation's most valuable resource—our citizens.

Quite the contrary, our health care system's focus, at every phase of its development, but especially since its expansion and increasing sophistication after World War II, has been on maximizing opportunities for profit and/or career advancement for the players within it. Which helps explain why we now have a health care lobby *four times* the size of the lobbying effort run by the defense industry.[13] Which also helps explain why it's easier to get an MRI than a home health aide, and why, according to a 2012 Institute of Medicine report, we as a nation lose roughly $750 billion annually to unnecessary services, administrative excess, lax preventive measures, and medical fraud.[14]

I've been a physician in private practice, a senior administrator at one of the country's premier academic medical centers, an executive at the country's largest pharmaceutical company, a medical reporter and commentator, and, during the administration of George W. Bush, a candidate for surgeon general of the United States. I've waded through the quagmire at every level, from the trenches to the command center, and I've had many years to reflect, research, and analyze—to try to make sense of my experience and put it in the broadest and most meaningful context.

Accordingly, this book is much more than a string of horror stories about soulless hedge fund managers buying companies to jack up prices of lifesaving drugs for children, or mold-contaminated steroids causing outbreaks of meningitis, or an absurd and wasteful insurance system that only Rube Goldberg could have dreamed up. The book will tell some of those stories, but only as a way of directing our attention to two basic questions: How did we get into this mess, and what do we do about it now?

To address the second question—what do we do now?—I believe we truly need to understand the first: the developmental steps, starting decades ago, that led to the structure we now find ourselves forced to muddle through.

In his epilogue to *The Big Short*, Michael Lewis said that the reason American financial culture was so difficult to change was that "it had taken so long to create, and its assumptions had become so deeply embedded."[15] I think the same can be said of the culture of American health care. It is a system that includes many caring and committed professionals who labor tirelessly in the trenches; yet at the highest levels, that culture has become a self-serving network of vested interests that is, if anything, more dangerous and more harmful than the cabal of defense contractors, hawks, and saber-rattlers that, nearly 60 years ago, President Eisenhower labeled the military-industrial complex. The network of mutually beneficial relationships in health care weaves back and forth across the boundaries of big business, academic medicine, patient advocacy organizations, and government to create a fabric with the strength of Kevlar—a fabric I call the *Medical* Industrial Complex (MIC).

My focus is on examining how that fabric operates today, but I believe that understanding the weave requires seeing the present in a historical context, which means following the trajectory of medical care from the domain of patient, physician, and local pharmacist into the domain of global corporations, Wall Street mergers, K Street lobbyists, Byzantine insurance programs, political logrolling, and rampant greed with hidden profit-sharing tactics worthy of a crime syndicate.

My focus is on US health care, but here, too, it's only reasonable to widen the frame and look at other systems to compare and contrast. After all, there is no way to comprehend just how truly awful our system's performance is compared with that of other developed nations without some benchmark—in this case, the much higher population-wide levels of performance, patient satisfaction, and even physician income achieved at a much lower cost elsewhere.

This brings us back to the most fundamental question about a commitment to the people's health as a matter of national purpose. In France, the United Kingdom, Canada, Germany, Scandinavia, and almost anywhere else in the developed world, when an individual has a medical issue, he or she engages with the system without question or concern, knowing that access to care is a basic right of citizenship, the same way that police protection or protection by the nation's embassies for travelers abroad is a right. Individuals in other nations get this kind of access. So does a small segment of our population with resources and the good fortune of having insurance and high-quality health services nearby. But population-wide, medical services in other nations on the whole are both far superior and considerably cheaper than ours, because each of these societies made a determination that a healthy population was essential to the country's economic well-being, as well as to the national identity.

At a certain point, such a determination created the obligation to define what "a healthy population" means, and this led to the setting of priorities, which often included ways of promoting health that extended beyond the scope of health care per se, integrating planning for housing, education, jobs, nutrition, the environment, safety, and security. After establishing such goals, these countries set about budgeting and allocating resources in order to meet them.

In the United States, we never made that commitment. Instead, as we gained increasing leverage in our ability to fight disease, we simply doubled down on a prior commitment to preserve the widest range of entrepreneurial opportunities, believing somehow that market competition would save the day and produce the most modern, efficient, streamlined system possible.

Today's health care status quo was born in the immediate aftermath of World War II, as a product of American health care's original sin. Without undertaking dialogue or planning to support population-wide health, as the Canadians did, or the build-out of a universal health care system, as our military did under the Marshall Plan for our recently vanquished adversaries in Germany and Japan, our political and medical leaders gave way to the conceit that scientific ingenuity and innovation could defeat disease the way we had just defeated the Nazis. They believed that when disease was defeated, good health for our citizenry would be left in its wake. Profiteers chose cure over care and embraced federal funding, over-the-top advertising, and the overpromising of scientific discoveries. When costs exploded and discoveries lagged, they fanned the fear of "socialized medicine," eroded regulations, and finally supported a partial expansion of health coverage, but only after being granted concessions to ensure that the private-market status quo would remain intact. And with health care expenditures approaching one of every five American dollars, they offered to manage the burgeoning health care data and cost-control enterprise for a price, and quietly dealt every health sector player in—except the American patient.

Unfortunately, that American bias toward health care as a business rather than as a human right produced a system with unconscionable disparities between the haves and have-nots. But what locked a bad system in place was that, by the time policymakers got around to trying to mitigate some of the worst excesses in the 1970s and 1980s following the passage of Medicare, the entrepreneurial wheels were humming, and the foxes—if you'll forgive the mixing of metaphors—were already in charge of the henhouse. Endless special arrangements and inside deals led to a mind-boggling level of complexity and the institutionalization of blatant conflicts of interest that undermined even the best intentions.

If you want to understand how we fail in quality and excel in cost when our health care system is compared with that of almost any other developed nation—and why drug prices jumped by nearly 20 percent in 2017 alone while the general inflation rate for the same year was 1.7 percent—the Medical Industrial Complex is the place to look.[16] If you want to understand why the level of National Institutes of Health (NIH) research funding rises and falls in direct response to aggressive lobbying, while health insurers and health professionals actively question the integrity of medical research, the independence of the US Food and Drug Administration (FDA), and the safety, effectiveness, and affordability of pharmaceuticals—again, check out the MIC.

It's not just the high cost and inadequacy of health insurance that should alarm us, or drug companies' price gouging, or our nation's third-world rates of infant mortality, or the fact that by some estimates 250,000 Americans die of medical errors in our hospitals each year,[17] or that a teenage girl in Mississippi is 15 times more likely to give birth than her counterpart in Switzerland,[18] or the barriers to abortion being erected in some states, or why we can't get the same drug prices that are available in Canada for drugs manufactured in the United States, or why we keep seeing fraud by overly ambitious scientists in biomedical research labs. It's also the prescription opioid epidemic, hospital chains buying hugely expensive ads while costs skyrocket, cancer centers hustling patients out just before they die to keep the institutions' mortality ratings low, and drug companies engaging in pay-for-delay collusion to slow the introduction of lower-cost generics. And serving as croupiers at this casino are the insurance companies, which assign critical decisions to patients despite a 2016 Yahoo Finance–PolicyGenius survey showing that only 4 percent of Americans understand the following four terms: "deductible," "co-payment," "co-insurance," and "out-of-pocket maximum."[19]

The strength and durability of the Medical Industrial Complex lie in the fact that strange bedfellows from each of these domains—medicine, insurers, hospitals, pharmaceuticals—long ago developed interprofessional relationships, creating an integrated career path that allows individual players to slide easily from academic medicine to government to corporations and back again, always aware that their willingness to go along to get along in one arena can improve the quality of their placement in the next.

For more than a half century, the MIC elite have engaged in a twisted dialogue excoriating government intervention at the same time that they scramble for government subsidies, creating a new reality where health care "nonprofits" pay multimillion-dollar salaries to their CEOs to engage in the same tactics as the most ruthless corporate titans. At every turn, the potential rewards for the successful few are so great that any concept of the greater good seems quaint, if not subversive.

Cozy relationships and generous gratuities have demonstrated a remarkable ability to corrupt even those we would instinctively put on the side of the angels, including members of the biomedical research community, deans of medical schools, directors of continuing medical education programs, officers at the NIH and FDA, and even seemingly altruistic patient advocacy organizations like the American Cancer Society.

A theologian looking at all this might conclude that American health care has lost its soul. A behavioral economist would point us toward studies showing that the exercise of moral judgment in a business context draws on a completely different cognitive framework from the one we use in making such decisions in our personal lives. What was intended to be a meritocracy has morphed into a self-serving aristocracy. Unfortunately, health care is now seen by most of its decision-makers as all business all the time.

When you combine that outlook with the B-school mantra that "the CEO's only responsibility is to maximize shareholder value, period," you get Kent Thiry, head of the nation's largest chain of for-profit dialysis centers, DaVita Inc., who told UCLA business students in 2009 that he saw essentially no difference between running his business and operating a string of Taco Bells.[20] (It is worth noting that DaVita paid almost $1 billion to settle allegations of kickbacks and overcharging in 2015.)[21]

Perhaps an even more apt poster boy for the Medical Industrial Complex is Raymond Gilmartin, former CEO of the drugmaker Merck & Company. Between 1999 and 2003, 93 million prescriptions were written for Merck's painkiller Vioxx. The drug was taken by about 20 million Americans—sales averaged about $2.5 billion a year—even as Merck knew and concealed the fact that high doses of Vioxx tripled the risk of heart attack and sudden death. In fact, the Merck team continued to aggressively sell the drug not only for pain but also for a variety of off-label uses. The FDA estimated in 2004 that Vioxx may have resulted in 27,785 heart attacks, causing analysts to project $20 billion in liability.[22] After losing four of its first nine court cases, the company managed to settle claims at $5 billion.[23] CEO Gilmartin took an early retirement from Merck in 2006 with an undisclosed settlement. Where did Ray land? Teaching a course titled "Building and Sustaining Succesful Enterprises" at the Harvard Business School.[24]

In our society it is commonplace to go on about the need to promote a "healthy business climate." But the health and well-being of our citizens are an absolute necessity for the country's well-being, for a productive and secure workforce, and for a healthy America. The US is the only country in the world that spends more on health care than it does on all other social services combined. The good news is that we already commit enough dollars and human talent to create what could be the best health care system in the world—a single-payer/multi-plan system that is universal and holistic, and that efficiently distributes our vast resources fairly and equitably in a manner that supports healthy families in healthy homes, rather than simply chasing cures. Far from being socialized medicine, this system asks that as individuals and a nation we use valued resources responsibly, and that we invest in strategic health planning to ensure our citizens are productive and have the opportunity to reach their full human potential.

Showing how we might get there is what this book is all about.

Chapter 2

Intertwined

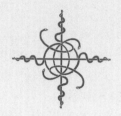

For more than a century, the most common symbol for all things medical in the United States has been the caduceus, the familiar winged rod with two snakes twined around it. It was adopted by the US Public Health Service in 1871 and incorporated by the US Army Medical Corps in 1902. The image was well intentioned but based on a shaky knowledge of the ancient Greeks. The more obvious symbol for medicine—also used today but not nearly as often—is the rod of Asclepius, a simple staff (no wings) with a single snake. Asclepius, son of Apollo, was the demigod of medicine. In contrast, the caduceus was the symbol of the messenger god Hermes, patron of commerce and trade—as well as thieves, liars, and gamblers.[1]

If there's irony here, it's a sad one, especially given that the joke would be on the American people. But when we assemble all the facts, it may be that using the caduceus, emblem of commerce and traders, to represent American medicine isn't so far off the mark after all.

Consider President Trump's second nominee to serve as the head of the US Department of Health and Human Services, Alex Azar. At a time when public anger at drug companies and at soaring drug prices has never been higher, Azar, the immediate past president of Lilly USA, was picked to oversee much of America's health care.[2] During his tenure at Lilly, the company dramatically raised the price of insulin in the United States—by 20.8 percent in 2014, 16.9 percent the following year, and 7.5 percent the year after that. Lilly's biggest insulin product, Humalog, costs more now than it did when it was introduced in 1996, even though its brand-name exclusivity has expired. In 2007, the price was $74 a vial. In 2017, it was $269. Rounding out the picture, Azar's Lilly also spent $5.7 million lobbying Congress and the Department Health and Human Services in 2016 alone.[3]

To take the symbolism further and associate all pharmaceutical executives directly with the snakes—or with the thieves, liars, and gamblers represented by the caduceus in ancient Greece—would be a clear overstatement. In fact, in my decade as a Pfizer employee, interacting with thousands of colleagues from the company and its competitors, I found that most believed their daily labor improved the lot of humanity. However, following through with the image of "intertwining"—as in the comingling of lobbying, political contributions, doctors, compliant politicians, and health care policy—the hidden realities are much different and provide a deeper understanding of what the Medical Industrial Complex is all about.

While pharmaceutical executives are certainly near the top of most Americans' list of the "archvillains" of health care, singling them out exclusively would be grossly unfair. We need to understand how their behavior intertwines with the behavior of other players in this system.

My own tribe, physicians, deserves its share of blame, but it's as a collective rather than as individuals that doctors have done the most to ensure the MIC syndicate's stranglehold on the nation's health. The biggest collective of physicians is the American Medical Association, and it is at the very center of the Medical Industrial Complex coil.

Often thought of as a bland and stodgy country club, the AMA is known to weigh in occasionally, to put its "Good Housekeeping" seal of approval, on this or that policy or procedure. In 2010, when the organization agreed to support the Patient Protection and Affordable Care Act, also known as Obamacare, it seemed to be taking an uncharacteristically progressive tack, but when we look through the lens of intertwined commerce, there is nothing surprising in this very conservative organization making a deal with a liberal president. The AMA's support for the Affordable Care Act was a quid pro quo for specific givebacks or assurances, such as resolving physician billing concerns and protecting historic federal funding of medical education and research. Suffice it to say that the average physician's salary climbed by 43 percent in the subsequent six years.[4] Then in 2017, returning to its historic, laissez-faire roots, and in a triumph of ideology over logic, the group threw its weight behind Donald Trump's first secretary of Health and Human Services, former orthopedist and congressman Tom Price, the leader of seven years' worth of legislative moves to destroy that selfsame Affordable Care Act.[5]

In resolving this seeming contradiction, bear in mind that both poles of the inconsistency are very much in keeping with the AMA's most fundamental purpose, which is to represent what it sees as the financial interests of its more than 200,000 members.[6] To understand the AMA's behavior, remember that it is a trade organization—not unlike the American Restaurant Association or the Screen Actors Guild—only with a membership that makes life-and-death decisions for the rest of us.

To serve the financial interests of its members, not primarily the health and well-being of the American people, the AMA maintains a political lobbying budget second only to that of the US Chamber of Commerce. As a trade organization, it publishes the *Journal of the American Medical Association* (*JAMA*), the largest-circulation medical weekly in the world, and also issues the Relative Value Scale Update, advising the US Centers for Medicare and Medicaid Services on appropriate billing amounts for medical procedures.[7] In this instance, the AMA, which throughout its history has railed against government involvement in health care, helps the government determine how much to pay its own members, providing the basis for allocating roughly $70 billion a year for physicians' patient-care services.

This strange-bedfellows relationship is but one small example of the intertwined threads of self-interest and the blurring of boundaries that are the heart and soul of the Medical Industrial Complex.

Code Blue will follow these basic threads—physicians, hospitals, drug companies, researchers, political influence—from where they originated to where they began to come together and reinforce one another. Later chapters will explore how government regulators, the insurance industry, aggressive marketers, expansion-oriented hospital chains, tobacco companies, religious zealots, and even nonprofit advocacy organizations were added to the weave, layer by layer.

But deep down in the heart of the tangle is the AMA, wielding tremendous power not just because of its political influence but because of its long-standing and well-cultivated prestige.

The AMA's imprimatur in and of itself bestows legitimacy, so the organization's approval has always been eagerly sought. But in keeping with a consistent pattern we'll see again and again, the purity of that imprimatur is not as carefully protected as it should be. In fact, the tacit approval implied by an affiliation with the AMA comes pretty cheap.

Any subspecialty organization, whether legitimate or scurrilous, can become a fully accredited satellite of the AMA by meeting a ridiculously low bar focused mostly on the parochial "trade organization" interests of the mother ship. The only concrete requirements for coming under the AMA aegis are that the applicant medical group must have been in existence for five years, at least 20 percent of its physician members must be members of the AMA, and the newly sanctioned affiliate must pledge to abide by AMA ethics and "cooperate with the AMA toward increasing its AMA membership."[8] Thus the AMA's acceptance of an affiliate requires no prospective quality evaluation, no oversight of any supposedly peer-reviewed journal, no assessment of the legitimacy of tax-deductible "continuing education" programs offered at luxury vacation spots, or any other meaningful appraisal of the affiliated organization's ethics or behavior.

It should come as no surprise, then, that the AMA Federation's institutional membership has ballooned to 121 societies. This list includes not only mainstay organizations like the American College of Surgeons and the American Academy of Pediatrics, but also recent, less notable entrants such as the American College of Mohs Surgery (dedicated to advancing the skin cancer treatment approaches championed by Frederic E. Mohs, MD), the Spine Intervention Society (dedicated to the practice of interventional procedures in the diagnosis and treatment of spine pain), and the Undersea and Hyperbaric Medical Society (dedicated to the science of undersea diving activities and hyperbaric oxygen therapy).

But as is so often the case within the MIC, seemingly small lapses in ethical safeguards can lead to serious consequences. Consider the American Association of Pain Medicine (AAPM), a fully accredited subspecialty organization under the aegis of the AMA.[9] It was created in 1983 with financial support from a company called Purdue Pharma, maker of what it had just introduced as the first "extended release" opioid pain pill. Partnered with a sibling institute at the University of Wisconsin, also supported by Purdue,[10] this AMA affiliate over the following decade and a half vigorously and all too successfully promoted the theory that chronic pain was being seriously undertreated and that Purdue's newest opioid product could be used liberally without fear of addiction. (How that product came to be approved by the FDA will come up later in the book.) To reinforce its selling proposition, and under AMA cover, the AAPM established its own specialty journal to publish "scientific" papers often written by Purdue-sponsored academicians.[11] These same individuals were then handsomely paid to speak at dinners sponsored by Purdue to promote the notion that aggressive prescribing of painkilling opioids was not only justified but essential.

But the AMA's collusion in enabling doctors to widely overprescribe a drug that was, in fact, highly addictive wasn't merely passive. Every medical student in the United States is assigned a lifetime identification number at the outset of training on entry to medical school. Whether a new physician is an AMA member or not, that identifying number becomes the property of the AMA. The AMA not only controls this Physician Masterfile database of 900,000 physicians but, for a healthy sum, licenses the information to a company that tracks physicians' prescribing behavior in a process known as prescription profiling, "unless an individual physician contacts the AMA and specifically 'opts-out.'"[12] The company then sells that information to every drug company in the United States. In fact, sales and royalties for proprietary data of this sort provide more than twice the revenue collected through membership dues.[13]

Using this precise, AMA-enabled tracking data, Purdue was able to direct its sales effort toward high prescribers of pain medications, enabling an army of 1,000 Purdue reps, backed by a first-year marketing budget of $200 million, to descend on these soft targets.[14]

Purdue's supposedly nonaddictive painkiller OxyContin is also known as "hillbilly heroin." According to a 2016 study by Yale University School of Medicine researchers, the drug is largely responsible for a 205 percent increase in hospitalization for toddlers, a 176 percent increase for teens, and the first widespread decline in longevity of white, middle-aged males in American history.[15]

How the AMA, with its maxim "First, do no harm," its Hippocratic oath, and its image as the prudent guardian of standards to protect Americans' health, came to play such a prominent role in creating an epidemic of addiction was neither an uncharacteristic ethical lapse nor an instance of a formerly noble organization being duped just this once by a commercial huckster. Rather, this example of "following the money" was merely the logical extension of the AMA's longtime modus operandi.

When the AMA was founded in 1847, the organization cloaked itself in virtue and set out under the banner of "scientific medicine" to expose medical charlatans. Admittedly, there was no shortage of hucksters and quacks to expose in the middle of the 19th century. However, given that, even among AMA adherents, drilling a hole in a patient's skull was accepted treatment for severe headache, and bloodletting was indicated for just about everything, "scientific" was a relative term. Thus, on closer examination, the way the AMA wielded "scientific" as a cudgel to restrict competition and to promote the financial interests of its own member doctors seems somewhat disingenuous. In certain lights, the AMA efforts in the late 19th century appear less a battle over scientific rigor and more an economic turf war, a conflict that, not surprisingly, had unintended and not entirely beneficial consequences.

The AMA admittedly did much good in establishing a code of ethics and nationwide standards for attaining the degree of medical doctor.[16] It also set out early on to determine the value of anesthetic agents in medicine, surgery, and obstetrics; to expose the dangers of patent medicines;

to advance public health standards; and to recommend that state governments register births, marriages, and deaths.[17]

But in its self-protective zeal, the AMA also greatly restricted the number of avenues that medical progress could take. In the AMA's view, the "one true church" of healing was established in the 18th century by the followers of Dr. Benjamin Rush, who, during the Philadelphia 1793 epidemic of yellow fever, promoted what was called "heroic medicine." The term was meant to suggest not that doctors were running into burning buildings to save their patients, but rather that they embraced a therapeutic model of aggressive treatment focused less on care than on cure, which included not only bloodletting and trepanation (drilling holes in the skull) but purging and sweating.[18] According to this school of thought, illness was caused by an imbalance among the "four humors"—a holdover from medieval medicine—and symptoms such as fever were not the body's attempt to fight the disease but rather complications that would only make the patient's condition worse. Thus practitioners believed that a fever should be suppressed with powerful drugs given in large dosages. With the medical elite promoting such aggressive interventions throughout the 18th and much of the 19th centuries, even treatments that had been found effective in the past, including healthy doses of supportive care, were relegated to the realm of dangerous and backward folklore.[19]

Some have observed that the odds of actually benefiting from an encounter with a physician tilted in the patient's favor around the year 1900, and certainly the "heroic" approach is one reason that before the 20th century, patients would have been wise to keep the doctor at bay. "Heroic" doctors subjected women to bloodletting even during childbirth and intentionally blistered the skin of febrile patients and viewed the second-degree burns that quickly became pus-filled as drawing infection from the body.[20] Even George Washington, lying on his deathbed in 1799, was bled repeatedly and given calomel and several blisters of cantharidin to induce sweating. Not surprisingly, the nation's first president died not long after the encounter.[21]

But beyond the brutalities inflicted on individual patients over the centuries—technical intrusions into childbirth and breastfeeding, frontal lobotomies, and radical mastectomies—the AMA helped reinforce the view that disease is an enemy to be fought, rather than a manifestation of natural processes that need to be redirected. This view persists to this day, especially in end-of-life care. Many doctors still consider death a defeat. Rather than extend comfort during the inevitable, they throw everything they've got into the battle, then abruptly walk away when "everything" begins to fail, severing whatever relationship they might have developed with the dying person. These "heroic" measures lead to emotional distress, phenomenal waste, and pointless suffering, especially inasmuch as studies show that even if the goal is to prolong life, no matter how compromised a life may be, the best way to do it is often by doing less, which is to say, by providing palliative care only.

But above all, the AMA codified a procedure-heavy, business-oriented view of medicine that involves protecting market share and a fee-for-service model, whether or not the service being provided is truly necessary, or even in the patient's best interest. Which brings us back to the idea of competition between conflicting medical models.

One of the AMA's primary targets in its nominal search for charlatans was a gentler, more holistic approach called homeopathy that arose in the 18th century as, in point of fact, a check on the ascendance of "heroic" medicine. Homeopaths argued that aggressive treatments meant to jolt the body back into health were often worse than the disease, and that the "heroic's" underlying theories, such as the belief that many diseases were the result of excess fluids, were way off the mark.[22]

Homeopaths—a term derived from the Greek words for "same" and "suffering"—called heroic medicine allopathic, a term derived from the Greek for "different" and "suffering." Homeopaths believe that the body should be returned to its natural state of health by applying techniques and medications that work in alignment with the body's natural healing processes (i.e., the symptoms of the disease being treated).

The German physician Samuel Hahnemann, who coined both terms, was the major rival of Benjamin Rush during colonial times. His challenge to Rush's emphasis on invasive cures was unambiguous. During the yellow fever epidemic, he said, "My sense of duty would not easily allow me to treat the unknown pathological state of my suffering brethren with these unknown medicines. The thought of becoming in this way a murderer or malefactor towards the life of my fellow human beings was most terrible to me."[23]

Hahnemann was the lodestar for physician followers who founded the American Institute of Homeopathy in New York City in 1844, after which schools of homeopathy began to pop up everywhere.[24] By the close of the 19th century, 22 such institutions and more than 100 homeopathic hospitals were treating approximately 15 percent of all Americans, while the allopaths banded together under the AMA banner were working diligently to put homeopaths out of business.

The AMA also attacked a third approach, called osteopathic medicine, founded in 1874 by Andrew Taylor Still.[25] Dr. Still pioneered wellness and whole-body medicine that championed the use of hands-on treatments for diagnosis, pain relief, and improved blood flow and an expanded range of motion that today sounds about as wacky and threatening as yoga or Pilates.

Many of these "unscientific" notions, driven underground by the AMA, especially the notion of wellness and prevention advanced by functional-medicine internists, have now reentered the mainstream and are seen by many as valuable supplements, if not alternatives, to the brand of expensive, invasive, and mechanistic high-tech medicine long championed by the AMA. But on an even more sophisticated level, today's renewed focus on the microbiome—meaning the patient's own specific ecology as it responds to and at times collaborates with microbes or invasive agents, including cancer cells—along with the new, comprehensive, uniform theory of inflammation, especially in autoimmune disease, could be said to draw directly on concepts promulgated by Hahnemann when he first came into allopathic medicine's crosshairs.

The point is not to say that homeopathy was right and that the AMA's stated goal of greater scientific rigor was wrong. But a case can be made that biomedical science might be further along in dealing with cancer, autoimmune disease, and so many of the ailments we associate with an aging and stiffening body if our search image had not been restricted by the AMA's self-serving insistence on suppressing all alternative approaches.

Unfortunately, the AMA saw itself, its new *Journal of the American Medical Association*, and its state and county medical societies and credentialing bodies as the sole guardians of scientific truth. The organization, funded by member dues and burgeoning advertising fees from growing pharmaceutical, chemical, tobacco, and food industries, teed up the historic alignment of money, power, and product that persists uninterrupted to this day.

At the dawn of the 20th century, the AMA began to consolidate its influence over American medicine by taking charge of physician training. In 1904, when 28,000 students were enrolled at 155 different medical schools, the AMA created the Council on Medical Education (CME) as the certifying body for all training leading to the degree of medical doctor.[26] The CME's first recommendation established minimal entry requirements; the second codified the course requirements for the first two years of classroom instruction and insisted that these years be followed by two more years of intense learning with direct patient exposure.

These recommendations had very little impact until 1908, when the CME, funded by the Carnegie Foundation, hired the renowned educator Abraham Flexner to complete a formal study of medical education in the United States and Canada.[27] Flexner visited all 155 medical schools and found that only 16 required applicants to have completed at least two years of university education before admission. The quality of the professors' medical knowledge was highly variable, which was not surprising given that many of the schools were proprietary ventures run to make a profit.

Flexner recommended, among other things, that 124 of the 155 schools be closed, that prerequisites for medical training be greatly expanded, that training in the scientific method and research be emphasized, that medical schools assume responsibility for in-hospital clinical training, and that state medical licensure become standardized nationwide.[28]

By 1920, the AMA, aggressive and organized, was firmly in charge of American medicine. Seventy of the country's 155 medical schools had disappeared, and the number of medical students, at 13,800, had been cut in half. By 1935, only 66 schools remained, and 57 of those were part of a university.[29,30]

All this was definitely progress, spearheaded by the AMA, but to some extent the doctors' organization had thrown several babies out with the bathwater. Eventually the AMA succeeded in putting most homeopathic physicians out of business (at least in the US; in Europe, homeopathy is very much in the mainstream), and homeopathic health systems either disappeared or converted to allopathic. The AMA's campaign to discredit osteopathic medicine was less successful, and the osteopathic schools, which granted the degree of doctor of osteopathy (DO), held on.[31]

In the 1930s, showing consistency in its guildlike effort to limit competition, the AMA was less than helpful in assisting foreign-trained medical professionals fleeing Nazi Germany.[32] The organization's attempt to prevent its members from working for early health maintenance organizations that briefly flowered during the Great Depression, like the medical cooperative established to help struggling farmers by Dr. Michael Shadid in Elk City, Oklahoma, in 1929, earned it a federal conviction in 1943 for violating the Sherman Anti-Trust Act.[33,34] Even AMA's support for the concept that certain medicines should be by prescription only had a business component that served its pharmaceutical allies, providing a legal fig leaf for the drug companies to use the intervention of a "learned intermediary" as a plausible defense against corporate lawsuits.[35]

During World War II, the AMA and everything else gave way to the primacy of FDR's war effort. But with the peace, the AMA quickly reasserted itself in opposing President Harry Truman's effort to create a single-payer system of national health care. Seven months into his presidency, Truman proposed a national health care plan focused on the needs of children and rural Americans, arguing that health care, like education, "should be recognized as a definite public responsibility." The AMA was quick to respond, going on the offensive and hiring the public relations firm Whitaker and Baxter to manage a $4 million public campaign funded by a $25 special fee levied on each of its physician members. Truman challenged the organization, saying, "I put it to you. Is it un-American to visit the sick, aid the afflicted or comfort the dying? I thought that was simple Christianity."[36] But the AMA had no compunction about exploiting America's newly rekindled fear of communism to attack the plan as "socialized medicine." Prefiguring Joseph McCarthy's witch hunts just a few years later, the AMA went so far as to target members of Truman's White House as being followers of "the Moscow party line," and the proposal went down in defeat.[37]

The AMA's red-baiting scare tactics, much like the NRA's gun hysteria today, prevailed through the placid 1950s. But when pressure for federal health insurance resurfaced as part of John F. Kennedy's New Frontier, the doctors promoted what they called "spontaneous" activism to fight the advent of Medicare and Medicaid, describing these now popular and successful programs in apocalyptic terms. AMA spokesperson Dr. Edward Annis stated at the time, "We doctors fear that the American public is in danger of being blitzed, brainwashed, and bandwagoned."[38]

Not until 1962 did the organization tacitly acknowledge the equivalency of an MD and a DO.[39] In the following decades, homeopathy began to reassert itself in the form of natural medicines and healing techniques, as well as an emphasis on consumer-driven health and prevention. Similarly, a new awareness of the benefits of movement therapies and massage made ordinary citizens far more willing to consult an osteopath and a range of other hands-on functional healers.[40]

Out of touch with larger societal trends, the AMA began to lose membership in the 1970s. Currently, less than one-quarter of America's physicians belong to the organization; yet its influence today is stronger than ever, in part because of its remarkable political dexterity funded through nonmember revenue streams, including the journals and databases it licenses to generate more than 50 percent of its revenue.[41]

The legacy of the AMA in establishing a more empirical medicine is, of course, a huge positive. Yet in so doing, it also ensured that American medicine would narrowly adhere to an "industrial model" with a sometimes dehumanizing reliance on technology, when the incorporation of more humanistic and holistic approaches could have taken us further, faster, and accomplished more. The AMA's narrow and aggressive approach also established medicine as first and foremost a business, and like any business, one that must focus on profitability by selling products and sophisticated procedures to continually expand market share.

In selling products, the AMA's foremost partner would be America's drug manufacturers.

At first a competing power center, but now a close ally within the Medical Industrial Complex, the American drug industry arose in the same 19th-century milieu that gave rise to the AMA. These were the days of medicine shows featuring snake oil salesmen who traveled from town to town to hawk commercial elixirs. By the turn of the 20th century, this form of swindling and chicanery began to coalesce into a reputable industry. But the prior preponderance of dubious "patent medicines" was such that when legitimate medicines came along, provided by corporate-minded chemical manufacturers like Eli Lilly, George Merck, and Charles Pfizer, these manufacturers began to refer to their products as "ethical drugs" in order to create distance from all manner of cures being peddled at the time. Even so, the 1897 Sears, Roebuck catalog still offered a syringe and a small amount of cocaine for $1.50; and laudanum, a "whole opium" preparation, was seen as an all-purpose remedy and consumed the way Advil is these days.[42]

Today, the manufacturing and the sale of pharmaceuticals are a heavy industry, tightly regulated by the government, and yet the degree to which it has fundamentally risen above its snake oil roots is open to debate. This sector of the Medical Industrial Complex employs something on the order of 1,100 highly trained federal lobbyists, more than two for each member of Congress. The Center for Responsive Politics estimates that the drug companies spent $280 million on Capitol Hill in 2017 alone, a 12 percent increase over 2016 spending. They also poured $58 million into the 2016 election.[43] All of which adds up to a very persuasive "medicine show."

During the era when the AMA was founded, pills and tailored doses were still largely made by hand, tinctures were created by maceration or percolation, and ointments were combined with a mortar and pestle. Chemists and druggists developed their own specific products such as cough syrups or worm eradicators or ointments for scabies. But then technical innovations created incentives for large-scale production, beginning with the soft gelatin capsule, introduced in 1834; cocoa butter, introduced in 1852, which launched a worldwide surge in suppositories; and especially the subcutaneous injection, introduced in 1855, which allowed rapid absorption of medications like opioids and heroin.[44]

The pioneers who moved the drug industry from fly-by-night to a more secure place in the community were often chemists like the young German immigrant cousins Charles Pfizer and Charles Erhardt, who arrived in Brooklyn in 1849 with a plan to make products that were safe and effective.[45] They launched their enterprise with an antiparasitic compound called santonin that paid the bills, but then they reached an entirely new level of success in 1880 when they began to produce citric acid, a natural preservative found highly concentrated in lemons, oranges, and limes that extended the shelf life of foods and beverages. By 1917, when WWI all but eliminated the supply lines for natural fruit, an American food chemist named James Currie was experimenting with the mold *Aspergillus niger*, and he published a paper proving that it was an extremely efficient driver of citric acid production.[46] Pfizer scooped up Currie after the war, and by 1919 the company was making a fortune producing the stuff, much of it being sold to makers of sugary beverages like Coca-Cola to balance the sweetness and create a tart, refreshing flavor.[47]

Pfizer applied the same fermentation techniques to producing gluconic acid (used as a food preservative and cleanser) as well as ascorbic acid (vitamin C).[48] Its expertise in fermentation grew, as did its plant, with deeper and larger fermentation tanks replacing shallow pans and flasks—knowledge and facilities that would come in handy 20 years later when the world was once again at war and looking to scale up production of a different mold that would serve as the world's first "wonder drug," penicillin.[49] By then, the world of "ethical drugs"—those with ingredients displayed on their labels and distributed by the medical profession—was crowded with competitors.

In 1873, another chemist, Eli Lilly, set up a medicinal wholesale company in Indianapolis, Indiana. With three employees, including his then 14-year-old son, Josiah, Lilly expanded his business rapidly, with a sixfold increase in sales in his first two years.[50]

A few years later, Lilly sent Josiah off to the new Philadelphia College of Pharmacy and Science, and the young man graduated in 1882, just as the company gained the rights to produce and sell its first proprietary medicine, Succus Alterans, used for the treatment of venereal disease. When Eli died in 1898, Josiah became president of the company. In 1907, Josiah's son, Eli Junior, joined as the head of finance.[51]

Eli Lilly's first serious breakthrough came in 1895, when he discovered gel capsules as a way to package medicines for easy consumption. The capsules not only preserved the dose until it was ready to be consumed; they also served therapeutic purposes by allowing timed release and improved absorption. By 1917, the company had mastered and refined the same straight-line production techniques that were being employed by Henry Ford—techniques capable of producing 2.5 million capsules a day.[50] Raw materials came in at one end, and with the aid of conveyers, chutes, and pulleys, they exited at the other end in seven different sizes as finished products.[51] Supply, as Lilly saw it, was now properly positioned to keep pace with growing demand.

Despite the distance companies like Lilly and Pfizer had traveled from the world of snake oil, they were still largely on the sidelines when it came to basic scientific research during the first three decades of the 20th century. This was partly the result of the AMA's proprietary attitude regarding who was qualified to contribute. In 1915, the AMA's Council on Pharmacy stated, "It is only from laboratories free from any relation with manufacturers that real pharmaceutical advances can be expected."[52] In typical "we alone are keepers of the flame" fashion, the physician leaders held to—or at least espoused—the belief that profit and research didn't mix.

But medicine was undergoing a revolution, and Eli Junior saw no reason why drug companies shouldn't be a part of it. In 1910, Sigmund Freud had organized the International Psychoanalytical Society.[53] In that same year the US Bureau of Mines, with the US Public Health Services, began a study of lung diseases in miners.[54] Sickle-cell anemia had just been described as a disease.[55] The AMA began to attribute death by heart attack to "hardening of the arteries."[56,57] The American Society for the Control of Cancer (the forerunner of the American Cancer Society) was established with the aid of John D. Rockefeller, and the first X-ray machine was put into use.

Offsetting these medical advances, World War I killed 16.6 million people, including 6.8 million civilians.[58] The Spanish flu followed, killing in 1918 and 1919 nearly 5 percent of the entire human population.[59] Cholera, malaria, the plague, polio, smallpox, diphtheria, syphilis, gonorrhea, hookworm, and typhus struck millions more. And while infectious diseases and traumatic injuries took the greatest human toll, and consumed the majority of public resources, by 1920 changing survival rates caused entrepreneurs like Eli Junior to start focusing on the chronic diseases that afflicted those well along in years. Life expectancy for newborns in the US, with improvements in water, food, transportation, and housing, had risen from 47 years to 57 years in the two decades between 1900 and 1920. Eli Junior envisioned acute diseases giving way to those that would require long-term management and, most important, long-term intake of prescription medicines.[60] He was fond of saying, as he did in December 1918, "Ideas don't cure people. Drugs cure people. That's why we must bring the research scientists and the drug manufacturers together."[61]

He was also keen on starting a medical research arm inside the company, and the man he found to drive the effort was George H. (Alec) Clowes, a bench scientist who had spent the previous eighteen years at Roswell Park Memorial Institute, a cancer laboratory and hospital in Buffalo, New York.[62,63] Eli Junior hired him and gave him free rein to find the next big discovery in medicine.

Almost immediately, on December 28, 1921, Clowes sought out J.J.R. Macleod and Frederick Grant Banting at the American Physiological Meeting in New Haven, Connecticut. The diabetes researchers from the University of Toronto had been working with an extract secreted by the islets of Langerhans, groupings of specialized insulin excreting cells within the pancreas.[64] By injecting this extract, called isletin, into a lab animal whose pancreas had been removed, they had managed to lower soaring blood sugar levels by 40 percent. The only catch was that purifying eight ounces of isletin, later known as "insulin," required two and one half tons of beef or pork pancreas just to get started.[65]

Clowes made the case that the scientists needed the resources of a commercial firm, and that Lilly would be more than happy to partner with this academic lab, bankrolling the research with full support not just for purification and large-scale production, but for dosage setting and marketing as well. As Clowes put it, "This will take corporate horsepower"—an observation that would be repeated ever after as the mantra for the Medical Industrial Complex.[66]

The scientists rejected Clowes outright. Unfazed, he rushed to the nearest Western Union office in New Haven and wired his boss a three-word report: "This is it."

Hoping to provide their discovery at low cost to those needing it, the scientists had already sold the patent to the University of Toronto for one dollar. For almost a year, the university tried to scale up production on its own and failed miserably. Faced with unprecedented demand and little if any supply, the university called Clowes, who had been waiting patiently in Indianapolis. The university worked out a deal with Lilly to become sole distributor for one year, royalty-free, in exchange for 28 percent of each batch.[67] Again, the hope was that if drug companies acquired the rights at little or no expense, they would keep their prices low and even the poorest would benefit.

Accordingly, in those early days of insulin therapy, price was not a major concern, but the larger issue arose almost immediately and haunts the Medical Industrial Complex to this day—the question of fair and equal access to lifesaving medicines.

In April 1919, a young girl named Elizabeth Hughes was diagnosed with diabetes. She was not just any Hughes—she was the daughter of Charles Evans Hughes, two-time governor of New York and an associate justice on the US Supreme Court, who had resigned from the bench to become the Republican Party candidate for president in 1916.[68]

The girl's condition had grown perilous just as word of Banting and Macleod's remarkable new drug got out. Judge Hughes went directly to University of Toronto president Robert Falconer and begged for a special privilege. Hughes, who would later return to the Supreme Court as chief justice, wanted this drug for his daughter no matter who else had to do without, and he was not above calling attention to the million-dollar grant made to the university by the Rockefeller Foundation, whose board included Hughes's friend and church mate John D. Rockefeller Jr. Elizabeth Hughes was the third patient treated.[69]

The relationship between Lilly and the University of Toronto established the precedent of academic research institutions and pharmaceutical companies partnering to create massive supplies of high-quality medicines. What lagged behind was the creation of a body of law that would protect patients from abusive or fraudulent treatment while also ensuring equal access to the new medicines coming.

By the time Elizabeth Hughes died in 1981, at age 74, she had received more than 42,000 insulin injections, yet she expunged all references to diabetes in her father's papers. Both to protect herself and to protect her father's reputation, she went so far as to destroy all pictures of herself taken during the period of her declining health in childhood.[70] In Judge Hughes's official biography, a two-volume comprehensive summary of his life published under Elizabeth's supervision, there is no mention of her illness whatsoever.[71,72]

For Justice Hughes, a student of ethics, law, and religion, this represented an uncharacteristic ethical lapse. For the Medical Industrial Complex, his placement of personal needs and priorities above established rules and norms was just a small taste of the many lapses to come, when conflicts of interests—whether personal, financial, or political—would color life-and-death decisions.

Today, price is the greatest barrier to equal access to medicines, and price gouging is a fact of life—and often a matter of life and death—even with hundred-year-old medicines like insulin. Americans with diabetes pay more than the citizens of any other country, spending an average of $571.69 per month on diabetes costs.[73] Even with insurance, this means that some Americans spend almost half their income just managing their condition. There are documented accounts of diabetics setting up GoFundMe campaigns to pay for insulin, then dying when they came up short. In 2017, a 26-year-old diabetic was found dead in his Minnesota apartment after rationing his insulin because he had "aged out" of health coverage under his parents' plan.[73]

Multiple state attorneys general are currently investigating charges of price-fixing by the original producer, Eli Lilly. The company is also named in a class-action lawsuit alleging that it colluded with two other drug companies, Sanofi and Novo Nordisk—the three together controlling more than 90 percent of the global market—to artificially inflate US prices of insulin. One issue under examination is a pay-for-delay scheme in which Sanofi paid Eli Lilly to hold off launching an insulin similar to its Lantus brand.[74]

You would think that patient advocacy groups would be up in arms, but as will be explored later in *Code Blue*, many of these groups are, in fact, heavily subsidized by drug companies. And the most chilling aspect of all this appears when drug companies defend their policies with the term "value-based pricing." In other words, these are lifesaving drugs, so it only makes sense to charge an arm and a leg. You want to stay alive, you pay the price. But then the Medical Industrial Complex is all about the health of the industry, not the health of all Americans.

Chapter 3

Government Steps In

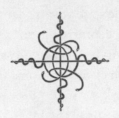

When investigators entered the lab on October 2, 2012, they found dirty floor mats and ventilation hoods, guck floating in vials of medicine, and a "clean room" infested with bugs and mice. The sterilization equipment was coated with a greenish-yellow residue; mold and bacteria seemed to be just about everywhere; and even though quality control required consistent temperature and humidity, the air-conditioning was shut off every night.[1]

According to the Centers for Disease Control and Prevention, these were the conditions that led the New England Compounding Center (NECC) of Framingham, Massachusetts, to expose some 13,000 people to fungal meningitis. In all, 732 people were made sick by contaminated injections of steroids, and 64 died.[2]

Compounding pharmacies like NECC are authorized by a confusing combination of federal and state authorities to mix and match existing medicines to create tailor-made capsules and injectable medications at precise dosages for individual customers, but regulation is left largely to the states' pharmacy boards. Originally focused on fulfilling small customized orders from physicians or retail pharmacies, compounding pharmacies in increasing numbers have enlarged their operations and extended well beyond good manufacturing practices.[3] As with everything else associated with the Medical Industrial Complex, boundaries tend to slip and slide, and these institutions have grown over the years to become, in effect, full-scale drug manufacturers, only without federal oversight.[4]

The unfortunate lesson of the NECC disaster is that the moment regulation slips up and relies on the varying good intentions of financially strapped and highly variable state governments, we find ourselves back in the Wild West of the 19th century, where "anything goes" was the only rule for drug manufacturing, and snake oil salesmen made quick profits by fleecing the gullible with claims, potions, and miracle cures that could just as easily do nothing or kill you.

Leading the charge to corral the Wild West for the better part of a century has been the Food and Drug Administration. Housed within the Department of Health and Human Services, the FDA oversees everything from food safety to sperm donations to tobacco products, dietary supplements, prescription and over-the-counter drugs, vaccines, biopharmaceuticals, blood transfusions and medical devices, electromagnetic-radiation emitting devices, and cosmetics, as well as animal foods and feed.[5] The commodities under its purview represent more than $1 trillion in annual consumer spending, and its 2017 budget was $5.1 billion.

Yet the FDA is often no match for the forces working against it from within the Medical Industrial Complex, a syndicate of overachievers who, in the words of Yale Law School professor Daniel Markovits, have turned America's meritocracy into a "modern-day aristocracy."[6] The FDA has headquarters in White Oak, Maryland, as well as 223 field offices and 13 laboratories nationwide. It also posts employees to foreign countries ranging from China to Costa Rica.[7] It sends consumer safety officers from its Office of Regulatory Affairs out to inspect production and warehousing facilities and to investigate complaints, illnesses, or outbreaks. Investigators from its Office of Criminal Investigations—the officers who carry guns—focus on criminal cases such as fraudulent claims and knowingly shipping adulterated goods in interstate commerce.[8] These are the agents that some say should have been more vigilant in shutting down the compounding pharmacy in Framingham before it exposed 13,000 people to meningitis.

In fact, the FDA had been asking Congress for years to give it stronger, clearer authority to police operations just like the Framingham compounding pharmacy, but the free-market mantra has always been that the agency "has enough power as it is" and that states can manage the rest. After the meningitis outbreak, though, leaders of every stripe pilloried the FDA for failing to act on reports of unsafe practices at the facility dating back as far as 2002.[5]

Waiting until *after* a catastrophe seems to be an all too familiar pattern in the US government's effort to regulate anything that might conceivably interfere with the health of the health care business itself. From the very beginning of regulation, players within the Medical Industrial Complex have submitted only when forced by some egregious crime or calamity, and then done everything they could, including falsifying and manipulating research and evidence, to wiggle out from under any constraints on business as usual. And when it comes to drug regulation, progress, as we will shortly see, often requires not only a disaster, but one that involves the nation's children.

As early as 1820, the US Department of Agriculture's chief chemist, then Peter Collier, encouraged federal legislation to address the widespread food adulteration he had uncovered. But over the next 25 years, more than 100 attempts at corrective legislation were defeated by a coalition of food and drug producers, as well as the magazine and newspaper publishers who benefited from the producers' advertising dollars. The collusion was blatant, but sometimes hard to sort out because of all the overlapping threads.

Now, 200 years later, those threads have become even more numerous and more complicated, involving multiple layers of regulation, lobbyists, and corrupted legislators intent on skirting consumer protections. A recent example involves the Drug Enforcement Administration (DEA), which operates under the US Department of Justice and is tasked with combating drug smuggling, the use of illegal drugs, and the illegal sale of prescription drugs, a role that puts it on the front lines against the rampaging opioid epidemic.

One technique used by the agency is to monitor suspicious shipments of opioids being moved by distributors—huge truckloads of resalable drugs going to out-of-the-way places that couldn't possibly have a legitimate need for so much medication. In one case, the sole pharmacy in Kermit, West Virginia, population 392, received nearly 9 million pills of hydrocodone (OxyContin) during a two-year period. The *Charleston Gazette-Mail* reported that between 2007 and 2012, out-of-state distributors poured nearly 800 million painkillers into West Virginia—a state that has borne the brunt of the opioid crisis. These were clear red flags that warranted the attention of the DEA.[9]

But Congressman Tom Marino (R-PA) objected to aggressive enforcement when it came to such massive and highly irregular shipments, and he sponsored legislation to, in effect, put blinders on the DEA and slow it down.[10] In 2016, Congress passed his bill, which was nobly called the Ensuring Patient Access and Effective Drug Enforcement Act. In describing the legislation, the DEA chief administrative law judge John Mulrooney wrote, "If it had been the intent of Congress to completely eliminate the DEA's ability to ever impose an immediate suspension on distributors or manufacturers, it would be difficult to conceive of a more effective vehicle for achieving that goal."[11]

Later, it came to light that Congressman Marino had received $100,000 in donations from political action committees aligned with drug wholesalers. Marino's chief of staff, who shepherded the bill, was Bill Tighe, who went on to become a lobbyist for the National Association of Chain Drug Stores. The actual author of the bill was D. Linden Barber, an executive at Cardinal Health, a major drug distribution company at the center of mega-sales of opioids. Equally disturbing, Barber had previously served as associate chief counsel for the DEA, and thus knew exactly how to throw a monkey wrench into the enforcement machinery.[11,12]

Adding insult to injury, in 2017, President Trump nominated Congressman Marino to serve as head of the White House's Office of National Drug Control Policy, often referred to as "American drug czar," and thus the go-to guy for all matters drug-related. Fortunately, when the backstory of the Ensuring Patient Access and Effective Drug Enforcement Act was exposed by *60 Minutes* and the *Washington Post*, Marino withdrew his name from consideration.[12]

*   *   *

Whether blatant or subtle, corrupt or aboveboard, resistance to regulation has been standard operating procedure within the Medical Industrial Complex since the government first tried to rein in the pharmaceutical free-for-all in 1848. This was the year when Congress authorized the underfunded and undermanned US Customs Service to inspect imported drugs and homegrown remedies, and to destroy those found to be dangerous or adulterated.[13] Unimpressed by this limited effort, the Women's Christian Temperance Union continued to push for stronger and more expansive legislation, and between 1870 and 1900, 190 bills were proposed in Congress to give the government real power to ensure the purity and safety of food and drugs.

To no one's surprise, all but a meaningless handful of the propositions were defeated by a coalition of wholesale and retail pharmaceutical firms, along with news outlets and journals that benefited from unregulated advertising.[13] As an FDA historian recounted, "In the same era, thousands of so called 'patent medicines' such as 'Kick-a-poo Indian Sawa' and 'Warner's Safe Cure for Diabetes' reflected both the limited medical ability of the period and the public acceptance of the doctrine that the buyer could and should look out for himself." Attempts at regulation were met with "strenuous opposition from whiskey distillers and patent medicine firms who were then the largest advertisers in the country."[14]

The US Public Health Service was coming into its own during this same period, but its focus was on epidemic diseases, not drugs. John Adams created the service's predecessor, a series of maritime hospitals for sick and disabled seamen, in 1798. Outbreaks of yellow fever and smallpox eight decades later had led to quarantines and calls to organize something more substantial. In 1889, Congress created the US Public Health Service Commissioned Corps. By 1900, with the encouragement of the AMA, it had expanded its focus to include sanitation and hygiene but still had no involvement in monitoring the safety of medicines or the rampant abuse of alcohol and narcotics.

Selling toxic drugs had never been a good business model, but in fact the practice was not actually prohibited until Congress passed the Biologics Control Act of 1902, and even then the death of a five-year-old

St. Louis girl was needed to spur action.[15] At that time, diphtheria, a
bacterially transmitted disease, was the leading killer of young people,
with 200,000 cases and 15,000 deaths in 1900 alone. The little girl had
come down with tetanus a few days after receiving a diphtheria antitoxin.
This drug had been prepared by injecting horses with progressive doses
of diphtheria toxin, then harvesting the horses' antibody-rich serum and
purifying it, for injection into humans to produce immunity. Shortly after
the girl's death, her two siblings met a similar fate, and an investigation
revealed that a donor horse had tetanus.[16]

These deaths caused an uproar, and ensuing public pressure led
to the 1902 law that regulated the sale of serums and toxins involved
in interstate or foreign commerce. An ill-prepared US Public Health
Service was put in charge of licensing all producers of biological products applicable to human disease, but then the uproar died down and
the pressure ceased. Besides, as further tragedies would show, including the 1938 death of 104 children who ingested a poison-laced elixir
of sulfanilamide for strep throat, the 1902 law was a fairly toothless
attempt at control.[15]

All the same, this was the Progressive Era, when crusading jour-
nalists known as muckrakers tried to expose the outrageous practices of
corrupt politicians and the robber barons of big business. One of the
movement's great successes was Ida Tarbell's book *The History of the
Standard Oil Company*, in which she condemned overachiever John D.
Rockefeller's ruthless business tactics. Congress by then had passed the
Sherman Anti-Trust Act of 1890, which effectively split up Rockefeller's
monolithic oil empire.[17]

Less well known was the 1905 book *The Great American Fraud*, by
Samuel Hopkins Adams, which exposed bogus endorsements and worth-
less claims made by drug companies as to the potency of their medicines,
drugs, and tonics. In tandem with Upton Sinclair's book *The Jungle*, which
exposed conditions in the meatpacking industry, Adams's journalism, following in the wake of the tetanus mess in St. Louis, led to passage by the
Senate and the House of Representatives of the Pure Food and Drug Act
and the Meat Inspection Act, both of which were signed into law in 1906.[18]

The Pure Food and Drug Act established the Food, Drug, and Insecticide Administration (later shortened to Food and Drug Administration), but otherwise it was little more than a truth-in-labeling law. It prohibited the manufacturing and interstate sale of adulterated or misbranded foods, drugs, and liquors; required that quantities and proportions appear on labels; and provided for the seizure of misbranded products, with fines and even imprisonment for violators. What the legislation did not require was pretesting of new products for safety, or prescriptions for the sale of drugs.[19] In fact, five years later, the Supreme Court ruled in *United States v. Johnson*, a case involving the shipment from Missouri to Washington, DC, of bottles of medicine bearing labels claiming to cure cancer, that the Pure Food and Drug Act specifically did *not* prohibit false therapeutic claims about what a drug could do, but prohibited only false and misleading statements about the ingredients or identity of a drug.[20]

In 1912, Congress enacted the Sherley Amendment to overcome *United States v. Johnson*, but this law was limited to prohibiting the labeling of medicines with false therapeutic claims *intended* to defraud the purchaser—a standard of proof that was very difficult to reach.[21] For the next half century, Washington's attempts to regulate drugmakers would remain similarly timid and reactive, and almost always in response to a human tragedy.

An exception to the rule was the Harrison Narcotic Act of 1914, which required prescriptions for products exceeding an allowable limit of narcotics, and it mandated increased record-keeping for physicians and pharmacists who dispensed such drugs.[22] Before Harrison, the right to prescribe came with the license to practice medicine, which was a state-granted affair. The federal government now wanted to prevent doctors from treating addicts simply by piling on the opioids, and to prevent them from selling drugs and remedies out of their own offices. Several physicians appealed their convictions under the Harrison Act, but two 1919 Supreme Court cases upheld the government's right to regulate physician prescribing.[23] The cases involved the egregious abuse of physician prerogative. In one case the doctor had literally sold for 50 cents apiece 4,000 prescriptions for opioids over an 11-month period. Unfortunately, though the legislation required physician prescriptions and an orderly paper trail, regulation alone can't completely stop sloppy prescribing, as the modern-day opioid epidemic well illustrates.

Over the next 15 years, with World War I, the Roaring Twenties, and the coming of the Great Depression, food and drug safety was not a priority issue for any branch of government.[24] There was progress, but not in health care. In pushing his New Deal agenda to lift the US out of the Great Depression, Franklin Roosevelt enjoyed a number of early victories—the Emergency Banking Act, the creation of the Federal Deposit Insurance Corporation, and the creation of the Civilian Conservation Corps. But these efforts were overshadowed by the New Deal innovation destined to have the most dramatic effect on the lives of ordinary Americans (and on the expansion of the Medical Industrial Complex): Social Security.[25]

On August 14, 1935, the Social Security Act became law. But tighter restrictions on drug manufacturing were still a long way off when a synthetic chemical shown to act strongly against the streptococcus bacteria first arrived from Germany that year. Derived from a compound called prontosil, the medication was called sulfanilamide. Medical journals warned that this was strong medicine—in the wrong dose and in some people, it could injure the liver or kidneys, or cause the skin to blister— but at a time when any infection could prove fatal, a drug to kill deadly bacteria was considered worth the risk. The likes of Merck, Squibb, and Eli Lilly began to produce more than 100 different formulations, available in both powder and tablet form. Usually the doctor would provide instructions for the pharmacists on specific components to be mixed and dosage requirements, but no prescription was absolutely required, and people could get it over the counter.[26]

Thus in the spring of 1937, the head of sales for S.E. Massengill Company in Bristol, Tennessee, went to the company head, Samuel Evans Massengill, with an idea generated by customer feedback. Massengill salesmen were passing along reports from doctors that there was demand among parents of young children suffering from strep throat for a liquid version of the new drug.[27]

Massengill, with 1,500 products in its catalog and $300,000 in assets, placed the challenge of creating a liquid sulfanilamide in the hands of the company's chief chemist, Harold Cole Watkins, who quickly homed in on finding an effective substance in which powdered sulfanilamide could be dissolved.[28] His choice was diethylene glycol, which smoothly dissolved sulfanilamide powder and led to a concoction that was 10 percent sulfanilamide, 72 percent diethylene glycol, and 16 percent water. Flavored with raspberry extract, saccharine, and caramel, it passed the taste and smell tests, but in keeping with then current federal regulations—or lack thereof—there was no test for safety. In fact, no one did even a rudimentary check of the literature on diethylene glycol, which would have quickly shown that it was a highly toxic component of brake fluid, wallpaper stripper, and antifreeze that had caused a fatality in 1930.[29]

Instead, perhaps sensing that its competition would be right behind, Massengill rushed its "Elixir Sulfanilamide" into production, then shipped 240 gallons of the red liquid to 31 states through a network of small distributors in early September 1937.[30]

Within two weeks, children began to die. Then on October 11, 1937, six Oklahoma physicians raised the alarm with Dr. James Stephenson, president of the Tulsa County Medical Society, who promptly asked the AMA for help. The doctors' organization contacted the Massengill Company and requested a sample for chemical analysis. Within days, the analysis confirmed the presence of the deadly toxin diethylene glycol.[31]

The company was already aware of a problem with the liquid medication through internal feedback from employees in the field, and it had sent telegrams to 1,000 salesmen, doctors, and druggists. But in a classic dodge, the telegram only weakly requested the return of the product without informing the recipients of the danger. By then, reports of deaths were flooding in from all across the country, and a later analysis would show a correlation between high mortality and large numbers of enthusiastic and trusting physicians.

In all, more than 100 children died, but only after going through 7 to 21 days of wrenchingly painful illness including "stoppage of urine, severe abdominal pain, nausea, vomiting, stupor, and convulsions."[27]

To give credit where credit is due, the response by the AMA and the FDA prevented a much greater tragedy. When the medical association sounded the alarm, FDA director Walter Campbell dispatched inspectors to Bristol to inspect the Massengill factory, its products, and its sales records. On October 15, 1937, at the FDA's insistence, company officials sent out a second set of telegrams raising the alarm to all. These read, "IMPERATIVE YOU TAKE UP IMMEDIATELY ALL ELIXIR SULFANILAMIDE DISPENSED. PRODUCT MAY BE DANGEROUS TO LIFE. RETURN ALL STOCKS, OUR EXPENSE."[27]

FDA inspectors also descended on Massengill's branch offices in Kansas City, San Francisco, and New York, where they identified more than 200 salesmen, many of whom were at addresses different from those provided by the company. Adding to the challenge, some doctors were less than forthcoming, and druggists' records were not much help. One East St. Louis pharmacy identified a patient simply as "Betty Jane, 9 months old." Eventually, FDA investigators tracked down nearly 228 of the original 240 gallons of Massengill's Elixir Sulfanilamide and pulled it off the shelves.[27,31]

The whole disaster was vigorously reported in the press, and drug safety soon inched its way up the list of New Deal priorities, with Senator Royal Copeland, a New York physician, and Commissioner Campbell joining forces to craft an adequate and comprehensive national Food and Drug Act. Campbell took the lead, linking the disaster to the absence of adequate consumer protections. He also cited many deaths and cases of blindness from the use of another new drug, dinitrophenol, and liver damage due to the use of cinchophen, a drug often recommended for rheumatism. The AMA, the American Pharmaceutical Association, women's groups, and the national press all closed ranks in support of a new, stronger law to address the problem.[32,33]

Senator Copeland wrote an impassioned editorial in *Scientific American*, detailing the deficiencies of the 1906 law and itemizing the resulting medical disasters, including horse liniment marketed as a miracle cure, and radium water treatments that disintegrated skull bones.[34] On November 16, 1937, Copeland took the Senate floor to formally address the sulfanilamide tragedy, requesting that the Department of Agriculture, which had jurisdiction over the FDA, issue a formal investigative report. Four days later, the FDA presented Congress with a 34-page summary.[33]

On December 1, 1937, Senator Copeland submitted an updated bill in which "manufacturers were required to furnish the Secretary of Agriculture with records of all the tests regarding a drug's safety that had been conducted; a complete list of the drug's ingredients; a description of how the drug was to be manufactured, processed, and packaged; and specimens of all projected labels the drug would carry. In addition, if requested, the manufacturer would be obligated to supply samples of the drug to the FDA. The secretary would then either certify the drug as safe for sale to the public or, if no certificate were issued, provide the reasons detailing why it was refused."[34]

By June 11, 1938, bills from the Senate and House of Representatives had been reconciled, and on June 25, 1938, President Roosevelt signed into law the 1938 Federal Food, Drug, and Cosmetic Act.[35] Its new, gutsier provisions included the following:

• Extending oversight control to chemist-produced cosmetics and therapeutic devices.

• Requiring new drugs to be shown as safe before marketing. This requirement started a new system of drug regulation.

• Eliminating the Sherley Amendment requirement to prove an intent to defraud in drug-misbranding cases.

• Providing that safe tolerances be set for unavoidable poisonous substances.

• Authorizing standards of identity, quality, and fill-of-container (a reasonable standard of identity and quality) for foods.

• Authorizing factory inspections.

• Adding the remedy of court injunctions to the previous penalties of seizures and prosecutions.

Samuel Massengill belatedly issued a statement on behalf of his company: "My chemists and I deeply regret the fatal results, but there was no error in the manufacture of the product. . . . I do not feel there was any responsibility on our part."[36] Unfortunately, Massengill's morally blind position reflected the letter of the law at that time. In short, the absence of effective legal sanctions meant that a company or an individual could indeed sell a deadly medication and get away with it.

Despite the death of more than 100 people and an assault on the health of hundreds more, the company was criminally prosecuted on only one small technicality—the word "elixir" was misused on the product label, since the product did not contain alcohol. Accordingly, the company pleaded guilty to 164 counts, each carrying a penalty of $150, yielding a total government fine of $24,600. As for consumer liability, Massengill's lawyers quietly settled all cases for a reported $500,000. Chemist Harold Cole Watkins, on the other hand, was less hard-hearted than the founder. He committed suicide shortly before the Massengill trial began.[37]

This family-run drug company continued to operate for another 30 years until it was sold in 1971 to Beecham Pharmaceuticals. The Massengill name, originally retained as Beecham-Massengill Pharmaceuticals, was subsequently deleted. Clearly its value as a brand had been tarnished. A few years later, Beecham was bought by SmithKline, which in turn was purchased by Glaxo Wellcome in 2000. Cleansed from the website of GlaxoSmithKline (GSK), the name Massengill lived on, now a half century after the disaster, as a trademark for several women's health care products until December 20, 2011, when that business unit was sold by GSK as part of a consumer products package to Prestige Brands Holdings.[38]

Massengill's manufacturing facility in Bristol survived as well, being purchased and repurchased by middle-level pharmaceutical manufacturers until ultimately it was acquired by Pfizer.[39]

During the 18 years following passage of the Federal Food, Drug, and Cosmetic Act, there was explosive growth in new vaccines, blood products, and antibiotics as part of the war effort, accompanied by a slow accretion of further regulations:

In 1941, the Insulin Amendment required the FDA to test and certify the purity and potency of the drug.[40]

In 1944, the Public Health Service Act was passed, covering a broad spectrum of concerns, including the regulation of biological products and control of communicable diseases.[41]

In 1945, the Penicillin Amendment required FDA testing and certification of the safety and effectiveness of all penicillin products. Later amendments extended this requirement to all antibiotics.[42]

In 1950, a federal court of appeals ruled in *Alberty Food Products Co. v. United States* that the directions for use on a drug label must include the purpose for which the drug was intended.[43]

In 1951, the Durham-Humphrey Amendment defined the kinds of drugs that required medical supervision, restricting their sale to prescription by a licensed practitioner rather than availability over the counter.[44]

But then a new disaster struck, showing once again the limits of regulatory progress.

Poliomyelitis, often called polio or infantile paralysis, is a viral infectious disease that causes debilitating muscle weakness, most often in the legs. It's an ancient scourge depicted in Egyptian tomb paintings, and it's no respecter of caste or class. President Roosevelt was stricken at the age of 39 and had to rely on crutches and braces or a wheelchair for the rest of his life. I was also a victim at age 4 but, fortunately, without lasting effects.[45]

Shortly after World War II, the University of Pittsburgh virologist Jonas Salk set out to find a way to prevent the disease. He succeeded, and by 1955 the Salk vaccine was in wide distribution. Unfortunately, Cutter Laboratories, one of three companies producing the medication, inadvertently released several batches of the vaccine contaminated with live virus. The net effect was that 79 vaccinated children needlessly developed polio.[46]

This was a disaster not only for the reputation of the company but for the industry as a whole, as well as the government, which had been working to establish public support for mass immunization programs.

Oregon's Republican senator Wayne Morse, addressing his colleagues in 1955, laid the blame at the government's feet for "simply turning over" the entire vaccine process to a cartel of drug manufacturers.[47] Making matters worse, a concurrent investigation revealed price-fixing and collusion. The government procurement office documented that the childhood vaccine, produced at multiple sites from different companies, had provided the government with "hundreds of bids which were identical to a fraction of a cent."[48]

The specter of corruption, combined with contaminated vaccines, played into a narrative already unfolding in Washington.

Five years earlier Tennessee senator Estes Kefauver, chair of the Senate Subcommittee on Antitrust and Monopoly, had begun an investigation of organized crime in interstate commerce that became one of America's first televised spectacles, with an estimated 20 million to 30 million viewers. Before it issued its final report on April 17, 1951, the committee visited 14 cities and interviewed nearly 600 subpoenaed witnesses under oath, and 71 percent of all Americans said they were familiar with its work.[49]

Soon thereafter, Kefauver's investigation of monopoly practices expanded to include the rising cost of drugs.[50] In 1956, the year after the polio vaccine debacle, Smith, Kline & French, as it was then known, was called on the congressional carpet for a 40 percent increase in the price of its new tranquilizer, Thorazine, at a time when drug company revenues were on track to triple by the end of the decade.[51] Witnesses began to broaden the scope even further, telling Kefauver's committee about unscrupulous practices such as an ad for nitroglycerin that cited an article in the *Journal of the American Medical Association*, despite the fact that the study cited as evidence had used the drug in an entirely different dose. Following the money, the committee drew a direct line between journal advertising and AMA profitability.[52]

The antibiotic market had rapidly expanded. By 1956, penicillin sales of $70 million had been far outstripped by $180 million in sales of newer broad-spectrum antibiotics. Subsequent investigation of the more than $250 million antibiotic market resulted in a Federal Trade Commission investigation of tetracycline pricing, which alleged that six major pharmaceutical companies had colluded to create prices that were "arbitrary, artificial, non-competitive and rigid." The firms—Pfizer, Bristol Myers, American Cyanamid, Bristol Laboratories, Olin Mathieson, and Upjohn—were found guilty, but their convictions were overturned on appeal.[53]

But financial improprieties did not excite the emotions quite the way harm to children did. What truly captured the public's attention, and ultimately led to further regulatory change, was yet another childhood catastrophe.

During World War II, the Germans had tested a compound called THA-LOMID, α-(N-phthalimido) glutarimide, as an antidote to sarin nerve gas. After the war, the patent rights wound up with Chemie Grünenthal, the company that had first introduced penicillin into the German market.[54,55]

The compound was also licensed to US-based Smith, Kline & French, which, in 1956 and 1957, began to explore the drug's effectiveness as a sedative. The company conducted a clinical study of 875 Americans, including some pregnant women.[56] After analyzing the results, and noting the birth of at least one deformed baby, they quietly buried the findings, behavior that would not be discovered until more than a half century later, when it was dug out by plaintiffs' attorneys.[57]

Grünenthal, meanwhile, went all out on the product. Within four years, it achieved approval of thalidomide as a tranquilizer and painkiller throughout Europe, Africa, Australia, and Canada. Compared with other barbiturates and tranquilizers, this agent appeared to have limited risk of overdose, and Grünenthal was able to sell it over the counter, aggressively marketing it as a "wonder drug" for coughs, colds, headaches, and insomnia. By 1961, 14 distribution companies in 46 countries were selling the product under 51 different names.[54]

As use expanded, though, reports began to trickle in about peripheral nerve damage associated with the product. Even Grünenthal research director Heinrich Mückter became alarmed. In 1958, he was reported to have said, "If I were a doctor, I would not prescribe Contergan [thalidomide] any more. . . . I see great dangers."[55]

Despite such concerns, doctors were actually broadening the indications for use. One such physician was a well-regarded Australian obstetrician, William McBride, who noted that thalidomide appeared effective in limiting "morning sickness" in first-trimester pregnant women.[55] Once his finding became public, use of the drug exploded.

Grünenthal's marketing strategy was to license local distributors around the world, but the US remained untapped. When Smith, Kline & French relinquished its license in 1957, Grünenthal provided exclusive licensing to Richardson-Merrell (a company incorporated in Florida and later absorbed as part of Sanofi) and began working to get thalidomide approved for the American market.[55,57]

The FDA at the time was hardly a force to be reckoned with. Budget cuts had left the agency hamstrung, with only 26 drug investigators on staff—fewer than in the 1940s. Moreover, Senator Kefauver's investigation into price-fixing within the drug industry had uncovered issues of efficacy, safety, advertising, and irregular research protocols, which had led to accusations of collusion between the FDA staff and the drugmakers.[55,57] One notable case involved George Larrich, a former food inspector, who had assumed the helm of the FDA in 1954 with the active support of the pharmaceutical industry. Subsequent investigations revealed that FDA doctors had been ordered by Larrich to assist in preparing drug promotional articles and "to certify a new drug on the grounds that the drug company itself was the best judge of safety."[58]

In standard Medical Industrial Complex style, when Richardson-Merrell presented its application for approval of thalidomide to the understaffed FDA in 1960, it was backed by an army of lobbyists and plenty of friends in Congress. Everyone expected quick approval, especially considering that the drug was already widely used in Europe, Canada, and Australia.[55,57] Fortunately, even if the FDA as a whole was mostly a paper tiger, the examiner it assigned to the case was an indefatigable lion.

Frances Kelsey, born in British Columbia in 1914, had a master's degree in pharmacology from McGill University, and a PhD in pharmacology from the University of Chicago. She had also assisted the FDA in the investigation of Massengill's elixir in the 1930s.[55] With a healthy skepticism about European regulators, she was not overly impressed by the product's widespread use overseas. Moreover, while studying malaria transmission in the Pacific, she had discovered not only that quinine passed through the maternal-placental barrier but that fetuses were highly sensitive to drugs administered at maternal-dose levels, which made her especially attuned to the possibility of drugs taken by the mother affecting the developing fetus. She also had input from her husband, an experienced pharmacologist who was a hyperalert *JAMA* peer reviewer; he had already expressed concern about "dressed-up" articles submitted by academic researchers supported by clandestine drug-industry money.[55]

When Kelsey examined the portfolio submitted by Richardson-Merrell in August 1960, she immediately realized that the company had offered little more than a series of testimonials. And its data, although limited, showed subtle differences in the drug's action in animals versus humans. She was also disturbed by the lack of long-term testing and by the absence of specific data on women of childbearing age.

Any FDA examiner at the time labored under a rule that mandated automatic approval after 60 days absent a negative response from the agency. Coming in under the wire in October 1960, Kelsey stamped the file "incomplete," which forced the company to resubmit and the 60-day clock to be reset.[55]

Caught off guard, Richardson-Merrell turned up the heat. Over the next 19 months it had 58 documented interactions with Kelsey and the FDA. The company pressured her directly, impugned her reputation by challenging her professional qualifications, and went over her head to register protests with her boss.[55] Then in February 1961, she happened upon a report in the December 1960 issue of the *British Medical Journal* that linked thalidomide to damaged peripheral nerves.[59] The thalidomide file before her said nothing about this complication, leaving Kelsey to assume that the company had simply suppressed the information, which also suggested the possibility of more surprises waiting to be turned up. She officially requested more data on the neurologic side effects, as well as data to show that the drug was safe during pregnancy.

Despite Kelsey's vigilance, Richardson-Merrell had already exploited weaknesses in the 1938 legislation, which focused on minimal standards of safety rather than effectiveness, to distribute in the name of research some 2.5 million pills to 1,267 American physicians under the guise of a clinical test."[55] Subsequent lawsuits alleged that more than 20,000 Americans had received the product as a stress reliever, as an antinauseant in early pregnancy, or for headaches and insomnia. An estimated 3,760 women of childbearing age, 207 of whom were believed to be pregnant, were exposed. Ultimately, 17 US children were born with birth defects.[55] During this period, Kelsey continued to stonewall the Richardson-Merrell request while she monitored medical journals from around the world.

In the meantime, clinicians in Europe began to report clusters of the birth defect phocomelia, an absence of limbs resulting from the lack of fetal growth of the long bones of the arms and legs. The first known baby born with such defects—the child of a Grünenthal worker—had arrived on Christmas Day 1956.[55]

Two more cases were reported at a German pediatrics meeting in October 1960. In 1961, another pediatrician reported 13 cases referred to him in a 10-month period. In November 1961, German pediatrician Widukind Lenz wrote a paper describing the abnormalities and specifically implicated thalidomide. The following month, the Australian obstetrician William McBride—the same one who had recommended the drug for morning sickness—published a follow-up study that noted thalidomide's strong association with serious birth defects. He later theorized that the drug affected the DNA of dividing fetal embryonic bone cells, leading to the malformations.[55]

When West German authorities began to tally the numbers of deformities in eight pediatric clinics, they found no cases between 1954 and 1959—and then with the advent of thalidomide, a flood. In 1959, 12 cases were reported, a number which grew to 302 by 1961. West Germany pulled thalidomide off the market, with Britain following suit five days later, and other countries soon fell into line. Canada revoked the license on March 2, 1962, but not soon enough. The May 19 issue of *Maclean's*

magazine recounted the stories of eight victims of phocomelia, including the children of two doctors' wives who had taken thalidomide.[55,57,60]

In the US, Richardson-Merrell hung tough and didn't officially
withdraw its application before the FDA until the late spring of 1962. The
company then sent an anodyne communication to physicians participating
in its "clinical study," telling them to cease use of the drug. Kelsey and her
colleagues forced Richardson-Merrell to provide full contact information
for these physicians.[55]

Renowned pediatric cardiologist Helen Taussig, who had just completed a tour of Europe, met with Frances Kelsey and with Bureau of
Medicine official John Nestor to express her concerns about the disastrous
birth defects associated with the drug.[55] She then began to speak with
members of Congress. Several brief reports appeared in the *New York
Times*, as did a special communication in the June 1962 issue of *JAMA*.[61]

Senator Kefauver, who by now had a law languishing in Congress
that would require drug companies to prove that new drugs were both
effective and safe, saw all this and quietly contacted the *Washington Post*.[55]
On July 15, 1962, the *Post* ran a front-page article titled "'Heroine' of FDA
Keeps Bad Drug Off of Market."[60] It opened with four short, dramatic
paragraphs:

> This is the story of how the skepticism and stubbornness of
> a Government physician prevented what could have been an
> appalling American tragedy, the birth of hundreds or indeed
> thousands of armless and legless children.
>
> The story of Dr. Frances Oldham Kelsey, a Food and
> Drug Administration medical officer, is not one of inspired
> prophecies nor of dramatic research breakthroughs.
>
> She saw her duty in sternly simple terms, and she car-
> ried it out, living the while with insinuations that she was a
> bureaucratic nitpicker, unreasonable—even, she said, stupid.
> That such attributes could have been ascribed to her is, by her
> own acknowledgement, not surprising, considering all of the
> circumstances.

What she did was refuse to be hurried into approving an application for marketing a new drug. She regarded its safety as unproved, despite considerable data arguing that it was ultra safe.

With a little help from Kefauver, the article was republished coast-to-coast and around the world. Within days, the way citizens thought about pharmaceuticals' risk-benefit calculation had been inalterably changed.

Informed of Richardson-Merrell's end run to distribute 20,000 research samples of thalidomide, President John F. Kennedy opened his August 1, 1962, televised news conference by saying, "Every woman in this country, I think, must be aware that it is most important that they check their medicine cabinet, that they do not take this drug, that they turn it in."[62]

On August 7, in a very public ceremony, Kennedy gave Dr. Kelsey the President's Award for Distinguished Federal Clinical Service.[63] On August 10, the *Life* magazine cover story was titled "The Full Story of the Drug Thalidomide / The 5,000 Deformed Babies . . . The Woman Who Saved Thousands . . . The Moral Questions of Abortion and Euthenasia."[64] That same month, Dr. Helen Taussig published "The Thalidomide Syndrome" in *Scientific American*.[65]

By then, Senator Kefauver's bill had all the momentum it needed, but as was the case in 1906 and in 1937, it took a preventable and highly publicized health disaster involving children to get Congress to act.

On October 10, 1962, President Kennedy signed the Kefauver-Harris Amendment, which mandated methodical research protocols and provided protections for patients participating in clinical studies.[66] The law required a step-by-step process for new drug applications, with carefully reviewed dosage and toxicology studies in animals before human trials could begin. No products were allowed to reach the general public until full FDA approval had been granted, and all products had to be fully labeled and accompanied by a complete listing of the indications, benefits, and risks in language preapproved by the agency. And, mirabile dictu, for the first time, companies selling drugs had to prove that their products actually worked.

Drug companies were also required to track complications and report them during the life of the product, with deliberate non-reporting to result in significant penalties. All pre-1962 approvals of drugs then on the market were ordered to be reexamined according to these new regulations. No exceptions. No grandfathering. Finally, pharmaceutical companies had to allow their products going off patent to be produced by generic companies. Those patents then stood at 14 years from when the original application for a new chemical entity was submitted for review. In the future, those protections would be extended to 20 years on average. The FDA also now had complete jurisdiction over all drug advertising, which was required to list side effects.[67]

Not surprisingly, the Medical Industrial Complex was not pleased. The AMA had opposed the requirement to demonstrate efficacy, saying, "The only possible final determination as to the efficacy and ultimate use of a drug is the extensive clinical use of that drug by large numbers of the medical profession over a long period of time."[67] The editors of the *New England Journal of Medicine* opposed the patent provisions (calling them "arbitrary discrimination" against the industry) and the comparative effectiveness provisions necessary only if the manufacturer was actually claiming superiority.[68] The drug industry itself had weighed in with the claim that any determination of which medicines were "me too," meaning that the drug was essentially identical in function to an already existing compound on the market, would be arbitrary. Efficacy was hard enough to prove, the industry said. Proving *comparative* efficacy would be next to impossible.[67]

During the final negotiations for the bill's approval, President Kennedy's Department of Health, Education, and Welfare (HEW) felt that Kefauver had reached a point of obsession when it came to patents. The president had no interest in a protracted battle with the Republicans and their supporters, having squeaked out the slimmest of victories in 1960. With an eye toward a second term, he directed his HEW secretary, former Cleveland mayor Anthony Celebrezze, who had been sworn in on July 31, 1962, to prepare an alternative bill with the HEW seal of approval. His watered-down version of the bill was presented to Congress that summer. The legislative features that had focused on predatory pricing and excessive pharmaceutical pricing had been stripped away. What was left was a focus on safety and efficacy, not on economics or collusive practices between the medical profession and its pharmaceutical patrons. The legislation was passed unanimously by both houses of Congress on October 2, 1962, and was signed into law by President Kennedy eight days later.

In the final legislation, the major provisions that had been tied to patents—exclusivity, compulsory licensing, me-too drugs, brand names, and generic alternatives—were all deleted. As one perturbed legal critic stated at the time, "After practically a year and a half of worry by the drug industry, and the occasioning of tremendous expenses due to investigations by the trade and law associations, the traveling expenses to Washington, and the time of leading lawyers and business executives, and the taking of thousands of pages of testimony before a number of Senate hearings, an almost pathetically mild law . . . was enacted entitled 'Drug Amendments of 1962' which was free of any attempt to amend the Sherman Antitrust Law and similarly free of any attempt to affect the Patent Law."[69]

The Pharmaceutical Manufacturers of America (PMA) claimed victory, and Merck's CEO John T. Connor told a physician audience in Texas, "The new law—on the whole—is sound."[70] If Connor and the PMA were pleased with these regulations, then clearly the American public had no reason to be. The industry now recognized that government was where both the money and the power resided, and was determined to be part of the decision-making in the future.

In the near future, the geographic centers of power for the hospital, insurer, and pharmaceutical and medical industries would move from Boston, New York, Chicago, Philadelphia, and Hartford to Washington, DC, as the ranks of lobbyists exploded. While the new law expanded oversight of drug approval, and required evidence of safety and efficacy, the quality and integrity of the research that supported the evidence remained deeply flawed. And America's unfortunate history of needing a childhood disaster—as in 1901, 1938, and 1960—to prompt legislative action would repeat itself before the century drew to a close.

Chapter 4

The War of Science against Disease

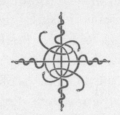

In the 1990s, James M. Wilson received a PhD and an MD degree from the University of Michigan, then completed an internal medicine residency at Massachusetts General Hospital and a postdoctoral fellowship at MIT. By 1997, he was one of the leading stars in the new gene-therapy movement, directing his own research institute at the University of Pennsylvania. The institute focused on adjusting the genes of children born with a hereditary disease called ornithine transcarbamylase deficiency (OTD), which prevents the normal removal of ammonia in the body. Wilson's experimental technique involved genetic engineering, splicing therapeutic genes into supposedly harmless viruses that, once injected into the body, could carry their payload to defective cells and repair the genetic errors.

Dr. Wilson was attempting to determine the maximum dose of genetically modified material that could be safely injected into affected youngsters. He had enlisted 18 participants, including a teenager named Jesse Gelsinger who had a version of the genetic disease in which some of his liver cells carried the genetic abnormality but other cells were entirely normal. Those who have the full-blown disorder die in early childhood. But with his mosaic, Jesse most of the time felt well, as long as he continued to take 32 pills a day.

Jesse and his parents heard about the experiments in nearby Philadelphia and were anxious to help those less fortunate who had the full-blown disease. When he arrived at the clinic on September 13, 1999, to begin the study, his blood ammonia levels were above normal, which in and of itself should have blocked his participation. Nonetheless, Wilson's team infused Jessie's bloodstream with 38 trillion colonies of a virus carrying genes engineered to reprogram his cells. Eight hours later, Jesse's fever hit 104.5 degrees. Two days later he was brain-dead.[1]

The patent for the technique of genetic modification being studied was owned by a company called Genovo, cofounded by the abovementioned James M. Wilson, the institute director. Wilson owned a 30 percent stake valued at over $30 million, and the University of Pennsylvania, which under the rules of the National Institutes of Health, was responsible for ethical oversight of the research protocol design and execution, was a hidden investor.[2] The informed consent Jesse had signed made no mention of Wilson's financial conflict of interest, or the university's, or the fact that some of the prior 17 participants had suffered significant inflammatory responses, or that two laboratory monkeys had died from massive inflammatory immune responses to injections of the very same agent.[1,2,3]

But the perverse financial incentives and conflicts of interest that led to such risk-taking went further up the academic food chain. Dr. Bill Kelley, an accomplished and aggressive medical researcher from the University of Michigan, had assumed the top post at the University of Pennsylvania in the early 1990s. Kelley's goal was to achieve dominance in a crowded and competitive local medical market that included six medical schools. The age of genomics was just gaining steam, and Kelley wanted Penn to lead the way and share the rewards. His rapid overexpansion and heavy investment in technology and personnel had resulted in a reported $198 million loss by the University of Pennsylvania's health system in fiscal year 1999.[4] No doubt Kelley harbored hopes that Penn's investment in Dr. Wilson's gene company, bolstered by NIH grants and private investors, might help balance the books. Jesse Gelsinger's death ended not only that research but Bill Kelley's tenure as well.

While someone like Charles Evans Hughes could compromise participation in and access to the fruits of medical discovery in making sure that his daughter got insulin, by the time of Jesse Gelsinger's death, big money had raised the stakes and blurred the line between academic and commercial interests so completely that the ethics of fair access to discoveries seemed like some primitive belief from a lost civilization. All scales had been tipped in the direction of American pharmaceutical innovation and the rapidly emerging field of biotechnology. Previous checks and balances had been deliberately supplanted by cross-sector partnerships, shared profits, and integrated career ladders.

Not all compromising academic-industrial entanglements were laboratory-based or involved such stark moral contrasts, however. The confusing gray areas where the interests of academics and the interests of commercial entities blur first hit home for me at the 2002 Winter Olympics in Salt Lake City. I was on a Pfizer trip, and my colleagues on our luxury bus were listening to a lecture by a former Olympic medal winner. Next to my wife and me was a well-dressed couple I didn't recognize. When I introduced myself, I learned that the gentleman was Antonio Gotto, MD, dean of Cornell University's Weill Medical College, who I naively assumed had been included in recognition of his status as one of America's premier medical educators. Only later did I learn that Gotto was not only past president of the American Heart Association; he was also one of the cardiologists who had led the landmark studies that had made statins the treatment of choice for lowering cholesterol. Moreover, Gotto had become a leading proponent of Pfizer's entrant to the market, Lipitor—a drug that for over 15 years would bring the company more than $100 billion in revenue.[5]

A trip to the Olympics is not such a big deal, and of course Gotto could accept the gift as an expression of gratitude and remain above reproach. Still, his ready acceptance revealed a high level of comfort with cross-sector entrepreneurism, a collaborative approach where who you know directly affects how far you go, and where the appearance of a conflict of interest was of no concern.

Science-based industries in the US once lagged far behind their European counterparts, in part because America was late to develop big research universities and the alliances they spawn. When those alliances began to form in the US, European transplants led the way, such as Merck, which by the late 19th century had set up a US branch to distribute the alkaloids, including morphine and cocaine, that were its stock-in-trade. In 1900, the company established a bacteriological laboratory in Rahway, New Jersey, to develop vaccines and diphtheria serum, and analytic laboratories to examine milk samples for tuberculosis bacteria and to test water supplies for typhoid.[6] Around the time that Lilly was signing papers with the University of Toronto for rights to distribute insulin in 1922, Merck's US branch was moving its research and development in-house, and beginning to collaborate with scientists at the University of Pennsylvania, which would later host the institute where Jesse Gelsinger was admitted to the study that killed him.

In the process of forming these new collaborations in the 1930s, negative feedback loops in academic research programs that had once allowed for caution and critical oversight were slowly being replaced by positive feedback loops that supported a self-serving meritocracy, sped up by rapidly expanding academic-business coalitions. World War II, and the challenge of defeating the Axis, provided more than ample justification for a no-holds-barred scientific plunge to ensure success. The end more than justified the means, and in pursuing victory, President Franklin Roosevelt was more than willing to set aside checks and balances.

After the war, separate, parallel tracks would in time give way to fully integrated career ladders with purposeful intermingling of professional, corporate, and governmental sectors. Increasing financial pressure meant that the risk-benefit curve in the testing of drugs would all too often be adjusted to play up benefits while downplaying risks.

The race to monetize molecules and introduce new treatments carried temptations enough, but the strong infusion of government money during and immediately after World War II tipped the scales sharply away from open, honest, and deliberate debate. With so much money at stake, even pure research would have an ever harder time remaining pure, and the distinctions between funding entities (both governmental and private), researchers, and other self-interested stakeholders would blur.[7]

Whether it involved materials, logistics, or coordinating laboratory studies themselves, the effort to put research on a war footing required a group of wily and innovative businessmen-scientists. Primary among them was the bespectacled gentleman who appeared on the April 3, 1944, cover of *Time*, leaning forward into the lens, tanned, in a light gray suit, with a crisp, white shirt and steel-blue tie, next to a ray-emitting radio microphone. The caption read, "Vannevar Bush: General of Physics."[8]

As overall head of President Roosevelt's Office of Scientific Research and Development (OSRD)—also known as the fifth branch of the military general staff, or G5—Bush coordinated 6,000 scientists working in some 300 laboratories, both university-based and commercial.[7] He had plenty of help at the top. Among others in his management team was one George W. Merck, a close friend and confidant since 1933. After Pearl Harbor brought the US into the war, Merck, who had already moved aggressively to centralize his own pharmaceutical company's research operations, became head of the US Army Biological Warfare Laboratories within Vannevar Bush's OSRD. The official policy was to develop weapons based on a wide range of infectious agents, primarily as deterrents but secondarily as offensive weapons if the US was attacked. They were never used during the war, and their existence was not revealed until 1946. As we'll see, the partnership between Bush and Merck outlasted the military effort and set the stage not only for academic-industrial partnerships to come, but for a highly profitable personal alliance as well.

Born March 11, 1890, in Everett, Massachusetts, the only son of a Universalist preacher and the grandson of a whaler, Vannevar Bush earned a math degree from Tufts, followed by a PhD in engineering from MIT.[9] From the beginning of his career he straddled the academic and the industrial in a way that anticipated the future of almost all scientific research. In 1917, he became head of the experimental laboratory for Tufts University's new radio station, owned by the American Radio and Research Corporation (AMRAD).[9] His work focused on wave disturbances in magnetic fields, which Bush and the US Army felt might help identify submerged German submarines. After World War I, he joined MIT's electrical engineering department, but he continued his affiliation with AMRAD, all the while codeveloping a thermostatic switch with another company that would be acquired 30 years later by Texas Instruments.[10] By 1924, he was working with AMRAD physicist Charles Smith, who invented the S-shaped gas rectifier tube to increase the efficiency of radios and eliminate the need for batteries. In 1925, its Metals and Controls Corporation was renamed Raytheon.[11] Obviously, Bush was well positioned to benefit from the long tail of his academic-industrial efforts.

In time, Bush left MIT to become head of the Carnegie Institute in Washington, DC, the most powerful philanthropic science organization in America, but he was already leading a shadowy second life helping design code-breaking automated machinery for the predecessor of our modern National Security Agency.[12] In 1939, with the Second World War consuming both Europe and Asia, Bush and James B. Conant, president of Harvard University, met with Frank B. Jewett, president of Bell Labs and of the National Academy of Sciences, to map out a strategy for overcoming our lack of scientific preparedness.[13] Out of that small meeting came a short, four-paragraph proposal for a centralized science operation—outside the control of the military—which Bush placed before President Roosevelt on June 12, 1940.[14]

The president read the report, seized his pen, and scratched at the top, "OK—FDR." With that stroke, the National Defense Research Committee (NDRC) was created, and with it, the fully codified and institutionalized era of academic-industrial partnerships in research.[15]

With a direct line to the president, the NDRC under Bush was charged with bringing together the best scientific minds from government, academia, the military, and private industry to meet the research needs of the US Army and Navy. Originally funded through the executive branch, it soon earned congressional support and was renamed the Office of Scientific Research and Development.[9]

Staffing up, Bush launched a nationwide talent search that ranged from Nobel laureates to high school chemistry teachers, compiling automated case histories on more than 200,000 individuals.[9] But the OSRD was most remarkable for being a government agency that, in a phrase that would become popular in Washington 50 years later, set out to "steer not row." Rather than build and manage large government laboratories, it contracted with universities and industrial laboratories, funding each lab to conduct research appropriate to its capabilities.[9]

The "total war" of the 1940s was a critical turning point for the advancement of science in general, and it led to such innovations as radar, the jet engine, and atomic energy. In biomedical science, the general advance in understanding and methods during the war led indirectly to James Watson's and Francis Crick's explication of the structure of DNA, as well as to the development of the CAT scan, amniocentesis, and ultrasound.

But the war also increased the threat of certain diseases such as influenza, smallpox, tetanus, typhoid, paratyphoid A and B, cholera, diphtheria, the plague, scarlet fever, pneumococcus infection, typhus, and yellow fever.[16] The danger of contracting these ailments was ever present on the battlefield, but the greater danger was in the gathering and movement of large aggregations of soldiers in barracks, ships, and hospitals. This spurred a policy that every soldier would be fully vaccinated, which encouraged the notion that, even in peacetime, every child entering public school should be vaccinated.[17]

When the war began, sulfanilamide was the latest addition to the medical tool kit. Despite the disastrous Massengill scandal in the late 1930s, the French Foreign Legion had demonstrated the value of sulfanilamide as an anti-infective on the battlefield in Nigeria in 1936, when an outbreak of bacterial meningitis had affected only 11 percent of the troops who had used the drug. That incidence climbed to 75 percent once the supply was exhausted. The drug found its way not only into Army doctors' medical kits but also into the first-aid pouch attached to the belt worn by every infantryman, inside which was an envelope of the sulfa powder and a gauze dressing for battlefield wounds.[18]

By D-Day, penicillin had become the leading advance, along with easily injectable morphine made possible by Squibb's invention of the syrette, a miniature tube filled with morphine that could be punctured by a delivery needle, inserted into a soldier, and squeezed to deliver the medicine. All medics carried it, and it was used in clearing stations strategically placed close to the battlefield. To avoid overdose, medics either drew an "M" on the wounded soldier's forehead or attached the used syrette to his clothing with a safety pin.[19]

Another lifesaving innovation that would carry over into peacetime was blood replacement. The American expert at the time was Dr. Charles Drew from Columbia Medical Center in New York. In 1938, Drew had developed the nation's first blood plasma system.[20] In 1940, before America's entry into the war, he established the International Transfusion Association to organize the Blood for Britain project. Within five months he had delivered 14,500 units of plasma, the liquid part of blood that, after all the cells are removed, still contains all the critical proteins necessary to control and stop bleeding.[21] As Roosevelt instructed the Army to prepare to mobilize prior to Pearl Harbor, Drew was appointed as the first director of the American Red Cross blood bank in February 1941. By the time the war ended, the Red Cross had delivered 13 million units of blood, much of it converted to plasma.[22]

Another threat that came with wartime troop deployment was venereal disease. The armed forces had long since resigned themselves to the reality that a sizable portion of homesick young men, lonely and far away from home, would figure out a way to contract syphilis or gonorrhea. During World War I, the US Army had lost the service of a startling 18,000 men in a single day to venereal disease. By WWII, the condom was standard issue, and therapy was close at hand. But still, as late as 1943, 606 US soldiers per day were reported to be "incapacitated by V.D."[23] This was no small problem, since standard-issue gonorrhea in 1943 demanded a 30-day course of treatment including pills and penile urethral injections of ointment. And that was mild compared with syphilis, which demanded six months of rigorous treatment. From the time US troops first shipped out, overseas soldiers were continually plagued with venereal diseases.[23]

Psychiatric illness was yet another huge area for medical attention during the war. Despite intense effort on the part of military leadership to weed out the vulnerable through a highly restrictive draft, more than a million psychiatric casualties occurred during World War II.[24] This wasn't just an issue of disease, stigma, or fault; it was a question of morale and productivity, and a chronic disease burden that continued to consume limited health care resources long after the war had ended.

During World War I, the psychiatrist Thomas W. Salmon, then medical director of the National Committee for Mental Hygiene, had recommended careful screening of new recruits to exclude "insane, feeble-minded, psychopathic, and neuropathic individuals," and approximately 2 percent of inductees were rejected on these grounds.[25] But even with these exclusions, "nervous breakdown" remained common enough to make clear that screening based on constitution, temperament, or perceived odd behavior was not an easy fix for the problem. Predicting how soldiers would react under the pressures of war was far from an exact science. Previously fit soldiers were coming in from the trenches stuttering and crying, deaf and mute, with hallucinations and amnesia, along with somatic vomiting and intestinal problems. "Shell shock" as it was termed, affected about 15 percent of all British troops.[26]

Salmon began to suspect environmental issues and recommended that psychiatrists be placed "as near the front as military exigency will permit."[27] He further recommended a three-tiered response: (1) Food, comfort, rest, and reassurance at the nearby aid station, which, alone, helped 65 percent of the men return to action in four or five days. (2) If needed, a three-week stay in a neuropsychiatric unit 5 to 15 miles from the front. (3) For soldiers still not capable of assuming duty (including noncombat duty), six months of treatment in a base hospital, usually 50 miles from the fighting. Only if this failed were they sent home.[25,28]

By the time Hitler's troops were marching across Europe, the notion of coddling soldiers with nervous conditions was out of vogue. In December 1940, two months after the draft had been instituted, psychiatrist Harry Stack Sullivan, a consultant for the Selective Service, advocated the screening out of all individuals suffering from mental illness, including maladjustment and neurosis.[29] Serving on the American Psychiatric Society's Military Mobilization committee, he did suggest that homosexuals be allowed to serve, but in the end, the committee rejected them as well. By 1941, Sullivan, a closeted gay man himself, resigned his post after a dispute with Selective Service director General Lewis B. Hershey.[30]

Sullivan's screening system did, however, prevail for the next three years, and it led to the rejection of 2 million men, a startling 12 percent of all applicants (six times the WWI rejection rate).[31] Of all men rejected for medical causes, more than one-third were released on neuropsychiatric grounds. And yet, the problem in combat—mental breakdown of all sizes and shapes—persisted. This became abundantly clear in November 1942, during Operation Torch—the invasion of Algeria, Morocco, and Tunisia. The high numbers of psychiatric casualties quickly grabbed the attention of Army Chief of Staff George Marshall. In spite of the heavy-handed selection exclusions, 34 percent of the battle casualties were officially labeled neuropsychiatric. The diagnosis was an automatic ticket back home to the States.[32,33,34]

At the time, one neurologist in North Africa, Frederick R. Hanson, discovered that a bit of kindness in the form of a hot shower and a warm meal, combined with sedation-induced rest, was remarkably successful in rehabilitating the majority of the "mentally incapacitated" men under his care.[35] Hanson's success did not go unnoticed by the Army's chief of the division of neuropsychiatry in the Office of the Surgeon General, William C. Menninger. After studying Hanson's results and reviewing all the information currently available to him, he decided that if psychiatric casualties in a standard unit exceeded one mental casualty for every four wounded in action, this was a harbinger of broader problems—like a breakdown in morale, leadership issues, prolonged combat fatigue, or a policy breakdown in the evacuation scheme.[29]

Other observations included the fact that new units with limited combat experience had a higher percentage of mental casualties than seasoned units did, and that the medical officers in these units were more inclined to ship out those with "normal fear reactions." On the other end of the spectrum, troops whose combat exposure exceeded 12 months began to experience a higher percentage of mental casualties.[36] In one study, the author observed, "It would seem to be a more rational question to ask why the soldier does not succumb to anxiety, rather than why he does."[37] This notion was reinforced a few years later with a new commitment by mental health professionals "to shift attention from problems of the abnormal mind in normal times to problems of the normal mind in abnormal times.[27]

The experience in North Africa had clarified for Army Chief of Staff Marshall that the plan for handling neuropsychiatric casualties in the field was seriously broken. At his request, Menninger came up with a plan that largely adopted Salmon's approach from WWI, reinforced by the heavy and liberal use of barbiturates and ether anesthesia if necessary for initial sedation of hysterical soldiers. In the most severe cases, other experimental treatments would be used, such as intravenous sodium pentothal, a.k.a. truth serum, to draw out (and ideally remove) the troubling traumatic memories of war.[32,37] A five-step echelon system would provide progressive evacuation of more serious cases, and the third echelon, still within striking distance of the battlefield, would be reinforced with special neuropsychiatric and convalescent hospitals wherever possible. However, there were not nearly enough psychiatrists to execute the plan, so Menninger came up with the idea of training a portion of the medical officers in what he called "forward psychiatry."[38] These officers, including my own father, who supervised a neuropsychiatric hospital for Patton's Seventh Army, were subjected to a 30-day immersion course to master Menninger's system and to become comfortable with the liberal use of barbiturates. They were thereafter labeled "30-day wonders."

Menninger and his allies also greatly liberalized the draft selection process for recruits, and even some of those previously rejected on psychiatric grounds were now readmitted, with studies later showing that more than 80 percent performed well when provided with the opportunity to serve.[39] As for the battlefield, Menninger saw to it that forward psychiatry, practiced by nonpsychiatric generalists, would become the rule. As his training film attested, "there are no specialists in the battlefield."

To do this he developed a system encoded in a diagnostic manual, Medical 203 (which was the basis of the *Diagnostic and Statistical Manual of Mental Disorders*, or *DSM*, released shortly after the war). Today, the bible of mental health, and now in its fifth edition, the *DSM* is a structured approach to the diagnosis and treatment of mental illnesses, including the use of wartime barbiturates and the many chemical children they spawned.[40] The pharmaceutical industry responded to all these developments with an aggressive search for "blockbusters" to capture the expanding market. Some of these new medicines were designed to treat very real ailments; in other cases, the drug came first, after which the drug company's newly energized marketing teams developed a problem for it to solve. By 1960, one out of every six American adults was being treated with pharmaceuticals for anxiety.

While the war changed American medicine's approach to disease, the war and the immediate postwar period also changed the disease profile of the American people, who were now better nourished and succumbed less often to infectious diseases, and thus had a lengthened average life expectancy. But the war had also led to an increase in smoking, and the postwar prosperity led to a richer diet weighted toward more processed foods and sugary beverages, as well as a generally more hectic and stressful environment with full employment and mass migration from south to north and east to west, all of which contributed to a sudden increase in diseases of affluence, which were experienced at every stage of that longer life span.

Meanwhile, a range of addictions, from cigarettes to alcohol to controlled substances—driven in part by wartime stresses—ensured an escalating number of patients with cancer, heart attacks, strokes, emphysema and bronchitis, ulcers, and liver disease. A small number of pharmaceutical powerhouses were ideally positioned to respond.

In 1940 there were several hundred pharmaceutical companies in the United States, none with a market share greater than 3 percent. By 1950, 15 large and highly innovative companies controlled 80 percent of sales nationwide and 90 percent of the profits.[41] What happened during those 10 years to effect this transformation had more to do with being in the right place at the right time, and less to do with wartime sales per se.

On one level, the demands of the rapidly expanding armed services did fuel spectacular growth, as drug companies ramped up to supply everything from barbiturates to merthiolate (the familiar red liquid anti-septic), and from morphine to sulfur bandages, all of which the government purchased eagerly with little negotiation at top prices.

But in terms of competition among the players themselves, the real game changer was participation in the 1942 War Production Board's penicillin project.[41] The 17 firms that were chosen by Vannevar Bush's leadership team had relevant expertise and the insight to respond to an open-ended government request for help to scale up penicillin production in the lead-up to D-Day. Being selected to produce the drug not only gave certain companies a huge influx of capital; it also put them in a vital information loop. Of the 10 largest pharmaceutical firms in 1979, 9 had participated in the penicillin program. By 2005, 12 of the 17 participants still existed, and they included all 10 of the largest American pharmaceutical firms.[41]

The bacteria-killing properties of penicillin had been known since 1928, when they were stumbled upon by a Scottish scientist named Alexander Fleming. Working at St. Mary's Hospital in London, Fleming had been researching *Staphylococcus*, a common pathogen that causes pus-filled eruptions called boils on the skin surface, as well as deadly damage to vital organs if it gains access to blood circulation. When Fleming noted that the presence of the mold *Penicillium notatum* on the edge of the growth plate stopped staph cold, he published his finding in 1929 in the *British Journal of Experimental Pathology*, but the world hardly noticed.[42] Continuing his investigations, Fleming found that cultivating *Penicillium* was not easy, and that after he had grown the mold, isolating the antibiotic agent was harder still. His clinical trials were inconclusive—contributing to his belief that the active ingredient in the mold would not last long enough in the human body to kill bacteria effectively. He tried to engage a chemist skilled enough to further refine usable penicillin, but in 1940 he gave up—just as the British and US governments became intensely interested in finding a drug to treat battlefield infections.

With wartime funding, Howard Florey and Ernst Boris Chain at the Radcliffe Infirmary in Oxford took over penicillin research, as well as the effort to mass-produce the drug. One of the companies they commissioned was Pfizer, which employed the same deep-tank fermentation method it had used decades earlier to produce the preservative and flavor enhancer gluconic acid. Pfizer purchased huge 7,500-gallon tanks and bought an old ice plant in Brooklyn with special refrigeration equipment, then reopened it as a penicillin factory on March 1, 1944, just in time to supply more than 90 percent of the drug brought ashore on D-Day, June 6, 1944.[43] Fifty-five years later, this same Pfizer plant would take the lead in producing Viagra.[44]

By early fall 1944, the Allies had gained the upper hand on the battlefield, and President Roosevelt had the luxury of thinking about how the US could translate its now thriving wartime-research structure into a postwar world. On November 17, 1944, he wrote to Bush: "There is no reason why the lessons to be found in this experiment cannot be profitably employed in times of peace . . . for the improvement of the national health, the creation of new enterprises bringing new jobs, and the betterment of the national standard of living."

Roosevelt went on to speculate about how the experience gained through OSRD could be adapted "to the war of science against disease."

By the time Bush had formulated his response in July 1945, Roosevelt was dead of a cerebral hemorrhage at the age of 63. As a consequence, Bush submitted his report, *Science: The Endless Frontier*, to the newly sworn-in President Harry S. Truman.[45]

Truman agreed that the government needed to support science in the postwar period not only to boost the economy, but also as a bulwark of national defense in the Cold War that was then taking shape, a war in which East and West would become rivals in everything from nuclear weapons to piano competitions. Where Bush and Truman parted ways was on the precise role of government. The president saw Washington as being much more engaged, and the new organization as allocating America's treasure under direct government management.[46] Bush leaned heavily toward a more independent, business-oriented venture relying on cooperation among independent scientists, subject to arm's-length government oversight and funding.

In 1947, Congress passed a compromise bill creating a new organization called the National Science Foundation (NSF). Truman vetoed the bill because it provided for the NSF's director to be appointed by an independent board rather than by the president. Congress passed the bill again, and Bush would later say, "I managed to convince Truman he should not veto it again. But I did so on the basis that he was being given protection, a buffer against those coming to seek favor."[46] Until passage of the National Cancer Act in 1971, the top government science director was chosen by the surgeon general, who was appointed by the secretary of the Department of Health, Education, and Welfare. After 1971, the position became a presidential appointment.[47]

As the OSRD was morphing into a new National Science Foundation that would spawn the National Institutes of Health, a wide range of World War II science luminaries had been infiltrating the highest ranks of academia, industry, and government, then continuing to actively cross-connect with one another. This marked a critical juncture, because together these individuals would solidify the nascent Medical Industrial Complex.

This moment also marked a critical departure from the path taken by the rest of the developed world. As they rebuilt and reorganized after the war's disruption, other industrialized nations, rather than the US, followed Roosevelt's prescient directive to harness science to improve "the national health" by making the universal health of their citizens a national priority. As Canada was welcoming its soldiers back home, for example, the province of Saskatchewan had already begun discussing universal health care as an expression of postwar solidarity. Its simple question "How do we ensure a healthy Canada and healthy Canadians?" led to the eventual establishment of a national health plan for all citizens.

Adding to the irony, at the very same moment when the leaders of the Medical Industrial Complex were rejecting President's Truman call for a national health plan, a proposal for funding more doctors and hospitals, and a program of national health insurance for all to be run by the government, our military under the Marshall Plan was fast at work creating just such new, and ultimately highly successful, national health plans for our two main vanquished enemies, Germany and Japan. We were willing to allocate precious taxpayer resources to ensure the future good health of the Germans and Japanese while denying Truman's call to establish the same benefit for our own people.[48]

An analysis of the German and Japanese programs made some years later by the Rand Corporation summed up the idea nicely: "Nation-building efforts cannot be successful unless adequate attention is paid to the health of the population. The health status of those living in the country has a direct impact on the nation's construction and development, and history teaches us it can be a tool in capturing goodwill of the nation's residents."[48] But somehow these insights escaped our leaders back then. Seventy years later, while our politicians still dither, average Americans are increasingly questioning why Canada, Germany, and Japan regularly outperform the United States on a wide range of health outcomes delivered at much less cost.

In the immediate postwar period, the United States fully embraced the idea of a nationally led war against disease. In the context of a healthy business climate and federally funded American ingenuity, control over our national research enterprise was transferred to a mid-20th-century version of today's dynastic venture capitalists committed to eventually turning a budding meritocracy into a stable and everlasting aristocracy. Meanwhile, general public health planning and execution were thoroughly decentralized down to the state and county levels. In 1950, county health departments served nearly 90 percent of the US population and employed 35,000 workers nationwide.[49] They varied widely in funding, priorities, training, execution, and outputs, and their influence steadily diminished over the next half century.

But while public health was throttled down—not until 1992 would the Centers for Disease Control (CDC) grudgingly add the words "and Prevention" to its name—the spigots for research and development, or R&D, were wide open.[50] In 1940, the US government funded less than 7 percent of the nation's scientific research and development. By 1950, that share had grown to 50 percent of a much larger total. Most assumed that Vannevar Bush would be director of the OSRD's peacetime equivalent, the National Science Foundation, and many were surprised when Truman did not appoint him.[46] However, Bush was ready to move on, and he had no shortage of opportunities to translate his public-sector experience into a continuing stream of private-sector gains. Bush chose to join forces with his old colleague George W. Merck.

Merck was the largest vitamin producer in America and the second largest in the world when, in 1946, the company launched the new antibiotic, streptomycin, the first effective therapy for tuberculosis.[51] This was followed two years later by its proclaimed "miracle drug" cortisone.[52] But even with these successes, George W. Merck saw the company losing market share to Pfizer, which was going long on retail marketing and aggressively deploying "detail men" to doctors' offices. These detail men did much more than provide details of the products to the doctors and hospitals they visited. They acted as connectors, messengers, and fixers to the clinicians as well. Merck decided to follow a different path, one that emphasized the power of his experience in centralized research and that relied heavily on the science administrators he had rubbed elbows with in WWII.[53] These included the former OSRD Committee on Medical Research chair Alfred Newton Richards and the OSRD general counsel John T. Connor. He saw these individuals not only as valuable repositories of knowledge and experience but also as links in an equally valuable network of contacts throughout the public and private sectors.[54] As a foretaste of entanglements to come, both of these men had held government and academic posts throughout the 1930s and 1940s while at the same time collecting paychecks from companies like Merck.[55]

In May 1949, Vannevar Bush agreed to join the Merck board of trustees. Company colleagues advised that he had "special responsibilities among the Directors to get inside the minds of those in the scientific areas on whom the future success of the company depends."[53] Within one year, the company had adopted the same basic structure for research that Bush had set up for the OSRD. This included hiring eight specialty consultants embedded in academia, among them researchers covering the fields of nutrition, pharmacology, biochemistry, veterinary medicine, and pathology.[56] In addition to basic science insights and problem solving, these consultants gave the company access to academic laboratories and testing equipment, and to publications; links to colleague scientists overseas as the company went global; and identification of prospective new US employees who might fit into a corporate environment.[56] Merck also created a wide range of institutional grants, scholarships, and research fellowships.[57]

When George W. Merck died in 1957, Vannevar Bush became chairman of the company's board, a position he would hold until 1962. By then, his approach to integrating research, development, production, sales, patents, and engineering, along with contacts within the medical profession, had become standard operating procedure throughout the Medical Industrial Complex.[46] He still believed in high science. But as he watched the market share of Merck's earlier "wonder drug" cortisone slowly slip away, Bush realized that there was more to pharmaceutical success than science administration—in fact, much more than science per se.

The company had purchased the pharmaceutical marketing and sales whiz Sharp & Dohme in 1953. In 1958, after several years of messy integration, Merck released its second wonder drug, the diuretic Diuril (chlorothiazide), targeting hypertension, which had been identified as a major contributor to both heart disease and strokes. With the full support of numerous cardiology thought leaders, and a never-to-be forgotten product giveaway for prescribing doctors—the Diuril "invisible couple," two see-through clear plastic figurines, each seven inches tall and revealing interior organs in a manner considered pretty racy for the 1950s—the company went all out on marketing. It sold $20 million worth of Diuril that year.[58]

Through the early 1950s Merck also had been accumulating the same kind of aggressive sales force as archrival Pfizer. In return for products prescribed and sold, the pharmaceutical salesmen were committed to their physician customers' personal and professional success. Whether it be achieving goals in clinical care, medical education, or research; climbing the academic career ladder through publications, presentations, or acquiring positions on government advisory boards; filling leadership posts at medical centers; or securing locations and funding for family vacations, the detail men did whatever they could to make it happen. In this evolving meritocracy, they became the all-purpose facilitators, and the very glue of the Medical Industrial Complex aristocracy.

Between 1947 and 1959, research and development (R&D) investment throughout the drug industry in the US grew from $30 million to

$170 million, and sales grew from $890 million to $2.7 billion. By the time Bush retired as chairman in 1962, Merck was universally viewed as the world's number one drugmaker, with annual sales near $250 million.[59]

While the AMA's brand of heroic medicine had already defined "health" narrowly as the absence of disease, the successful outcome of the war strengthened the view that disease was an enemy to be defeated. Not incidentally, the Allies' success on the battlefield strongly suggested that the path to victory was through the same industrial model, and the same unencumbered, collaborative, free-enterprise approach to research that had triumphed over the Nazis. Thus the more "holistic" notion—that health was more than merely the absence of disease, that it was something to be nurtured and sustained by positive inputs, including societal commitments beyond specific medical goods and services—slipped further into the background.

In addition, the wartime mind-set of our "backs against the wall" that had rushed penicillin and streptomycin into widespread use ahead of extensive testing carried over into peacetime. Miracle drugs and scientific discoveries inspired, motivated, and excited Americans. But they also pushed ethical qualms, concern for individual rights, and procedural caution to the margins.

During the war, Allies carried out experiments, including exposure to known toxins and radiation, on the most vulnerable members of society, including prisoners, the poor, and the disadvantaged. Following the war, and spurred on by nearly a million psychiatric casualties, experiments with electric shock, insulin, and camphor-induced coma, as well as psychosurgery to cut away portions of the brain believed to be malfunctioning, were commonplace.

The war also helped redefine the way we would staff our health care system. In 1941, only 11,000 doctors were in the Medical Corps; by the war's end, the number approached 45,000, representing roughly 40 percent of the nation's physicians.[60] Meanwhile, special casualty hospitals were developed for heart and lung surgery, plastic surgery and burn care, neurosurgery, eye and ear surgery, and vascular surgery, staffed by highly trained teams that exposed those 45,000 physicians to these elite fields.

When the war ended, many generalist physicians took advantage of the GI Bill to fund additional residency training to enter these higher-paying, more prestigious specialties. With financial incentives aligned, the number of specialty training positions grew from 5,000 in 1940 to 12,000 in 1947, and hit 25,000 by 1955.[61]

Like psychiatry and the various surgical specialties, nursing was greatly enhanced by the war and moved toward specialization. The profession itself had developed on the 19th-century battlefields of Crimea when British social reformer Florence Nightingale organized the efforts of 38 volunteer women and 15 Catholic nuns.[62] Their work, focused heavily on sanitation and hands-on care, was said to have been responsible for significantly decreasing death rates. In 1855, she created the Nightingale Fund for the training of nurses and wrote the book *Notes on Nursing*, which would become the cornerstone of the nursing training curriculum.[63]

The day the Japanese attacked Pearl Harbor, only 1,000 nurses served in the Army Nurse Corps, even though no special training was required. Six months after the US entered the war, there were still only 12,000 enlisted nurses.[64] In July 1943, Lieutenant General Brehon B. Somervell, commanding general of the Army Service Forces, authorized a formal four-week training course, the Nurse Cadet Program, with full educational subsidies and officer rank upon completion.[65] By September 1945, more than 27,000 nurses had moved through the program.[66] By 1948, the program had swelled the ranks of nursing by 150,000, and experts had emerged in psychiatric nursing, surgical nursing, nurse anesthetists, rehabilitation specialists, and nurse managers running field medical facilities.[67]

With these increasingly specialized disease fighters now at the ready, what remained necessary was a structured setting to engage the battle against disease. That problem was solved in 1946, when Congress passed the Hospital Survey and Construction Act, also known as the Hill-Burton Act, named for Senate sponsors Lister Hill (D-AL) and Harold Burton (R-OH). The bill provided federal funding directly to facilities in return for their commitment to provide uncompensated free care to the poor for a period of 20 years after construction. The goal was to create 4.5 hospital beds per 1,000 residents nationwide.[68]

All the pieces were now in place for the consummation of a Medical Industrial Complex that would systematically pursue disease over wellness, seek profitability over health, and eventually morph into a loosely organized syndicate that now controls 20 percent of the nation's GDP.

As for the people who would be directly affected by these health policy decisions, they were absorbing a culture of rapid change and vastly increased mobility. Even before the war, Eli Junior, George Merck, and other pharmaceutical chieftains could see the winds shifting. Their planning in the early 1930s acknowledged that life spans were increasing as hygiene and sanitation improved and the understanding of infectious diseases expanded. At the same time, the basic science of cardiovascular disease had been delineated, and early warnings of tobacco-related increases in lung disease and cancer had begun to appear. A few years later, these same leaders gained a bird's-eye view of the health status of America's 12 million soldiers, riddled with disease, addictions, and psychiatric trauma, along with the plans to demobilize 90 percent of them by 1947. And as Eli Junior said, "Ideas don't cure people. Drugs cure people."[69]

If soldiers were on the move, so were Americans at home, and they would need drugs as well. During the war, 15 million people relocated, including 6 million mostly rural citizens of the South who moved to cities in the North. After the war, the continued movement from south to north, from east to west, from rural to urban followed the jobs, and changed both racial and gender politics forever. Women were initially encouraged to give their jobs back to returning soldiers, but the numbers of women in the workforce had rebounded by 1947 and exceeded wartime totals. And among high school girls graduating that year, 88 percent envisioned having a job in addition to raising a family in the future.[70]

The *Mad Men* era was still more than a decade away, but America had entered the era of *The Man in the Gray Flannel Suit*, the influential novel and movie depicting a nation that had lost its wartime sense of purpose and willing sacrifice and had replaced those virtues with the pursuit of material comforts and predictable personal security. These themes would play out in how the Medical Industrial Complex continued to expand.

Chapter 5

Advocates

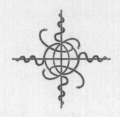

In addition to the more obvious players within the system, the Medical Industrial Complex's Kevlar strength depends on a network of connectors, messengers, fixers, and facilitators that often operate below the surface, in the cracks, and behind the scenes. These self-interested patrons include the patient advocacy groups that came of age at the same time as America's coordinated research strategy under Vannevar Bush. They have made a major contribution in raising both awareness and the funds necessary for research. But as an unfortunate corollary of their success, they wield a kind of "tail that wags the dog" power, which sustains a problematic status quo and often gets in the way of meaningful health care reform.

Not surprisingly, these organizations work hand in glove with the MIC's government-relations programs. A 2018 Kaiser Health News study showed that the pharmaceutical industry gave at least $116 million to 594 US patient advocacy groups in 2015. That amount far exceeded the $63 million posted for direct lobbying activities in the same year.[1]

Most of these patient advocacy groups not only accept funds willingly, deliver letters of support, and make congressional office visits on demand, but also compete with one another for the privilege. Since 1982, for example, the Susan G. Komen breast cancer foundation has rolled out a "Think Pink!" breast-cancer-awareness media barrage that now goes so far as to have NFL players wearing pink spikes.[2] But the eminent breast surgeon Dr. Susan Love not only criticizes this billion-dollar promotional effort aimed at awareness; she disputes the value of early detection and prefers to raise funds through her own nonprofit, which focuses on trying to cure the disease itself.[3] Breast Cancer Action, meanwhile, accuses both the Dr. Susan Love Research Foundation and advocates of screening and early detection of being complicit in "pink-washing"—taking funds from cosmetics companies and even automobile companies that want to divert attention from their dodgy records with regard to cancer-causing chemicals.[4]

But where the system of advocacy becomes most troubling is in its interaction with the governmental agency that allocates most of America's research funding, the National Institutes of Health. Highly publicized campaigns—like our "War on Cancer," "Be the Generation" to end AIDS, and "Genomic Revolution," with its promises of tailor-made personalized stem cell cures for all—begin and often end at the NIH without delivering the kind of widespread benefit to the nation's health that might be attainable through other methods.

Overpromising progress derived from NIH research, especially when it comes to cancer, has a long history. Richard Nixon predicted the imminent demise of cancer when he announced his "War on Cancer" in 1971.[5] Three decades later, Andrew von Eschenbach, head of the National Cancer Institute, told Congress that its funding would "eliminate the suffering and death from cancer, and do so by 2015."[6] In 2009, NIH director Francis Collins, cheerleader for the genomic revolution, confidently predicted, "We are about to see a quantum leap in our understanding of cancer."[7] But in 2018, the primary technique used to edit genomes and weaponize viruses to destroy cancer, CRISPR (Clustered Regularly Interspaced Short Palindromic Repeats), was found in some cases to actually trigger new cancers in affected cells.[8] The overall cancer death rate since 1990 has dropped by 25 percent, but only 1.5 percent of that drop has occurred in the past decade.[9] Adding to the irony, an American Cancer Society–supported research study in 2018 reported that prevention could outperform research, stating that deaths from cancer nationwide would drop by 22 percent if all Americans had universal access to high-quality health care.[10]

The research arm of the nation's Department of Health and Human Services, the NIH is housed in 75 buildings on 300 acres in Bethesda, Maryland. It consists of 27 different institutes and centers that together awarded over $37 billion in grant funding in 2018 to more than 2,500 universities, medical schools, and other research institutions in every state and many countries around the world.[11]

This government agency is not only highly susceptible to the influence of advocacy groups; it is guided by private citizen advisory boards whose members, more often than not, have a range of conflicts of interest derived from serving as consultants or employees in the very companies and academic organizations that benefit from NIH funding. This system of influential boards, pressure groups, and competing institutional fiefdoms means that who you know is often more important than what you know, and that the art of persuasion at times carries more weight than the supporting evidence. This cronyism has encouraged a culture of overpromising throughout the research establishment, as well as a focus on dazzling, high-tech cures rather than the fundamentals of public health and prevention.

Sadly, the United States has embraced this culture of big-ticket research and development as if it were a substitute for rational health planning and delivery, as if success in finding cures and developing new drugs and devices would preclude the need for services altogether. This is in marked contrast to the approach taken by nations such as Canada, Switzerland, and Germany, which treat research and development—R&D—as one element of a comprehensive national health plan. What all other developed nations know, and what we have yet to acknowledge, is that health is not just the absence of certain targeted diseases, and that the nation's health and well-being require a well-planned and universally available network of integrated health services, along with secure social services that can bolster our population's safety, financial security, nutrition, housing, and education.

The United States is the only developed nation that spends more on health care than all other social services combined.[12] For example, the nation invests very little in nutrition education, local access to healthy foods, aggressive taxing of unhealthy foods, school programs focused on nutrition and exercise, or general public-health campaigns, even as obesity rates exceed 40 percent in the US population. Obesity is now a contributing factor for 18 percent of deaths a year, including 40,000 cancer cases, and for rates of cardiovascular disease 2.5 times those in non-obese Americans.[13]

The same is true of childhood poverty, which cost the nation $1.03 trillion, or 5.4 percent of the GDP, in 2015, by promoting poor health, crime, and low productivity. For each $1 spent to ameliorate poverty, our nation would save $7 in the economic costs of poverty.[14] The top 5 percent of hospital users in the United States, who consume over 50 percent of the health care costs, are predominantly poor and housing insecure.[15]

Finally, consider the abysmal state of postpartum care for moms in the United States. The vast majority are discharged less than 48 hours after birth. As a mom quietly struggles to manage her new infant's needs, she ends up ignoring her own substantial recovery. If she were in Switzerland, the hospital stay would be longer. In England or France, a midwife would be by for a home visit in the first week. In Sweden or Norway, there would be a generous maternity leave. In the US, one-quarter of women go back to work less than two weeks after giving birth.[16]

This is why the National Academy of Sciences consensus report in 2017 stated, "The context in which people live affects health. There are numerous social determinants of health within one's neighborhood—concentrated poverty, crime, walkable neighborhoods, the ability to exercise, and access to healthy food."[12] Yet funding for NIH projects with the word "public" or "population" in the title has declined by 90 percent in the past decade. In contrast, $15 billion of the total $26 billion of extramural NIH funding in 2016 was awarded to projects that included one of the following four index terms: "gene," "genome," "stem cells," or "regenerative medicine."[17]

Given the role of overpromoting and overpromising in today's biomedical research establishment, it makes sense that the structure for advocacy was set in place by two well-meaning socialites who knew a lot more about throwing dinner parties and framing press releases than they did about science.

For more than half a century, Mary Lasker and Florence Mahoney, both born to wealth and social standing, managed to steer legislation and financial appropriations to reflect their own priorities: intervention over prevention, segmentation over integration, applied research focused on interventional therapies more than basic science research, active inclusion of industry in major policy decisions, and the establishment of an integrated career ladder that encouraged compromised ethics and the skewing of fundamental checks and balances.[18] With nothing but good intentions, these women worked in a way that all but guaranteed a system riddled with conflicts and unintended consequences.

Born in 1900, Mary Lasker was the daughter of Frank Elwin Woodard, the head of the local bank in Watertown, Wisconsin, and a shrewd businessman with Chicago connections. By her own account, she was a campaigner almost from birth, and she traced her interest in promoting medical research back to an event she experienced at the age of three or four. Her mother, a local community supporter and civic activist, took Mary to see their ailing servant, a Mrs. Belter, who had undergone a double mastectomy as treatment for breast cancer. "I thought, this shouldn't happen to anybody," Mary Lasker later wrote. "And when I stood in the room and [saw] this miserable sight with her children cowering around her, I was absolutely infuriated, indignant, that this woman should suffer so and that there should be no help for her."[19,20]

In her teens, Mary Lasker traveled with her mother to Europe, briefly tested (and rejected) the University of Wisconsin at Madison, embraced art history for her degree at Radcliffe, and then did a little résumé-buffing at Oxford University. From there she moved to New York City, where she met the highly successful art gallery owner Paul Reinhardt, worked for him, then married him at the age of 26.[19]

The timing wasn't perfect. The Depression was about to take its toll on the art market, and Reinhardt sank into a deep depression worsened by alcohol abuse. In 1934, after eight years of marriage, Mary cut her losses.[21,22] But her first husband had spawned her interest in psychiatry as well as art, and some years later she would become one of the largest private art collectors in America, as well as the country's foremost advocate for federal investment in the National Institute of Mental Health.

Freed from responsibility for her ailing husband, she was able to travel in the highest levels of society in New York City. She met not only the top politicians, leading philanthropists, and academic elites, but also the leading proponent of birth control, Margaret Sanger of the Birth Control Federation of America. Mary was hooked and soon signed up for service.[23]

Reaching out for financial support, she turned to a dynamic advertising man, Albert Lasker, who had launched some of America's most recognizable consumer brands, including Lucky Strike cigarettes, Wrigley's chewing gum, Pepsodent toothpaste, and Sunkist oranges. Known as the "father of modern advertising," Lasker was also politically connected, having helped engineer Warren Harding's successful presidential campaign in 1920.

Twenty years Mary's senior, Lasker admired her intensity and sense of mission, but at the time of their meeting, he was still recovering from the dissolution of his second marriage, to movie star Doris Kenyon. Even so, Lasker became deeply committed to Mary's activism, and he donated to the cause, though his most lasting contribution to Margaret Sanger's legacy undoubtedly was his suggestion that she change the name of her Birth Control Federation of America to the Planned Parenthood Federation.

By the late 1930s, though, Mary was ready to reset her health-advocacy priorities. She could see that Pope Pius XI's and the Catholic Church's strong opposition to "artificial birth control," as outlined in the 1930 papal encyclical *Casti connubii*, was going to be a near-impenetrable obstacle in her path.[23] And Margaret Sanger had become even more controversial with her ties to eugenics. Moreover, accusations were flying around that the organization's "Negro Project," designed to expand African American women's horizons in the South, was targeting minorities for birth control to limit their numbers.

When Albert asked Mary what she wanted to accomplish, she listed reforms in health insurance, cancer research, and research against tuberculosis. Albert responded, "Well, for that you don't need my kind of money. You need federal money, and I will show you how to get it." When she protested that she had no contacts in government, he said that was no problem.[24] Not only had he bought and sold the nation's largest advertising firm—twice—but he had been a prominent Republican political supporter, a holder of various government posts, and a friend of presidents and congressmen galore.[25]

When Mary and Albert married in 1940, the world was preparing for war, and Mary could see there was little interest in a domestic initiative like national health insurance. So she focused all her energy on medical research. Her father had died of a stroke in 1933, and when her mother succumbed to the same ailment a few years later, Mary asked medical experts at the AMA, the Rockefeller Foundation, and top academic centers about the underlying causes of such often fatal arterial obstruction. Nobody seemed to know, and no one believed it could be prevented, which triggered a reaction in Mary much like the outrage she had felt at the sight of her childhood servant suffering from breast cancer.[26]

Beginning in 1942, the Laskers began to cultivate science luminaries who shared their commitment to maximizing government funding of applied research focused on curing diseases rather than simply studying them. As Mary surveyed the American research establishment, the one name that kept turning up was that of Vannevar Bush. As she noted, "I read that the only research of any consequence that was going on, by the Federal Government for the war effort, was being done through the Office of Scientific Research and Development."[27]

The Laskers realized early that they would need a credible health-related national organization to anchor and launch their campaign for a federal role in medical research comparable to the effort in war-related science led by Bush. In 1943, they set their sights on the American Society for the Control of Cancer, an organization created in 1913 by 10 physicians meeting at the Harvard Club in New York City and led by Dr. Clement Cleveland.[28] The organization's mission at the time was to "disseminate knowledge about the symptoms, treatment, and prevention of cancer; to investigate conditions under which cancer is found; and to

compile statistics about cancer." By 1940, this doctor-controlled organization had 1,000 members and an annual budget of $102,000, none of which
was devoted to research. The leaders were more than happy to grant the
Laskers easy entry to their board in return for financial support. By 1944,
the Laskers had seized control of the board, largely dumped the doctors,
and renamed the group the American Cancer Society (ACS). Its leadership
was now composed of name-brand corporate heads, entertainment giants,
and advertising executives. Its purpose was also clearly restated: The goal
was now to *cure* cancer. The organization would do so by advertising to
the public to raise funds and promoting the glory of medical discoveries through the popular press. In 1948, the ACS received $14 million in
private donations and allocated nearly $4 million to research.[24,28]

To add further glory to the idea of Big Science, Mary and Albert
created the annual Lasker Awards, with the somewhat self-serving tagline
"Sometimes called 'America's Nobels.'"[29] As they chose recipients, they
consciously developed relationships and secured their recipients' commitments to support expanded federal funding in biomedicine. Luminaries from the Army Medical Corps, including cardiac surgeon Michael
DeBakey and psychiatrist William Menninger, were early honorees, as
was Sidney Farber, a Boston Children's Hospital expert on childhood leu-
kemia. The dollar award wasn't very large, but given Arthur's connections
and expertise, the publicity surrounding entry into America's new medical aristocracy was priceless. Not surprisingly, honorees were more than
happy to testify before committees in Washington on a moment's notice.

Albert had been happy to provide seed money and introductions and
to selectively engage his television and media friends like RCA's David
Sarnoff and *Reader's Digest*'s DeWitt Wallace to, among other things,
break the taboo around mentioning the word "cancer."[24,30] But he wasn't
prepared to be Mary's constant companion in Washington, DC. Luck-
ily, she met a like-minded friend with a slightly different style but equal
determination and strength to serve that role. Her name was Florence
Mahoney.

Born one year before Mary Lasker in Muncie, Indiana, Mahoney
was raised in a privileged family and embraced women's rights, health,

and exercise as a young girl.[18] She worked in a children's hospital, and her subsequent career as a teacher eventually morphed into journalism. This second career received a boost in 1926, when she met and married Daniel J. Mahoney Sr., the president of Cox Newspapers. The newspaper empire, which included the *Miami Daily News* and the *Dayton Daily News*, eventually grew into Cox Communications, under the leadership of former three-time governor of Ohio and 1920 presidential candidate James Middleton Cox. His running mate that year was Franklin Roosevelt. Ironically, they lost to fellow Ohio publisher Warren Harding, who benefited mightily from the support and guidance of the young advertising genius Albert Lasker.[31]

In addition to managing her family and an extensive social life in Miami, Florence, under the pseudonym Mary Marley, wrote a weekly column in the *Miami News* focusing on controversial issues of the day, including birth control and the treatment of the mentally ill. At the same time, she used her natural talents as a hostess to wine and dine a range of luminaries and politicians who visited the burgeoning city. Her efforts were augmented by the political and business contacts of both Mahoney and Cox.

Florence understood as well as anyone the power released by combining social graces, an understanding of the news media, and political connections, along with passionate advocacy for disadvantaged communities. She also had an eye for talent. The list of high-level contacts grew as the Mahoneys shuttled between homes in Miami, Washington, and New York.

In 1944, the Laskers came to Miami to explain their recent takeover and rebranding of the American Cancer Society, as well as the shift in focus toward finding a cure. The Mahoneys' response was to organize Miami fund-raisers that delivered $35,000 to the Lasker Foundation, a gesture that cemented Mary and Florence's friendship.[32]

While Mary and Florence shared a philosophy anchored in women's rights and family health, the two had somewhat different styles.[33] Mary was more direct and in-your-face, demanding, and not shy about self-promotion. Florence was the perfect hostess, a softer but no less deliberate sell, who proudly wore the label "unpaid lobbyist" until she died in 2002 at the age of 103.[18]

With birth control off the table, at least for the time being, the two women converged on their three areas of shared interest: national health insurance, national medical research, and mental health services. After Roosevelt's death, Lasker approached President Truman with an appeal for, and a willingness to support, a push for national health insurance. According to Mary's account, he allowed her to help write the proposal. "He was interested in the general idea of health insurance," she later said, "because he had been a county judge and he had seen a lot of trouble in families, troubled for lack of money for medical care."[34,35]

On November 19, 1945, seven months into his presidency, Truman sent a message to Congress saying, "The health of American children, like their education, should be recognized as a definite public responsibility."[35]

The Truman plan was comprehensive. It included a call for universal health insurance; an expansion of hospitals, especially in rural areas, with incentives for physicians to staff these; and the establishment of a national board of doctors and public officials to develop standards for quality and performance. But he ultimately backed away from the undertaking in the face of withering AMA opposition, which included labeling the undertaking as "socialized medicine" and branding the Truman staff as "followers of the Moscow party line."[36] As noted earlier, this was during the same era when, under the Marshall Plan, the American government was establishing exactly these types of plans for universal health care as an essential part of rebuilding the war-ravaged economies of Germany and Japan. Deterred by the vehemence of conservative opposition, Truman backed away from trying to provide the benefits the US was endorsing for our former enemies, ultimately focusing on constructing hospitals and expanding federal support for medical education and research.[37]

But Mary was above all a pragmatist. In the 1930s, she had backed away from the cause of birth control when faced with opposition from the pope and the Catholic Church. Now she recognized that Truman's push for national health insurance had met its match with the AMA. So she reset her sights on a new goal. During the war years, she was critical of the lack of government support for medical research. She did note, however, that Vannevar Bush had been able to accomplish miracles via the

Office of Scientific Research and Development. But Mary and Florence were concerned that, with the coming of peace, the agency was going to be dismantled.[38,39]

As she later recalled, "I felt that the United States should have an on-going scientific effort in all areas of science and a substantial one in the area of medical research. . . . At the same time, the United States Public Health Service had within its organization something called the National Institutes of Health, which was for research, and the National Cancer Institute, and these two organizations, between the two of them, had about $2 million all told for research, most of which was spent intra-murally, within the Public Health Service itself. For instance, in 1946, the Cancer Institute had only $70,000 to give in grants to outside institutions for cancer research, and at that time they thought $70,000 was plenty."[40]

Meanwhile, Florence had learned that the chairman of the Senate Subcommittee on Wartime Health and Education was Senator Claude Pepper, who resided in her district in Florida, and benefited from the support of Cox newspapers.

On September 17, 1944, Pepper held a hearing that revealed that, until recently, the US Armed Forces had been rejecting about a third of recruits as either mentally or physically unfit. In the Laskers' view, this troubling level of incapacity was "due to inadequate medical care, lack of treatment and cures due to insufficient medical research."[41]

The next day, Mary and Florence met with Pepper for lunch in the Senate dining room and convinced him of the need for substantial federal funds for medical research. Pepper agreed to further hearings on December 13, 1944, and asked the women to draw up a list of expert witnesses. This marked the beginning of an active, selective, and often secretive career ladder these two influential women could influence through the granting of the Lasker Awards, the selection of "scientific experts" for congressional testimony, and, in the future, identification of candidates for various applied research and NIH disease-specific advisory boards.

In the fall of 1944, Mary was focused on trying to preserve the basic function of Vannevar Bush's OSRD. She approached her close friend, Anna Rosenberg, Roosevelt's trusted adviser and head of his War Manpower

Commission, who instructed her, "Write me a memo about it." Mary Lasker described the influence of her memo this way: "Roosevelt handed it to Judge (Samuel) Rosenman, who also was a friend of mine. . . . Rosenman drafted a letter to . . . the head of OSRD, and . . . [he] wrote a very handsome and fine outline of what he felt was needed, called 'Science: The Endless Frontier,' in which medicine was to be part of whatever was to be done about science generally." In other words, at least according to Mary, the draft of Roosevelt's famous wartime letter to Vannevar Bush was actually a Lasker creation.[42]

After Truman became president, Mary secured his tentative support for medical science funding, and by August 6, 1947, the House and Senate passed the National Science Foundation Bill, which included federal funding for medical research with an autonomous NSF director appointed by an independent committee of scientists.[43]

Lasker and Mahoney first pushed for research institutes independent of the National Institute of Health (then still singular) before shifting their position in 1946 in favor of expanding its research capabilities. Several new research institutes were established with their support by 1950, including the National Heart Institute, the National Institute of Mental Health, and the National Institute of Neurological Diseases (now Disorders) and Blindness, each with the ability to award research grants to investigators throughout the country and the world. With lobbying support, the NIH budget grew 150-fold, to $460 million, between 1945 and 1961, and reached $1 billion by the late 1960s.[44,45]

Florence divorced Daniel Mahoney in 1950 and moved permanently to Washington, where she became well established as the "unofficial host of the health lobby."[38] She encouraged Mary Lasker to hire a full-time lobbyist, and their choice was 1948 Lasker Award winner Mike Gorman, an Oklahoma journalist who had made his name in 1946 with an excoriating series on the wretched condition of Oklahoma's mental hospitals.[46] In 1951, they arranged for Gorman to become a member of Truman's Commission on the Health Needs of the Nation. Two years later, he became executive director of their new creation, the National Committee Against Mental Illness.

As a lobbyist, Gorman remained in Mary's employ for the next four decades, including in posts heading up other Lasker nonprofit disease-advocacy organizations addressing hypertension and glaucoma, each of which thrived on drug company support. One of their advocacy organizations, Citizens for the Treatment of High Blood Pressure, established in 1973 under the guidance of Mary Lasker and Lasker Foundation chairman and cardiac surgeon Michael DeBakey, and managed by Mike Gorman, secured $120 million from the federal government to monitor blood pressure and promote the use of antihypertensives.[44,45,46]

From the late 1940s until 1960, the Mary Lasker lobbying team—derisively termed "Mary and her little lambs" by opponents at NIH who objected to her influence—focused heavily on two Democratic legislators: Representative John Fogarty of Rhode Island, chairman of the House subcommittee on health appropriations; and Senator Lister Hill of Alabama, chairman of the Senate committee on labor and public welfare and the appropriations subcommittee for health.

Lasker provided the committees with Gorman-written data reports on death, disability, and loss of income due to diseases. Then, in what has been described by NIH biographers as an annual "choreographed ritual," she provided testimony by witnesses drawn from the ranks of former Lasker awardees like DeBakey and Farber and Menninger, who were extensively coached by Gorman to speak in plain language and ask for more, not less. Critics of the budget expansions would then be castigated by Fogarty and Hill as shortsighted. Lasker and Mahoney would orchestrate well-timed editorials in news outlets, and the subsequent legislative reports would urgently call for large increases and succeed, as they did in 1962 when they secured $155 million more than expected.

The various elements of advocacy within the Medical Industrial Complex—the Lasker Awards, the hosting of dinners at Florence's house, the gathering of select members of their medical aristocracy for testimony or appointment to the ever-growing NIH and FDA disease-category advisory boards (on which Mary and Florence themselves served for four decades), the coordinated planting of supportive pieces in print and broadcast outlets, the focus on curing rather than just studying disease that was so well integrated with the approach taken by the pharmaceutical houses, the career-advancement ladder behind the scenes, and the mock-ups for enabling legislation and staging successful legislative campaigns—all of it was designed and largely executed by these two women with the help of one lobbyist.[38,47]

By 1970, there were 11 different disease-specific or population-specific institutes under the NIH, each with the ability to choose its own advisory board and research committee to control the steady outflow and direction of extramural research grants. Staying true to their original focus on a cancer cure, Lasker and Mahoney successfully lobbied to keep the National Cancer Institute segregated from the NIH, thus preserving its line of federal credit, which jumped from just over $1 million in 1946 to $110 million in 1961 and, with the passage of the National Cancer Act of 1971, secured $1.59 billion over the next three years.[48]

Mary Lasker's fierce advocacy was admirable on many levels. She once famously said, "I am opposed to heart attacks and cancer and strokes the way I am opposed to sin."[49] But her sophisticated, backroom promotion and single-minded focus on discovery overshadowed investment in public health and prevention that would have benefited from equal measures of advocacy and arguably provided more benefit to more people. And to the same extent that she was opposed to disease, she was markedly pro-pharmaceuticals. She loved corticosteroids, thorazine, and cardiovascular drugs of all shapes and sizes. She made enemies at the National Institute of Mental Health by accusing its grant operation of obstructing research on psychopharmacologic drugs. In later years, Mary came into conflict with NIH leaders like James Shannon, especially when, in December 1969, she ran full-page ads in the *New York Times* and *Washington Post* with the headline "Mr. Nixon: You Can Cure Cancer." She would later lean on her friend Ann Landers to write a column supporting the proposed Conquest of Cancer Act that would provide profuse funding and free Lasker and her preferred researchers from oversight by the NIH bureaucracy. Landers complied in a column that reached more than 50 million readers in 750 newspapers. In response, one senator, John Tunney (D-CA), received 25,000 pieces of mail in support of the act.[50]

Even Florence Mahoney often found Lasker's maneuvering to be over-the-top. She outspokenly labeled Mary's efforts to wage a war on cancer as "dumb," even though she and Mary were now best friends and joint owners of a ranch in Arizona. NIH director James Shannon agreed with Florence. Many in Congress knew the implied promise of a cure was undeliverable over the short term. They were also opposed to segmenting the NIH into a "disease of the month" club. One congressman remarked at the time, "One of these days, we'll have a left-eye institute, then a right-eye institute, and then we'll start on the ears." Shannon deeply resented what he saw as a policy takeover "by uncritical zealots, by experts in advertisement and public relations, and by rapacious empire builders."[24] Mary Lasker responded that he was "afraid of clinical research."[51] Over the years, even beneficiaries of the system, such as the Noble Prize–winning immunologist J. Michael Bishop, who was also a 1982 Lasker Award winner, expressed their ambivalence. At the time of his Lasker Award, Bishop wrote, "I do not believe that prizes are essential to science. There have been many moments when I feared that they are even detrimental, holding up a misshapen image of what science is about. Winning prizes is not the point of science; it is not the objective of most scientists."[47] But at the same time, he reflected, "to authenticate and embolden may be the most beneficial effects of prizes in science. Pathbreaking discoveries are rarely greeted with immediate acceptance. They disturb the established order by too much. They are achieved by taking the risk of failure and even derision."

As for his benefactor, he knew her well. "Mary Lasker was not one to fret about such things. She had yet another view of prizes. She saw them as advertisement—she was, after all, married to a legendary advertising magnate. The purpose of advertisement is advocacy: buy my product, support my cause. . . . They can indeed be good advertisements. Using the drama of personal achievement, they focus public attention on the benefits and further promise of science. They allow the general public to share in the thrill of discovery. They whet its appetite for more."[47] Exactly, modern critics might say, and all that drama is part of the reason health care costs continue to cycle out of control without a thoughtful debate on the nation's health priorities.

During the 1980s, the Lasker Foundation engaged Geto and de Milly, a top New York City PR firm that also represented the American Cancer Society, to maximize its reach. The firm's case study report headline read, "Heightening the Worldwide Prestige of 'America's Nobels.'"[52] The text below read, "Our efforts bolstered the brand of the Lasker Awards and generated outstanding coverage around the world, including prominent articles in *The New York Times*, *The Wall Street Journal* (front page), *The Boston Globe*, *The Washington Post*, *Chicago Tribune*, *USA Today*, and *San Francisco Chronicle*; in-depth stories in medical research and science-related media; and TV and radio features including a profile for the nationally-broadcast *CBS Sunday Morning*." Albert Lasker would have approved.[52]

Mary Lasker died in 1994, a controversial figure. In the assessment of author and political journalist Elizabeth Drew, "Mrs. Lasker has been considered an able woman who has done good things but is too covetous of power, too insistent on her pursuits, too confident of her own expertise in the minutiae of medicine."[53]

The National Library of Medicine profile written after Lasker's death noted, "Her impatience to speed the transfer of medical knowledge from bench to bedside brought her increasingly into conflict with scientists and lawmakers. Her opponents objected that establishment of separate NIH institutes by disease category rather than by scientific discipline, the rush for clinical testing of such experimental treatments as cancer chemotherapy, and heavily publicized campaigns to 'conquer' complex and poorly-understood diseases like cancer were unproductive because they ran counter to the thrust of basic research: to gain knowledge of the cellular and genetic mechanisms underlying disease on which effective therapies could be based."[49]

Florence Mahoney died eight years after Mary Lasker. In a *JAMA* article memorializing Mahoney's contributions, a former NIH official is quoted as saying, "We liked to call her the 'poor man's Mary Lasker,' since she seldom got credit for things because she preferred to work behind the scenes."[31] The *JAMA* authors obviously had a soft spot for Florence. In their final sentence, reflecting on which of the pair was the powerhouse behind the explosive growth of federal research funding, they commented, "However, the record shows that when a crucial vote was needed, the matter was often favorably settled over drinks and dinner at Florence Mahoney's."

Vannevar Bush, as much as anyone, understood the delicate balance between basic scientific research and applied scientific research. In *Science: The Endless Frontier*, he writes: "Basic research is performed without thought of practical ends. It results in general knowledge and understanding of nature and its laws. The general knowledge provides the means of answering a large number of important practical problems, though it may not give a complete specific answer to any one of them. The function of applied research is to provide such complete answers. . . . Basic research leads to new knowledge. It provides scientific capital. It creates the fund from which the practical applications of knowledge must be drawn. . . . Today it is truer than ever that basic research is the pacemaker of technological progress."[54]

As the NIH grew, so did the shadowy Medical Industrial Complex it enabled, which included both basic and applied research in academic medical centers and within the pharmaceutical industry (which absorbed Vannevar Bush himself) and ever-expanding hospital systems, bioengineers, and medical device inventors, as well as scores of nonprofit patient advocacy and health professional associations that followed the Lasker-Mahoney template in wielding influence often detached from data.

Which also leaves the question of the true legacy of these two women. Should they be measured by the money they raised, or the massive speculative and partially privatized government agency they helped create, or the discoveries of those researchers they helped select and advance? Or should they be judged based on those they excluded, or the absence of a national health plan as a result of resources diverted, or the spawning of future MIC profiteers and a health delivery system so strikingly inefficient as to threaten the future of America's entire economy?

On the liabilities side of the ledger, here are five lasting results of their advocacy that reinforce our conflicted and wasteful Medical Industrial Complex:

1. An NIH that favors applied science research over basic science research, with extensive commercial ties to the pharmaceutical, biotechnology, and device industries.
2. A deeply segmented NIH with 27 different fiefdoms, prioritized by favored "dread diseases," whose funding decisions are directed by statutory required advisory councils made up of members with significant conflicts of interest, as well as relatives of Mary Lasker who sit on NIH advisory boards today.
3. An NIH that overpromises whether on cancer or genomics or precision medicine. Former NIH director and cardiologist Bernardine Healey presciently stated to a roomful of academicians in 1993, "Research is medicine's field of dreams."[55]
4. An NIH that is focused on high-tech cures for diseases rather than on fundamental public health and prevention, that is rife with conflicts of interest, and that serves as the linchpin of nontransparent career advancement and entry into the medical aristocracy.
5. An NIH fiercely supported by a trail of privileged academic centers and institutional researchers, reinforced by industry-supported, disease-specific patient advocacy organizations with the capacity to influence funding amounts and priorities, as well as the trajectory of scientific careers, through nontransparent awards, appointments, and career assignments in government, medicine, and corporations.

Well-financed special pleading, now 75 years old, has fundamentally weakened normal checks and balances both in the NIH and in the functioning of the Food and Drug Administration. Access and standing help define who gets preference as we allocate health care dollars. Funding is determined not solely by data and evidence, but also by who has the most influence in an insider's game.

Four examples show how the Lasker-Mahoney legacy operates in practice today.

One of these involves the Parent Project Muscular Dystrophy, or End Duchenne.org., now parentprojectmd.org.[56] This is not the Muscular Dystrophy Organization that for years ran the annual Jerry Lewis telethon and is supported by a wide range of unions and non–health care corporations like supermarket chains.[57] This is a splinter organization founded in 1994 by a woman named Pat Furlong in the hope of finding a cure for her two sons afflicted with a specific genetic disease that accounts for a small segment of children with muscular dystrophy in America.[58] There are about 10,000 children in the US with Duchenne muscular dystrophy, which generally causes them to become wheelchair users in their teens and die in their 20s. Furlong's own children died in their teens, but she has labored on, though not without compensation. Her 2015 salary was just under $200,000.[59] She placed her hopes for a cure on NIH-supported academic researchers and turned to pharmaceutical and biotechnology companies to build her advocacy organization. They provided unrestricted funds for staffing and daily operations, support for special events and projects, marketing muscle, and focus on new and promising areas of research. In return, the nonprofit provided direct and implied endorsements, a board seat for major sponsors, supportive legislative letters on request, and direct lobbying in Washington as needed.[58,59]

On September 19, 2016, Pat Furlong joined executives of one of the organization's sponsors, Sarepta Therapeutics, to celebrate the FDA's approval of a new treatment for Duchenne's called eteplirsen, which carried a price tag for the patient of $300,000 a year.[60,61] The battle for approval had been going on for years, and the victory was hard-won. In fact, the FDA's own expert advisory committee had voted 7–3 against approval, believing that the small research trial performed had not proved the drug's effectiveness. But that was before Furlong unleashed armies of youngsters in wheelchairs on the halls of Congress following the arrival of thousands of letters, emails, and telephone calls. Ultimately, the FDA director overruled his own experts and granted fast-track approval of the medication, which sent the share price of Sarepta into the stratosphere.[61]

Pat's press release that day began, "Today my sons are dancing! . . . Tears are all too familiar to the Duchenne community. But today, I am crying tears of joy. I landed in Boston, the home of the extraordinary Sarepta team and so many wonderful industry partners, and turned on my phone to this incredible news!"[60] She thanked Sarepta leaders, congressional champions, her academic researchers, and a range of other pharmaceutical company sponsors. In addition, as a testament to Sarepta's altruistic nature and her own support for liberalizing the drug-approval process, she announced, "We also know that Sarepta received a rare pediatric disease priority review voucher, which comes from a program intended to encourage development of new drugs and biologics for the prevention and treatment of rare pediatric diseases."[60]

A priority review voucher can be used by a company to fast-track any future drug submission to the FDA whether the drug meets a special need or not. By speeding up the review process, the voucher may allow a new drug to get to the market for sale 10 months sooner that it might otherwise. But at the same time, the company is allowed to sell its voucher for cash to another company that may not otherwise qualify.[62]

Ten days after Furlong's glowing commendation of Sarepta, her praise was shown to be somewhat naive. Without warning, the company's chief financial officer announced that Serepta wouldn't be using the voucher for approval of any future special-need drug for Duchenne, but instead would sell it on the open market. The expected $100 million plus from the sale of the voucher would be used to help finance other drugs in Sarepta's pipeline, pay for the scaling up of its manufacturing operation, and support the company's entry into European markets.[62]

Obviously, Sarepta's interests were not completely aligned with Furlong's. The lingering question is how much the interests of either party in this story were aligned with those of the public at large. Even though Pat Furlong's efforts may have supported a research breakthrough, albeit of dubious merit, there is little value to her organization's members if the majority can't afford Sarepta's outrageous price tag.

"Insider trading" within the tight-knit MIC fraternity is not limited to favors and influence, especially not when it involves public servants who claim to be advocates of our health but, in fact, have an obvious financial interest.

New York congressman Chris Collins was accused by the Office of Congressional Ethics of breaking the law by advancing the cause of a company, Innate Immunotherapeutics, where he was the largest share-holder and also a member of the board.[63] In 2016, he admitted having up to $50 million invested in this one small company that pinned its hopes on a new treatment for multiple sclerosis. Another investor in the company was former HHS secretary Tom Price, who was forced to resign after using federal jets rather than the Metroliner to travel from Washington to Philadelphia.[64]

Collins was a major pitchman within the halls of Congress for Innate, encouraging other members and the congressional staff to become investors as well. Records going back to 2013 show that Collins advocated for the drug without disclosing his financial interest. When he at last met with NIH staffers and notified them of his personal involvement, he still appealed to one MS expert to advise the company on its planned clinical trial. In June 2017, Innate's stock lost 90 percent of its value when the clinical trial of its vaunted drug failed. In August 2018, he was indicted, and one month later, he abandoned his reelection bid for Congress, only to reverse himself the next month, and go on to win reelection in November 2018.[65]

Industry bias is also embedded within the NIH hierarchy. In 2014 and 2015, George Koob, director of the National Institute on Alcohol Abuse and Alcoholism, had actively solicited funds from the alcoholic beverage industry in return for conducting a study exploring whether moderate drinking was good for the heart. But then the beverage industry took offense upon discovering that the institute had also funded research by Boston University's Dr. Michael Siegel exploring the association between alcohol marketing and underage drinking. Koob called Siegel on the NIAAA carpet and told him that support for "this kind of work" was over. Later public disclosures uncovered an email from Koob to lobbyist Samir Zakhari of the Distilled Spirits Council assuring him, "Sam: For the record. This [meaning the research casting an unfavorable light on the alcohol industry] will NOT happen again."[66] As for the implications of the public health research being suppressed, Koob was said to have told a group of scientists at one point, "I don't f***ing care!" A subsequent review of NIAAA grants found that since 2014 the agency has not funded research by outside scientists on the impact of alcohol advertising.[67]

Finally, recall the case of Antonio Gotto, the cardiologist, statin enthusiast, and dean of the Weill Cornell Medical College. In 2011, a decade after joining Pfizer colleagues at the 2002 Winter Olympics, he announced his retirement. The medical enterprise he oversaw now ranked 35th in the contest for NIH grant funding. Sanford Weill, former chairman of Citigroup and namesake of the medical school, aspired to move up the ranking. His choice as Gotto's replacement in 2011 was Laurie Glimcher, a Harvard arthritis expert who had run an immunology lab under a three-year contract from Merck, owner of the $3-billion-a-year osteoporosis drug Fosamax. She also sat on the board of Bristol-Myers Squibb, where she earned close to $250,000 in compensation, not counting an additional $1.4 million in deferred stock awards in 2010. Add to this $238,545 in compensation that same year from lab-equipment manufacturer Waters Corporation for consultative services. Weill's selection of Glimcher from a 51-candidate pool likely was influenced by her favorable views of the MIC aristocracy. On election, she said she was committed to "leverage the strengths of everyone" including academic, pharmaceutical, and biotech scientists, and she reassured investors, "There should be no silos between all of these different strengths."[68]

Four years later, in 2016, Glimcher resigned her position after turning down the post of dean at Harvard Medical School, becoming instead the CEO of the Dana-Farber Cancer Institute in order "to harness the awesome power of the immune system . . . and genetics to fight cancer." In her disease-fighting role, she also oversees fund-raising for a well-known childhood cancer advocacy brand, the Jimmy Fund.[69]

What the Glimcher case and many others illustrate is that the MIC is no longer simply a loose association of health industry power players who go along and get along to help ensure one another's success. Rather, in the modern era, the various organizations have become Washington, DC–centric, with sophisticated government relations programs that include patient advocacy arms. As Mary Lasker and Florence Mahoney so well illustrated, advocacy within the MIC can create widely distributed benefits among the people who know people who promote people who support the syndicate.

Chapter 6

The House of God

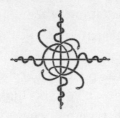

As we have already seen, the Medical Industrial Complex's complexity and opacity cover a multitude of self-serving schemes. Nowhere is this more evident than in the nation's hospitals, which account for one-third of annual US health expenditures. Hospitals are major employers in most communities, critical to citizens' sense of security, and yet maddeningly confusing when it comes to providing and being paid for care. Their billing procedures are often difficult to decipher, and highly publicized accounts of human error, which have increased over the years, have seriously undermined patient trust.

For example, in April 2013, at Regions Hospital, in St. Paul, Minnesota, Esmeralda Hernandez gave birth to a premature, stillborn baby boy she named José. After she cradled the tiny infant in her arms overnight, the hospital staff said that they would arrange to cremate the remains.[1] About two weeks later, though, the family heard some disturbing news: The body of an infant, still wearing a diaper and Jose's identification bracelet from Regions Hospital, had been found the day after his stillbirth amid dirty linens in a laundry facility 45 miles away. An employee at the facility had been opening bags of dirty hospital laundry when he felt something drop onto the floor. He looked down to see a baby lying on the metal grate beneath him. The laundry called the hospital, which sent the mortuary staff to pick up the body, but neither the laundry nor the hospital notified either the family or the police.

Swaddled in a sheet, the body initially had been placed on a shelf in the hospital morgue, and then an employee mistook the bundle for simply dirty laundry. According to Mrs. Hernandez's lawyer, insult was adding to injury in that Regions knew exactly what had happened but kept quiet about it until the family called to inquire. Meanwhile, gawking laundry workers had taken photos of baby José and circulated them on the Internet.

When contacted by the police, the office manager at the laundry said that it was "not uncommon" for its employees to find in the hospital's linens medical waste that might include discarded tissue, blood, and occasionally an arm or a leg.

Indeed, only a few days later, a baby named Chang was delivered to the same laundry service under the same circumstances. Nor is this a situation unique to one hospital in Minnesota. During the same 12-month period, similar mistakes took place in Miami, Florida; and in Lorain, Ohio. In 2008, in Fort Worth, Texas, a stillborn boy was accidentally sent to a laundry, and the body was later found crushed and disfigured.[1]

But indignity is hardly the only offense of which American hospitals are guilty. Shortly after Elizabeth Moreno had back surgery in late 2015, she received a bill for $17,850.[2] But that staggering hit to her personal finances was not for the procedure itself; it was just the bill for a follow-up urine test the institution had quietly made standard practice for surgery patients being discharged with a pain medication prescription.

The Houston-based lab that conducted the test charged $4,675 to check her urine for a variety of opioids; $2,975 for benzodiazepines; and $1,700 more for amphetamines. Tests to detect cocaine, marijuana, and PCP (angel dust) added another $1,275. The bill also included $850 to test for buprenorphine, a drug used to treat opioid addiction, as well as an $850 fee to verify that nobody had tampered with her specimen.

Moreno's insurer, Blue Cross and Blue Shield of Texas, refused to cover these costs, stating that the lab was not in her insurance network. In its "explanation of benefits," Blue Cross mentioned, incidentally, that it would have valued the lab work at $100.92.

Moreno's father, a retired physician named Paul Davis, accused the lab of "price gouging of staggering proportions" and complained to the Texas attorney general's office. In response, the lab's attorney said that, given the rise in opioid abuse, the testing was a justified public health initiative necessary to prevent further escalation of the nation's raging opioid epidemic. He also said that the lab was in no position to question a doctor's judgment, even if the doctor was under its employ.

When Dr. Davis went further up the line to ask for an explanation, the surgeon said that his actions were essentially "defensive medicine." He claimed he had ordered the tests fearing possible retribution from the state medical licensing board, but the Texas Medical Board doesn't require urine tests for patients receiving opioids for short-term pain.

Dr. Davis later discovered that the lab has an F rating with the Houston Better Business Bureau and that both the lab and the facility where the surgery was conducted are owned and operated by the same Houston anesthesiologist.

Complaints against America's hospitals go well beyond emotional injury and price gouging.

In 1999, the Institute of Medicine published a report on hospital safety that made headlines.[3] The carefully referenced piece claimed that hospital mistakes were responsible for a startling 98,000 deaths in the US each year. That made hospital error the sixth-leading cause of death in America. The report caused a wave of soul searching by medical leaders, and an equally large wave of hiring of high-priced consultants to correct the problem by designing safety into these complex human and technologic systems.

On September 23, 2013, hospitals received a grim updated progress report in the *Journal of Patient Safety*. Study author John J. James, PhD, now estimated the annual carnage to be as high as 440,000 deaths, elevating avoidable hospital errors to the third most common cause of death in America.[4] In the article, he pointed a stern finger at the self-important medical elite by quoting Sophocles's *Antigone*: "All men make mistakes, but a good man yields when he knows his course is wrong, and repairs the evil. The only crime is pride."

The performance of American hospitals is especially dire for women. Pregnancy-related death rates in the US have more than doubled in the past 25 years, placing the US last in this category among all developed nations. Three times as many moms die in childbirth in the US as do women giving birth in Canada or the UK.[5] But that's not the worst of it. In the US, for every woman who dies during the birth experience, 70 more nearly die.[6] Women of color have been especially affected. The maternal death rate for black women, according to the most recent government data, was 43 per 100,000 live births in 2015, compared with 13 per 100,000 for white women.[5] Since 2010, 5 percent of rural hospitals have closed their doors.[7] More than half of the remaining rural hospitals lack obstetric services, thus leaving 2.4 million women of childbearing age in the lurch. Native American hospitals functioning under the jurisdiction of the federally funded Indian Health Services are failing.[8]

In community hospitals, approximately 10 percent more elderly patients die within 30 days of hospital discharge when compared with those discharged from major teaching hospitals.[9] The list of factors contributing to poor performance among hospitals more generally is long and complex. It includes rapid changes in our knowledge base, the absence of a system of well-integrated workplace continuing education, out-of-date guidelines, staffing issues, the absence of optimal technology, poor handoffs between shifts, ineffective integration of outpatient and inpatient care, the pressure for early discharge, and an implementation of electronic medical records that lags behind that of other developed nations.

In 2017, the *Wall Street Journal* placed an accusatory spotlight on the independent and self-regulating professional organization responsible for quality control among hospitals, the Joint Commission on Accreditation of Healthcare Organizations (JCAHO).[10] The *Journal*'s article had been triggered by recent litigation involving the death of two babies within a period of six weeks early in 2014, as well as the concurrent death of a pregnant woman with preeclampsia from a hypertension-induced stroke, in a western Massachusetts community hospital. Hospitals formally review all unanticipated deaths of patients in physician-led mortality review committees. In addition, these unexpected deaths had been recorded in a review by the Centers for Medicare and Medicaid Services, but the Joint Commission made no change in the hospital's "fully accredited" status.

Since 1965, Medicare has required that health care facilities have Joint Commission or state accreditation to receive Medicare reimbursement, and the Joint Commission is now used by 80 percent of these, some 21,000 facilities.[11] These data-reporting requirements cover a range of quality measures as well as extensive documentation of cases of unexplained injuries or deaths of patients under a hospital's care. The organizations pay an annual fee that can vary between $1,500 and $37,000, depending on their size. The remaining 20 percent choose to be evaluated by their own state agencies. The federal government respects the findings of the Joint Commission, as do nearly all state agencies. But the *Journal* investigation found that 350 hospitals that were reported by accreditors to be out of compliance with standard quality measures, and thus in violation of Medicare rules, in their recent past still maintained JCAHO accreditation. Indeed, fewer than 1 percent of those that were out of Medicare compliance had had their accreditations revoked.[10] The Joint Commission, in fact, has a history of being remarkably supportive of institutions, even in the face of underperformance. As JCAHO CEO Dr. Mark Chassin says, "Our mission is to work closely with health-care organizations to help them improve the care they provide."[10]

When an institution receives JCAHO accreditation, it gets not only a pat on the back but also a media and marketing kit called the "Gold Seal of Approval." This includes "We Are Accredited!" pins and stickers for employees and a brochure for patient areas that says, "Whenever or wherever you receive health care, look for The Joint Commission Gold Seal of Approval."[12]

But critics, looking at the quadrupling of preventable hospital deaths due to human error over the past decades, point to the cozy relationship between the JCAHO and its hospital clients as one of the all too convenient interminglings of interests that pervade the Medical Industrial Complex. As health care business strategist Rita Numerof sums it up,

"It's industry insiders."[10] Thirty-two members of the Joint Commission's governing board are health system executives. Among the remaining 12 members are representatives of the AMA and the American Hospital Association, as well as several health care lobbyists.[13]

The Centers for Medicare and Medicaid Services (CMS) runs unannounced visits to check the Joint Commission's results, and in 2014, CMS found an alarming disparity between its own findings and the Joint Commission's in 42 percent of the visits to general hospitals and in 75 percent of those to psychiatric hospitals.[10] The same general disparity was evident in reports in 2015 and 2016.[14] As is so often the case within the Medical Industrial Complex, attempts to monitor quality or improve performance through regulation spawned entrepreneurial opportunity, and the JCAHO created a consultative subsidiary, the Joint Commission Resource, that charges hospitals to get them ready to pass their Joint Commission inspection.[15] This is tantamount to SAT test proctors running the SAT prep courses on the side.

Joint Commission services bring in close to $150 million a year, and easily help cover Dr. Chassin's million-dollar salary as CEO.[10] But if a patient wants to view a hospital's Joint Commission report, these are considered proprietary. The JCAHO website called Quality Check is not consumer friendly and is geared mostly to professionals.[16] CMS floated the idea of making the full results of Joint Commission reports public, but to no one's surprise, the JCAHO and its allies shot it down, claiming that "confidentiality of their inspections encourages candor."[10]

Though the Joint Commission was officially set up in 1951, its origins date back to the Flexner Commission in 1910, when the AMA and its allies trimmed medical schools and hospitals down to size and largely eliminated for-profit and homeopathic hospitals. That year, Ernest Codman, MD, a pioneering Boston surgeon, tracked each of his patients for at least a year, then shared his "End Results Cards" with colleagues. These contained each patient's basic demographic data including diagnosis, treatment, and outcomes. In 1911, he launched his own "End Results Hospital" and followed 337 patients over the next five years, recording and then publishing the 123 errors in practice that had led to patient harm.[17]

The fact that Codman was a surgeon as well as a hospital owner and director was not unusual during his era; many of the hospitals were physician dominated and run. Entry to join a hospital medical staff was by invitation and strictly limited, and these exclusive clubs were self-run and self-policed. The administration of hospital functions, including facility support, nursing, and pharmacy, was managed by a limited staff that answered to the hospital director, who answered to a board of supervisors or stewards made up of well-known public figures. Philanthropy was encouraged, and staff duties included a variety of voluntary coverage and charitable pursuits.

With Dr. Codman in the lead, the American College of Surgeons concentrated on the continuous improvement of hospital functions, and in 1917, the ACS developed the "Minimum Standard" for hospitals and instituted the first on-site inspections. A decade later, it released its first standards manual, which was considered voluminous at 18 pages.[18]

For the next 30 years, the growth of hospitals, like that of the research establishment, enjoyed a leisurely pace. At the end of World War II, however, 45,000 veterans of the medical corps and 60,000 wartime nurses returned home with an appetite for specialization and institutional solutions.[19] The government obliged with a GI Bill that led to greatly expanded specialized knowledge and skills, which were applicable mostly in hospital settings. Federal dollars supported training, research, and the goal of creating 4.5 hospital beds per 1,000 residents across the land.[20]

This tremendous growth in the number of hospitals and their increasing sophistication spurred the American College of Surgeons to approach the American Medical Association, the American College of Physicians, the American Hospital Association, and the Canadian Medical Association to form in 1951 the Joint Commission on Accreditation of Hospitals (JCAH). The new organization was to focus on implementation of the American College of Surgeons' new Hospital Standardization Program. Part of this effort meant replacing physician-directors with professionally trained hospital administrators.[21]

In 1965, with the advent of Medicare, the JCAH for the first time began to charge hospitals for its surveys.[22] Five years later, surveys of psychiatric hospitals were folded in as well. At about the same time, Congress, perhaps recognizing variability among the hospital reports, mandated that the secretary of Health and Human Services validate the JCAH findings. In the next 20 years, ambulatory facilities, dental services, and laboratories were added to the inspection list. The new name, the Joint Commission on Accreditation of Healthcare Organizations (JCAHO), adopted in 1987, reflected the broadening scope.[23]

But the Joint Commission's habit of relying on the active or retired hospital managers and physician leaders to conduct reviews has led to a great deal of carrot and very little stick. Institutions being surveyed usually have advance notice, and preparation for a JCAHO visit has spawned a wide range of consultancy operations that assist the hospital staff in reviewing guidelines, inspecting equipment, updating policy manuals and training, doing legal reviews, and staging mock surveys in preparation for the real thing. Critics contend that the resultant conditions on the day of a JCAHO inspection often don't reflect real-world conditions and that these institutions revert to business as usual once inspectors leave.

By 2003, the JCAHO had added a charm offensive that included not only its gold seal of certification, but also a wide range of awards and training initiatives, including National Patient Safety Goals, Speak Up, Disease-Specific Care Certification, the Franklin Award for Management Excellence, Primary Stroke Care Certification, and the Universal Protocol for Preventing Wrong Site, Wrong Procedure, Wrong Person Surgery.[23]

So, while the pursuit of excellence is certainly an admirable goal, it has been compromised by the embrace of the same intermingling of interests that we've seen throughout the Medical Industrial Complex. Rather than constituting the clear-cut checks and balances that one might expect in a regulatory environment, the inspectors and the inspected appear more like a well-coordinated, full-employment initiative. The collegial process rewards powerful collaborators that have the ability to skew the competitive landscape and not only control the standard of excellence but also grant exemptions when that standard isn't met.

Considering the organization's origins and leadership, it is not surprising that the JCAHO has been slow to respond to the current opioid epidemic, which was initiated in part by the overprescribing of narcotics in the nation's hospitals. In 2016, a coalition of clinical pain experts from public health associations and medical centers challenged the JCAHO's lagging standards on pain that had helped solidify pain's standing as the "fifth vital sign." In a letter to JCAHO president Dr. Mark Chassin, they stated what was already obvious to most other health professionals: "We believe the Pain Management Standards continue to encourage unnecessary, unhelpful and unsafe pain treatments that interfere with primary disease management. Pain is a symptom, not a vital sign. . . . Mandating routine pain assessments for all patients in all settings is unwarranted and can lead to overtreatment and overuse of opioid analgesics."[24]

The move toward specialization and increased sophistication that emerged after the war has led to a two-tiered system.

As of 2018, there are 5,534 hospitals in the United States, 87 percent of which are designated as community hospitals. These provide close to 90 percent of the nation's hospital beds and handle 92 percent of the admissions. Only 430 hospital institutions are designated as academic medical centers, and they are committed to a triple mission of education, patient care, and research.[25] These top-tier centers, labeled "awesome citadels of science" by Harvard sociologist Paul Starr in 1982, are richly endowed with technology, diagnostics, and specialists, and they are usually affiliated with schools and universities that train medical students, residents, and nurses, as well as a range of other health professionals.[25]

Roughly the top 10 percent of these 430 academic medical centers control 75 percent of the NIH grants and are about 30 percent more expensive on average than other hospitals. Almost all of these include a medical school that was an original survivor of Abraham Flexner's severe culling operation begun in 1910 to improve medical education. To get a sense of the current size and scope of these elite institutions, consider the granddaddy of academic medical centers, Columbia-Presbyterian Medical Center in New York City. It moved to 168th Street in New York in

1928 and laid claim to being "the world's first medical center to combine complete patient care, medical education and research facilities in a single complex."[26] On January 1, 1998, the Columbia-Presbyterian Medical Center merged with New York Hospital to form New York-Presbyterian Hospital. Their respective medical schools, the Columbia University College of Physicians and Surgeons and the Weill Cornell School of Medicine, remained independent. Since that time, the corporation has expanded its care network to include dozens of ambulatory care sites and smaller hospitals. In the first decade of the new century, it also launched the Herbert Irving Comprehensive Cancer Center, the Audubon Business and Technology Center, and a new research building on 165th Street. Those investments paid off richly. A comprehensive report on NIH funding in 2008 listed Columbia's College of Physicians and Surgeons as the recipient of $343 million in NIH grants. Academic medical centers throughout New York state received nearly 5,000 separate grants that year, totaling just under $2 billion.[27] By 2017, federal grants for Columbia University's life science projects had grown to nearly $600 million.[28]

According to 2012 IRS filings, the institution that year had some 22,000 employees servicing roughly 125,000 patients a year who occupied 2,500 hospital beds. Total revenue was in the range of $4 billion a year, with operating profits of around $500 million. Eleven skilled executives within the organization earned more than $1 million in annual compensation. At the top of the ladder was CEO Steven Corwin, MD, with a salary well in excess of $3 million a year.[29]

If you include all hospitals today, large and small, the average annual compensation of their CEOs is somewhere north of $600,000.[30] In general, those hospitals with more beds, more technology, more teaching, and more urban settings pay more. CEO compensation is often tied to patient-satisfaction scores, but not to quality outcomes. With 440,000 preventable deaths each year, according to the latest estimates, who exactly should we be holding responsible if not CEOs?

Dr. Corwin manages an enormous enterprise that is far more complicated than all but a handful of hospitals. But whether he should be the czar of an entrepreneurial research effort as well, while attempting to serve New York City's daily health and wellness needs, is a question worth asking.

The trajectories of the hospital and the employer-based insurance industry have been converging since the Nixon administration pushed cost containment, in the face of rapid heath cost inflation in the 1970s.[31]

Since WWII, employers have borne the lion's share of the costs of employee health insurance premiums. These plans exploded in the US after the National War Labor Board, which regulated wartime wage and price controls, ruled in 1943 that health insurance benefits would be exempt from the price controls. The board's action was a response to labor unrest tied to increasing productivity demands in the face of stagnant wages as America struggled to reach wartime manufacturing goals. Its action was subsequently reinforced by later IRS rulings that these fringe benefits would not be taxed as income. The net effect was that, by 1950, 77 million Americans had gained health insurance coverage, delivering a huge additional cash flow to hospitals. This was further augmented by federal dollars in the form of construction grants for hospitals from the Hill-Burton Act, as well as NIH research grants.[32]

Up until 1950, hospitals had been relatively stable nonprofit entities. They focused on service and relied on loyal community-based boards and philanthropy to support hospital construction needs. In the first half of the 20th century, physicians dominated, with reform of medical education and hospital care following the clear directives laid out in the Flexner Report. At the time of the 1929 Wall Street crash that began the Great Depression, the country had committed $3.5 billion, or 3.5 percent of its GNP, to health care. In light of the limited therapies available, this seemed reasonable. Physician wages at the time averaged 2½ times those of a skilled worker.

The focus on "care" not "cure" began to change with scientific advances during and after WWII.[33] Yet by 1973, the national debate had shifted again from cure to cost. The Health Maintenance Organization Act, signed by President Richard Nixon that year, rewarded insurers that created health maintenance organizations to manage both care and cost. The movement to managed care was further reinforced one year later when, as a by-product of the Employment Retirement Security Act (ERISA), corporations could self-insure their own employees with protections from liability.[34] Over the prior two decades, bed capacity in hospitals had increased by a third. But once employers took control of their own health care, they invariably became cost-conscious, with business coalitions suggesting a national goal of reducing the cost of care by 15 percent. Almost immediately occupancy levels and the length of stay in hospitals dropped precipitously. The recession of 1980–1981 reinforced that trend, as did advances in technology that promoted ambulatory procedures and less invasive interventions in nearly every specialty field.

In 1982, the National Commission on Social Security Reform quietly inserted an innocent proposal to reform hospital payments and delivered the package to the Reagan White House and Congress. In January 1983, Reagan approved the measure that all but eliminated cost-plus hospital reimbursement for Medicare patients, putting in its place a prospective payment system.[35] Before this, doctors and hospitals were able to establish their own prices for services and expect payment with submission of itemized bills. But now, episodes of care were bundled under 400-plus diagnoses or diagnosis related groups (DRGs). Under the new system, Medicare would pay a fixed amount for a given diagnosis regardless of how long a patient was in the hospital and regardless of how many resources were consumed. If the hospital was efficient and careful, it could make money. If not, the institution would eat the difference.[36]

At the time, the American Hospital Association did not object, because its analysis suggested that this system could be a winner for its members. Academic health centers were supportive because the new system included extra payments above and beyond those awarded to community hospitals as acknowledgment of these institutions' role as educators of medical students and residents, their treatment of more complex disorders, their service to the poor and uninsured, and the overutilization of resources that was part and parcel of an educational training environment.

But the law, along with the expansion of managed care and the self-insured employers' cost containment, fundamentally changed the hospital balance of power. For the first time, hospitals across the country were struggling each year to stay above water. Clearly, physicians could no longer receive carte blanche in managing their patients in the hospital. Cost now mattered, as did the numbers of tests and therapies ordered, the standardization of equipment in and outside operating rooms, and the length of a patient's stay. Suddenly physicians found themselves being evaluated for both the quality and the cost they were directing. As one analyst put it, "The quiet change in payment methods introduced a cascading set of changes—dramatically shorter hospital stays, fierce competition among health care payers, and new limits on physician autonomy." Another remarked, "How, where, and for how long patients would be treated is being circumscribed by new rules, regulations, and protocols."[37]

By 1984, the business community saw little relief as its health premium costs exceeded $100 billion nationwide. In response, employers experimented with more choice and lower-cost plans. Half of all employers changed their offered health plans between 1983 and 1985. Many went for restrictive networks that often limited use of expensive academic health centers.[38] Prior to this, the top 40 or so premier institutions had witnessed spectacular growth since the passage of Medicare and Medicaid, and the explosion of research funding from the federal government. The grants covered a wide array of services and facilities, including reimbursement for direct and indirect costs. But now, profits at elite hospitals had declined suddenly.

By the time the 1990s arrived, prospects for these premier institutions were looking questionable. The educational enterprise was increasingly underfunded. Inpatient reimbursement continued to decline alongside admissions and the length of stay. The extensive faculty hirings of the previous two decades left the institutions with an aging, top-heavy faculty and little room for young, research-savvy faculty members to advance. Care was increasingly shifting to an outpatient model, which complicated the training of residents and students. The focus now was on cost control and redesigning workflow to increase efficiency. In the decade ahead, fears of declining revenue would become reality. Medicare margins for the major academic teaching hospitals declined from 14.2 percent in 2000 to 2.3 percent in 2006 and –0.6 percent in 2009.[35] As a result, they began to pursue research dollars even more aggressively.

President Clinton's foray into health care reform, launched on September 28, 1993, offered academic leaders a seat at the table. In addition to proposing mandatory universal coverage, a generous benefit package, and protections for those with preexisting conditions, Clinton's 1,000-page proposal included the creation of a national health board to oversee quality, extra funding for physician training, the creation of medical information systems, malpractice and antitrust reform, and a Medicare prescription drug benefit. But one year later, it went down in defeat at the hands of a coalition of conservatives, libertarians, and the health insurance industry, which invested millions in a fictional TV couple, "Harry and Louise," who publicly despaired over the impending tidal wave of bureaucracy that was about to overtake their lives.

Fear of that impending tidal wave contributed to huge wins for Republicans in the 1994 midterm elections. With Republicans now in control of Congress, and health care costs continuing to escalate in the status quo environment, the Balanced Budget Act of 1997 incentivized the rise of managed Medicare, a partial privatization of the federal program that allowed commercial insurers to share in cost savings by instituting procedures such as restricted access to high-cost hospitals and providers.[39] The appearance of choice further strengthened the belief among employers that the health care benefits they provided to their employees should be repositioned as a "defined contribution" rather than a "defined benefit." In the past, employers committed to providing workers with health coverage and were willing to bear the brunt of rising costs from year to year. But now, they identified a maximum financial contribution they were willing to provide each employee for health care. Any cost above that maximum was now the employee's responsibility.

Along with these financial changes, employers moved to a menu of different health plans with varying benefits and costs in the belief that forcing workers to consider the value of various plans and make a conscious choice each year would result in lower consumption of health care services.

The Office of Management and Budget in 1984 predicted that the creation of alternative choices for the Medicare population would save $115 billion over the next five years. But hospital leaders felt the price for them would be high. Consumers were demanding more choice, less cost, more efficiency, more outpatient care, and more screening and prevention.[39] What followed was a buying spree as hospitals, surgical centers, long-term-care facilities, and health maintenance organizations began to merge with one another in a cascade of strategies designed to achieve geographic dominance over their competitors. Individual hospitals gave way to hospital systems with ambulatory-care facilities, diagnostic and treatment centers, and salaried physicians. To service these new networks, hospital systems invested in advanced information systems to link together partners in an explosion of data management designed to measure cost, quality, and patient satisfaction.

Only the strongest would survive. The 1980s had witnessed the closing of approximately 500 hospitals, a trend that would continue for the next two decades and involve large, city-run facilities as well as small hospitals in rural areas.[40] Many institutions merged or were acquired, and physicians continued to opt to be employees of these ever-growing health systems rather than compete with them as independent professionals. As these geographically linked health-delivery networks strengthened, the pressures on the top-flight academic health centers intensified, and they found themselves competing with increasingly sophisticated suburban hospitals staffed with physicians and nurses they had trained.

Once more, academic institutions doubled down on their differentiating strengths: biomedical research, specialty medical training and care, and complex, high-tech interventional medical and surgical procedures, as well as care for urban, poor, and very sick patients, in the hope that supplemental funding would be provided. To do this, they signed cooperative research agreements with industry, constructed research buildings, opened clinical research units, created specialized patent offices with intellectual property lawyers, and encouraged faculty members to pursue federal grant money. Local government was more than willing to incentivize their entry into the tech economy, viewing this as the wave of the future and a rich source for future high-wage jobs.

Academic medical center CEOs like Steve Corwin also figured prominently in the negotiations with the Obama administration that led to support for the 2010 Affordable Care Act from the American Hospital Association and the Association of American Medical Colleges, a teaching hospitals group.[29] The American Hospital Association agreed to financial pricing concessions for Medicare and Medicaid of $155 billion in return for the new hospital business generated through expanded insurance coverage, as well as an agreement with the Obama administration that federal funding for research and medical education would not only continue but expand.[31] Opportunity abounded at the crossroads of medicine and technology for leaders like Corwin.

A *New York Times* headline on March 22, 2017, said it all: "Where Halls of Ivy Meet Silicon Dreams, a New City Rises." The article cataloged a series of investments by major academic medical institutions in the city over the prior 15 years that were just now reaching fruition. Having witnessed Stanford University's accumulation of over $1 billion in science-related royalties, New York City had decided to go full Silicon Valley. With the encouragement of its tech-savvy mayor, Michael Bloomberg, who provided seed money, rezoned land, and spurred competitive zeal with a contest he called "Applied Sciences NYC," funds flowed in during the first decade of the new millennium.

Michael H. Schill, the founder of New York University's Furman Center for Real Estate and Urban Policy, recalled the beginning of the movement: "A lot of universities for which the words 'applied sciences' and 'entrepreneurship' were dirty words now are jostling with each other to get a piece of the game." In May 2017, Columbia University opened a 17-acre, $6.3 billion campus on a former industrial site featuring the Jerome L. Greene Science Center. Cornell University followed in the summer with a 12-acre, $2 billion campus on Roosevelt Island in the East River featuring a science-technology partnership with the Technicon–Israel Institute of Technology. The scientific powerhouse Rockefeller University signed a deal with technology leader Carnegie Mellon University. Not to be outdone, NYU successfully floated a nearly $1 billion bond to expand its Tandon School of Engineering with a focus on high-tech and biologic devices.[41]

The success of each of these ventures leans heavily on health system leaders like Steve Corwin and the faculty, students, and staff of the affiliated medical schools and health systems. Those evolving systems now include a range of outpatient care organizations and an array of network hospitals. They have profit-sharing deals with pharmaceutical and medical device companies, many of which reside in new campus-based laboratories. They have also been on a physician-practice buying spree, pushing their medical staff to be more productive. The proportion of hospital-employed physicians was just under 40 percent in 2015 and by 2017 had passed 50 percent.[42]

While the medical staff's independence and control of its destiny have been steadily declining over the past quarter century, the loss of power has not been evenly distributed. The battle to attract top-admitter physicians and surgeons and maintain them on the hospital medical staff has increasingly devolved into open warfare between competing systems.

Pennsylvania Hospital, where I served as top academic officer from 1991 to 1997, was founded by Benjamin Franklin and Benjamin Rush, and was the nation's first hospital. With pride, it traced its roots back to ancient traditions of sanctuary, charity, and mercy.[43] But beginning in 1990, it was forced to function more like one of the scheming characters on a reality-TV show. Oversupply, and the competition it spurred, was a large part of the reason.

Pennsylvania Hospital had always provided selective surgery for a wealthy clientele from Philadelphia's Main Line, as well as instruction for medical students and residents from the University of Pennsylvania—an affiliation that had been in place for 250 years. But Philadelphia has six different medical schools within a stone's throw of one another, and 350 doctors per 100,000 in population—close to double the number required—at a time when the city is losing population to outlying suburban areas. Two-thirds of those doctors are specialists whose pay is tied to the number of patient procedures they perform. It is one of the most powerful medical training sites in the US, with roughly one in five doctors in America having acquired some portion of their training in the city.

In 1991, a single orthopedic surgeon, Dr. Richard Rothman, and his small group generated directly or indirectly a majority of the hospital's revenue.[44] He accomplished this feat by individually performing more than 20 hip or knee replacements a day through a process the American College of Surgeons calls "concurrent surgery."[45] The group selected four fellows each year to do an extra year of specialized joint-replacement surgery following a residency in orthopedics. These were fully licensed orthopedic surgeons who performed the noncritical portions of Rothman's surgeries. Running four cases side by side, two more than even the most aggressive surgeons were willing to attempt, he would move from room to room overseeing the cases and scrubbing in at critical moments. The process was technically legal and approved by the American College of Surgeons, but it clearly pushed the limits of acceptable surgical standards within the community. The hospital turned a blind eye as long as the outcomes remained stellar, and they were.

As the hospital's chief rainmaker—in medicine they're called "heavy admitters"—Rothman had enormous power, which he was said to have tried to parlay in 1990 into his own specialty hospital with management oversight, as well as the kind of aggressive marketing campaign that would put his picture on billboards. A tug-of-war ensued that did not resolve the issue but instead hastened the resignation of the hospital's longtime and beloved CEO Robert Cathcart. My arrival there as a partner of the new CEO was part of the immediate fallout.

What followed came to be known as the Philadelphia "hospital wars."[46] Dr. Rothman and his partners were tightly aligned with a group of surgeons at Pennsylvania Hospital that was inclined to vote as a bloc and exerted tremendous financial clout over the institution. During his long career as CEO, Cathcart had kept this group roughly in check. But with his retirement, the power shifted.

The University of Pennsylvania Health System's residents in training rotated through Pennsylvania Hospital, and its residency programs were certified through the university. The powerful surgeons had unpaid academic titles and standing at the university, which helped with publications and national recognition for their roles as educators and researchers. Furthermore, Pennsylvania Hospital's board of managers was stacked with University of Pennsylvania loyalists.

But for years, the nearby Thomas Jefferson University medical school had been locked in a battle with the University of Pennsylvania for dominance in the city of Philadelphia and the surrounding eight counties. Both institutions were aligning with community hospitals and physician groups to ensure patient flow into their premier teaching hospitals. While the population in Philadelphia itself was declining by about 3 percent a year, the surrounding counties were growing at a 6 to 7 percent clip. Clearly, in the city at the time, there were just not enough patients to go around.[47]

University of Pennsylvania president Bill Kelley was a specialist in rheumatology whose management team was busy buying up generalist physician practices on the Main Line to expand the health system's primary care base and ensure a continued heavy stream of referrals to specialists in the university's prestigious academic health center. He was a hard charger, known when he was an administrator at the University of Michigan as "Neutron Bill" for his propensity to blow up organizations' leadership ranks, leaving only the buildings standing.[48]

Jefferson was led by Paul Brucker, a well-respected founding father of the discipline of family medicine, who had a softer but no less determined style.[49] He favored loose associations and relationship-based referrals. He wanted Pennsylvania Hospital in his health system and had begun making overtures. To its advantage, Jefferson was located only two blocks from Pennsylvania Hospital, whereas the distance between Pennsylvania Hospital and the University of Pennsylvania was two miles.

Beginning in 1994, the outreach from Jefferson was increasingly visible. First came invitations to various educational programs. Then, as manager of the hospital's Academic Affairs department, I became involved with its admissions committee and was on the dean's committee for hospital affiliates. A mingling of our academic databases followed, allowing

Pennsylvania Hospital clinicians access to a wide range of additional online educational services. But most important—and this was a poorly kept secret—Jefferson's dean, Joe Gonnella, had been quietly courting Pennsylvania Hospital's highly regarded power bloc of surgical chairmen, encouraging them to switch their academic affiliations and move their practices to Jefferson.[49]

The board of managers at Pennsylvania Hospital had no interest in seeing a 250-year affiliation with the University of Pennsylvania go down on their watch. When they faced off with the surgeons, the stakes were high, the tempers were hot, and neither side budged. Rothman and the others crossed over to Jefferson, and in 1995 the board of managers of Pennsylvania Hospital entertained and eventually agreed to an offer from the University of Pennsylvania to sell their much devalued enterprise.

A decade after the surgeons assumed their new leadership positions at their new academic home, Richard Rothman had his own freestanding Rothman Institute at Jefferson, along with billboards throughout the region. The institute has generated an ever-growing bank of patient-care and research-grant dollars. In 2016, Dr. Rothman, now in his 80s, continued to perform 15 to 20 joint replacements a week. His institute employed 140 physicians and had an annual revenue of $475 million. Any link between this and the ancient tradition of "houses of God" for healing, as imagined by the heroic Benjamin Rush, who, along with Benjamin Franklin, created the historic Pennsylvania Hospital in 1751, is long forgotten.[46,50,51]

Throughout the country, similar top-admitter turf wars continue to rage. Hospital beds nationwide have decreased by 200,000 during the past decade, and yet occupancy rates, the actual proportion of times the beds are in use, still hover at only 65 percent. So top admitters are more valuable than ever. We now have 2.8 beds per thousand citizens nationwide, somewhat short of the original 1946 Hill-Burton goal of 4.5 beds per thousand, but that appears to be more than enough, especially if they are properly distributed geographically. In 2017, America's hospitals cared for more than 35 million inpatients at a cost of about a trillion dollars, paid by insurers and patients. Thus, hospitals represent roughly one-third of all health care expenditures nationwide.[25]

When patients confront this cost on an individual basis, it's in the form of a bewilderingly opaque document we call the hospital bill. *New York Times* columnist and author of *An American Sickness* Elisabeth Rosenthal wrote: "Only in America do medical treatment and recovery coexist with a peculiar national dread: the struggle to figure out from the mounting pile of bills what portion of the fantastical charges you actually must pay. It is the sickness that eventually afflicts most every American."[52]

In Rosenthal's view, "excessive testing and sky-high charges" have been "aided and abetted by the complex system of billing and coding that underlies bills."[52] Systems that define disease entities actually date back to 17th-century London, but they first became seriously codified in 1890 by a physician, Jacques Bertillon, who created the Bertillon Classification of Causes of Death. (He also contributed mightily to forensics by introducing new methods of detection, such as the fingerprint.) Bertillon's system stood until 1940, when the World Health Organization adapted it and renamed it the International Statistical Classification of Diseases, Injuries and Causes of Death (ICD).[53]

Four decades later, the US government, under Ronald Reagan, adopted the coding, by then in its ninth form, as the basis for its new prospective-payment billing system. The now famous ICD-9 codes were the functional underpinning for the diagnosis related groups or DRGs in the Medicare hospital-reimbursement plans, which instituted bundled payments for entire episodes of care. Medicare and private insurers, which tend to follow the government's lead when it comes to the mechanics of billing, now have moved on to the ICD-10 version, but in the meantime, private insurers have created their own arcane and increasingly complex versions.[54] It speaks volumes that not one but two codes exist for earwax-removal and are used by both government and private insurers—one for manual manipulation and another for removal by way of irrigation.[52,55]

As with most other forms of complexity in our increasingly complex health care system, the coding and billing system rapidly attracted profiteers. A cadre of consultant experts spread out across the nation, calling on not just hospitals but doctors' offices as well, offering—for a fee—to help organizations maximize their billings. As simple a maneuver as weighing a patient in the office can bump him or her up from a Level 3 visit code with a $175 payment to a Level 4 payment of $225. Thousands of dollars in reimbursement separate code 428 (heart failure) from 428.21 (acute systolic heart failure). And coding incentives add not merely costs but perverse incentives. For example, an emergency department can boost reimbursement coding if it provides a prescription for a narcotic painkiller to a patient whose broken finger it just repaired, which has no doubt played a role in our deepening opioid epidemic.[52,55]

Before long, the ad hoc consultancy that expert coders provided evolved into an actual decree, spawning coding-program graduates who anxiously joined their new national association, the American Academy of Professional Coders, now nearly 200,000 members strong.[56] All of this is fine with the American Medical Association, which owns the 1966 copyright and exclusive distribution rights for Current Procedural Terminology (CPT) codes, which define the billable services that marry with the ICD diagnosis codes available in print and electronic formats, and the resource-based relative value scale (RBRVS), the physician payment system codes required by the Centers for Medicare and Medicaid Services. The AMA collects approximately over $80 million a year in licensing and royalty fees from those who purchase the codes and other data products that are required for all providers participating with the Centers for Medicare and Medicaid Services. Sales of these and other regularly updated information products, like the physician master file database that enables that prescription profiling of individual physicians by drug companies, now account for more than twice the revenue derived from membership dues.[56]

The coding workforce in hospitals and offices, which aims to expedite and maximize reimbursement, is now opposed by an at least equal force of coding experts employed by the insurance companies to slow down and minimize payments. Insured patients are caught in between, presented with confusing bills from doctors and hospitals that catalog what insurers have refused to pay and what the patient is expected to make up. When patients contact the doctors' and hospitals' billing offices, they are directed back to their insurers. By then a portion of the confused and exhausted patients just give up and pay up rather than commit to an often months-long dispute to receive the full coverage they deserve. But even so, they are in a far better position than the millions of uninsured Americans. For these "self-pay" patients, bills, which are on average two and a half times the discounted rate that hospitals and doctors charge insured patients, arrive at their doorsteps before they have had time to recover. Hounding by remarkably aggressive bill collectors follows in lockstep. Injuries compounded by disease and stress bring many to a common destination—medical bankruptcy.[58]

In 2017, past-due medical debt in the US exceeded $75 billion and weighed down 43 million Americans. But for some hospitals, it has become a profit center. Dallas-based Tenet Health Care is in the process of selling off some of its 77 hospitals to relieve a $15 billion debt load. As part of its financial recovery plan in 2008, Tenet created a subsidiary called Conifer that has 15,570 employees. While representing only 5 percent of Tenet's total earnings, Conifer's profit margins are twice those of Tenet's health services. Conifer provides bill-collecting services not only for all of Tenet's hospitals but also for more than 700 other for-profit and nonprofit hospitals, including many Catholic nonprofit institutions.[59] Englewood, Colorado's, Catholic Health Initiatives has a 24 percent stake in Conifer and in 2017 was responsible for 34 percent of its revenue.[59] This calls to mind the words of Sister Irene Kraus, the first woman and member of a religious order to be chair of the American Hospital Association's board of trustees, who in 1980 famously said, "No margin, no mission."[60]

With the addition of some 20 million previously uninsured to the Obamacare-insured ranks, the already expanding health care sector, challenged by the health demands of an aging population, added 394,000 new jobs in 2016 to its existing ranks of nearly 16 million. Doctor hires are a small portion of the overall hospital workforce expansion nationwide, which helps explain why hospitals and health care operations maintain top-perch honors as job makers in most communities. Even so, health care corporations now employ over half of the doctors practicing medicine in the US, a movement away from independence fueled in large measure by the sheer difficulty of managing billings and payments.[61]

Insurance coverage had a documented impact on the expansion of health care services and participating health institutions' revenue. For example, hospitals in rural states that participated in the Obamacare Medicaid expansion increased revenues by 18 percent under the program, while revenues of those in nonparticipating rural states declined by 14 percent. This 32 percent gap well illustrates the degree to which hospitals rise or fall based on case mix and insurance profiles. Had the repeal-and-replace efforts of 2017 prevailed, operating margins in participating states were predicted to decline by over 5 percent by 2026.[62]

The explosion of complexity helps explain why there are now 16 health care workers for every physician in America, and why half of these workers have no clinical responsibilities. While one man's wasteful bureaucracy is another man's job, there is no denying that complexity breeds inconsistent performance, which in health care can be life-threatening. As a recent *New York Times* headline blared, "Go to the Wrong Hospital and You're 3 Times More Likely to Die."[63] It turns out that the "wrong" hospital also delivers a 13 times greater complication rate when compared with the "right" hospital.

In 1984, Jack Wennberg, a Johns Hopkins–trained physician at Dartmouth, was the first to bring this variability of medical practice decisions and outcomes to light. Tracking national diagnostic related groups databases on patients in New England, he was able to demonstrate a wide variability in the number of surgical procedures traced to choice of doctor and hospital in the same basic geographic markets, and in the process unleashed the field of medical outcomes research. Tonsillectomy varied from a low of 8 percent of all children in one location to a high of 70 percent in another. Prostate surgery varied from a low of 15 percent to a high of 80 percent in elderly men. And hysterectomy in women by the age of 70 was only 20 percent in one locale and 70 percent in a neighboring community. While the results could not provide the correct number for each procedure—the number that should have been done—they exposed the variability that was a function of individual physician preferences and hospital policies or lack thereof.[64]

Twenty years later, Wennberg was unable to demonstrate much improvement in medical performance. In one study that analyzed Medicare claim forms in 77 different hospitals nationwide, he demonstrated "striking variations in resource inputs and use of services in the last six months of life."[65]

Since Wennberg's retirement in 2007, attempts to engineer variability out of health care systems across the country have been only modestly successful. Death rates in hospitals have nearly quadrupled in the past 15 years. Health-policy guru Don Berwick, a former Health and Human Services secretary, believes the problem is structural. He advocates a "Triple Aim," asking health care organizations to focus simultaneously on care, health, and cost. His proposed solutions rely heavily on careful coordination of staff and facilities using electronic health records and actual human institutional "integrators" committed to connecting the dots for individual patients receiving complex care. In his mind, "that role [of integrator] may be within the reach of a powerful, visionary insurer; a large primary care group in partnership with payers; or even a hospital, with some affiliated physician group."[66]

He has all the options above in his hometown, Boston. But even in a city renowned for its health resources, the environment can feel chaotic. For example, in 2017, the renowned Brigham and Women's Hospital carried out a round of cost cutting. In addition to the normal draws on its financial accounts, the hospital had absorbed losses associated with a heavy snowfall in 2016, a remarkably high $400 million expenditure for a new electronic health record system, and a $24 million consultancy expenditure to ward off a nurses' strike.[67]

The organization's 18,000 employees were asked to cut $50 million from the hospital's $2.6 billion budget, while also increasing revenue by 4 percent. Most of the ideas were tried and true, including an incentive buyout offered to 1,000 long-term workers whose jobs would be eliminated or filled by younger, less experienced employees. Seven percent of the nursing staff took the deal. Exactly what this will do for the care and health arms of Berwick's Triple Aim remains to be seen.

Other premier academic institutions are going down the same path as Brigham and Women's. The Mayo Clinic has recently reached its goal of cutting a total of $1 billion in annual costs over a decade-long effort. Ironically, at the same time, the clinic is at the center of a glitzy $5 billion Rochester, Minnesota, development plan called the Destination Medical Center, designed to "secure Minnesota's status as a global medical destination." With 32,000 workers, Mayo is already the state's largest employer. But the addition of new health facilities, technology, research labs, and entertainment, education, and transportation-support facilities in Rochester may lead to approximately 40,000 additional jobs.[68]

In 2009, the former president of the American Hospital Association, Rich Umbdenstock, cautioned hospital leaders to focus on patient wellness over entrepreneurial research patents and ultramodern cancer centers like the one at New York-Presbyterian Hospital.[69] But hospitals and their CEOs and boards have always had a penchant for brick and mortar. Add to this new-tech entrepreneurial zeal, flogged by industry and politicians pursuing technology palaces and job creation, and the promises of patents and profits that might accompany genomic-laced personalized medicine, and you get a better picture of why we pay so much for complexity within the Medical Industrial Complex. With an estimated 440,000 preventable US hospital fatalities a year, it is easier to understand why the label "hospital safety," now associated with the third-leading cause of death in the US, is increasingly a contradiction in terms.

But the biggest contributor to health care dysfunction is our Byzantine system of private insurance.

Chapter 7

Insuring Complexity

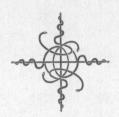

One of the great ironies of US political culture is the fear among many Americans of having our health care dictated to us by Big Government and yet our willingness—in the absence of a comprehensive, societal approach—to subject our health care to the dictates, whims, malfeasance, and greed of Big Business.

In 2003, when Medicare was facing a $13 trillion funding gap, the government handed over part of this federal program to private insurance companies to manage under the rubric of Medicare Advantage. The goal was to stem the costs of the then 38-year-old government insurance program for the elderly by incentivizing private insurers to utilize managed-care principles to curtail costs. The government offered the participating insurance companies a predetermined amount for each enrolled senior and added a bonus payment for patients with more complex medical conditions. But as we've seen repeatedly, almost no well-meaning initiative within the Medical Industrial Complex goes uncorrupted. In 2018, the Justice Department began an investigation of at least five of the Medicare Advantage insurers—UnitedHealth Group, Aetna, Humana, Health Net, and Cigna's Bravo Health—for making patients appear sicker than they were, thereby earning higher fees, while bilking US taxpayers to the tune of $10 billion a year or more.[1]

Our antipathy toward government control has given rise to a private insurance industry that directly and indirectly employs more than 500,000 people, a payroll burden that helps explain why more than 25 percent of every health care dollar goes to managing the business side of health care operations.[2] These large margins help explain why the five largest publicly traded health insurers—Aetna, Anthem, Cigna, Humana, and UnitedHealth Group—saw their stock value quintuple between 2010 and 2017.[3] Yet a large portion of the work these people do serves no direct medical or social purpose. Instead, in office parks across America, health insurance companies pay workers—whose salaries are supported by patient premiums—to deny or delay the medical claims made by those selfsame patients.

When the companies do agree to pay, getting the money is a Whac-A-Mole process whereby the insurer picks up this percentage up to that maximum for some aspect of these particular conditions, after co-pays and possibly deductibles. Which is why doctors and hospitals must employ the additional staff on their end to handle billing codes and other forms of busywork, thus creating additional overheads. This explains in part why, in 2016, 28 percent of Americans with insurance were paying more than 10 percent of their household income, above their health care premiums, for bills not covered by their insurance plans. This earned them the title "underinsured," and led to a situation in which 52 percent of them were unable to manage their medical debt and 42 percent avoided needed care for fear of going broke.[4]

Obamacare was added on to this existing system in a convoluted attempt to finesse our aversion to government control and our penchant for private enterprise. It was a plan developed in a Republican think tank, the Heritage Foundation, and first put into practice at the state level in Massachusetts, where it continues to work well, by Mitt Romney, a Republican governor.

On the national level, the Patient Protection and Affordable Care Act was endlessly attacked during Obama's entire second term by Republicans in Congress, evidently because this Republican idea was instituted at the federal level by a Democratic administration.[5] As their leader Mitch McConnell (R-KY) stated on the eve of the midterm election, on October 23, 2010: "The single most important thing we want to achieve is for President

Obama to be a one-term president." A few days later he added, "Over the past week, some have said it was indelicate of me to suggest that our top political priority over the next two years should be to deny President Obama a second term. But the fact is, if our primary legislative goals are to repeal and replace the health spending bill . . . the only way to do these things is to put someone in the White House who won't veto any of these things."[6]

President Obama served two terms as McConnell and the Republicans battled on. With Donald Trump elected president, McConnell failed by one vote to finally kill Obama's Affordable Care Act. Since then, the White House and its congressional allies have labored on, sowing complexity and confusion, while the general public increasingly seeks simplicity and standardized benefits at affordable rates.

The essential fact of our uniquely American, uniquely profit-driven, uniquely wasteful and dysfunctional system of health insurance is that, like almost every other element in the Medical Industrial Complex, it evolved through add-ons, accidents, and compromises rather than as a rationally formulated plan.

This is not the case in most other highly industrialized nations, and Canada is a good example. When Canada first came together as a nation under the Act of Union in 1840, the words "peace, order, and good government," often abbreviated today by the initials "POGG," were used to define the principles upon which the new country's government would be based. These descriptors are an interesting counterpoint to our own "life, liberty, and the pursuit of happiness."[7] Canadians' expectations were made clear in the Constitution Act of 1867, which stated that, under POGG, the health of the population was an expectation of government. For nearly a century politicians debated whether this responsibility lay with the national government, the provinces and territories, or both, but by the middle of the 20th century large majorities believed that a healthy and productive Canada was dependent on healthy Canadians, and that this required universal health insurance.

Action in this direction began initially in the province of Saskatchewan in the immediate aftermath of World War II, as soldiers returned home, and leaders explored how best to ensure that all their citizens would be healthy and productive in the future. A decade later, that debate had spread to all of Canada, and by 1965, Canada passed its own "Medicare," but the plan covered all Canadians regardless of age, while ours covered only citizens over age 65.

The concept of health insurance originated in the 1880s as a defensive move against Karl Marx. Workers in Europe were restless, and Otto von Bismarck, the Iron Chancellor of Germany, needed a way to take the wind out of the Marxist sails.[8] His solution was to give the poor a social safety net that included health care as well as public education. Overnight, it became mandatory for all workers above a certain income level to purchase health insurance through one of the nonprofit "sickness funds" subsidized by the government that sprang up across the country. The poor received subsidies. This near-universal coverage through privately purchased care was a tangible expression of the nation's social solidarity.

The German approach became the benchmark throughout Europe's social democracies and was also the model for the Japanese. In 1905, the Kanegafuchi Textile Company was the first to establish limited benefits for Japanese workers.[9] Other corporations followed suit, and between 1922 and 1938 a national health insurance act was progressively phased in, mandating that employers offer health insurance benefits and committing the government to provide health insurance to Japanese citizens not receiving an employer benefit.

As noted earlier, the unprecedented destruction of WWII left the Allies' two primary enemies wasted. But in a stroke of pure irony, the pathway we chose to reconstruct Germany and Japan to spur prosperity as a bulwark against communism was never applied at home. In a deliberate, well-planned, and well-financed approach to nation building—the stated objective was to create "peace, democracy and economic stability"—the US military, as part of the Marshall Plan, supported national health plans for our former enemies Germany and Japan. Their main conclusion, as experts at Rand Corporation later testified, was that "nation-building efforts cannot be successful unless adequate attention is paid to the population's health. In addition, efforts to improve health care can be a powerful tool for capturing the goodwill of the residents."[10]

Our own experience with organized health insurance was much more haphazard and chaotic. In 1929, administrators at Baylor Hospital in Dallas came up with the idea of offering employees the opportunity to pay a small monthly premium to cover the cost of a range of hospital services should they be needed in the future. This was instituted as a way to increase the occupancy of unused hospital beds.[11] They called the program Blue Cross, and they offered physician services a year later under the banner Blue Shield. When the Depression caused occupancy rates to plummet further, other hospitals adopted similar programs in other states. By 1939, 3 million citizens had purchased coverage.[12]

When President Franklin Roosevelt first itemized his priorities for New Deal legislation, a more systematic, national approach to guard against the devastating cost of medical calamity was on the list, but it was soon buried by the political realities and challenges of more pressing issues such as Social Security.[12]

In 1935, only 2 million Americans had any kind of health insurance. Across the country, only 48 employers provided this benefit, and most of these were small. One such employer was Henry J. Kaiser, who in 1938 hired a doctor to care for workers who were injured or became sick during the construction of the Grand Coulee Dam.[13]

As noted, the National War Labor Board in 1943 capped wages to control inflation, but as a way to placate dissatisfied workers, it left "fringe benefits" untouched. As an added incentive, the Internal Revenue Service later made employer-provided health insurance tax-free, a benefit that continues to this day.[14]

With the US and its allies victorious, and with Roosevelt elected to an unprecedented fourth term in 1944, supporters of a national health insurance program felt their moment had finally arrived. But then Roosevelt died suddenly, and Harry Truman was left to push for universal health insurance, a collective system of shared risk in which the high costs of the sick would be counterbalanced by the low costs of the healthy. The larger the pool of contributors, the lower the overall risk to the plan.

Studies at the time had confirmed and reconfirmed the weaknesses in the American health care system, in particular the fact that the poor and the aged, a rapidly increasing segment of the population, were especially vulnerable. Doctors and hospitals appeared to be inadequate, both in their numbers and in their distribution. Chronic disease was on the rise, and recent progress in new scientific treatments promoted by academicians of the day suggested that "disease could be eliminated" if only more research were funded.

Truman presented Congress with proposals for comprehensive national health reform. On November 19, 1945, he addressed Congress and said, "The health of American children, like their education, should be recognized as a definite public responsibility." He addressed five pressing health care challenges: (1) the lack of adequate numbers of health professionals in rural areas, to be addressed through federal subsidies; (2) the poor quality of hospitals in rural and low-income areas of the country, to be addressed by establishing national quality standards; (3) the lack of national health leadership, to be addressed by establishing a national board of doctors and public officials to guide health planning and ensure high standards of care; (4) the need to maintain wartime progress in scientific discovery, to be addressed by federal funding of research projects identified as worthy by his national board of doctors and public officials; and (5) the absence of universal health insurance, to be addressed by the creation of a national health insurance fund run by the federal government and open to all Americans but still optional. Enrollee premiums would cover the costs of hospitalization, and the government would pay the doctors' fees. In addition, lost wages of those with illnesses would be paid by the insurer.[15]

He met stiff resistance from the AMA, which labeled his call for national health insurance and the creation of a national medical board "socialized medicine." Truman was forced to accept a partial victory with the construction of new hospitals through the Hill-Burton Act, the expansion of federal funding of the NIH and government-sponsored research, and the creation of new medical schools and the number of doctors they trained. All this unfolded as the profession of medicine continued to evolve toward hierarchical specialization and cooperative power sharing between academic and corporate elites in the name of medical progress. Even so, in 1949, still only 9 percent of Americans had any form of health insurance.[15]

This was the year when the Toledo autoworkers union began to lay the groundwork for a regional pension and health benefit plan for its members and for the workers at their parts suppliers. At the time, unions were flexing their muscles, and strikes were common and occasionally violent. General Motors responded defensively with a health benefit program of its own, and after that, large companies competing for workers rushed to follow suit, even as they continued to oppose a national plan.[16] Corporate leaders saw nationalizing health care as an affront to free enterprise and a stepping-stone toward socialization of the workforce. Like most members of his class, then GM president Charles E. Wilson feared one thing above all others, collectivization; and he felt that GM was large enough to manage its own workers' risk. In dollars and cents, it didn't make sense to take on the cost. But in terms of long-term risk, and at a time when the cost of providing the popular benefit seemed no more than was manageable, Wilson opted to go it alone, and other corporate leaders followed. As a result, by 1962, GM was providing benefits to 462,000 employees as well as 40,000 pensioners, a healthy ratio of workers to retirees that meant the contributions of 11.6 employees were flowing into the GM system to support the needs of each aging pensioner.

A half century later, the tables had turned. In 2006, GM had 141,000 workers to support the needs of 453,000 retirees—a death-spiral reverse ratio of 3.2 pensioners for every worker! Had Wilson still been around, he might have realized that by opposing a national system at midcentury, he had undermined the long-term economic interests of himself, his company, and the nation.[16]

When President Truman retired to Missouri, conservatives like the leaders at GM, as well as those in organized medicine, generally breathed a collective sigh of relief. Dwight D. Eisenhower was now president, and his greatest passion was fiscal discipline. In his mind, the federal government was a last resort, although he understood that to be a successful politician, one had to respect certain boundaries. These included Roosevelt's New Deal, of which he wrote, "Should any political party attempt to abolish Social Security and eliminate labor laws and farm programs, you should not hear of that party again in our history."[17] But the winds were clearly changing. The very sick were increasingly arriving on the doorsteps of the nation's hospitals, desperately ill but unable to pay for their own care. As the costs became overwhelming, the nation continued to rely on the goodwill of public-spirited, community-based health facilities, hospital boards, and physicians who had taken the pledge to serve.

President Eisenhower believed in free markets, individual innovation, small budgets, state control, and political moderation. He was famously quoted as saying, "In all things which deal with people be liberal, be human. In all those which deal with the people's money or their economy, or their form of government, be conservative."[18] When it came to health care, he vocally rejected Truman's call for national health coverage and planning while, at the same time, agreeing with Truman's assessment that there was much work to be done in health care, especially in rural communities.

As a token of its trust in the new president, the AMA supported Eisenhower's creation of a new cabinet-level Department of Health, Education, and Welfare (HEW) in 1953, although it had blocked Truman's similar proposal. Eisenhower nominated his head of the Women's Army Corps, Oveta Culp Hobby, a Democrat, as secretary of the new agency. Her first action was to reject the AMA's handpicked nominee for chief health aide to the agency. But dustups like these were few and far between.[17]

Then in 1958, just when the American Medical Association felt it had the issue of national health insurance under control, the third-ranking member of the majority in the House Ways and Means Committee, Aime Forand (D-RI), introduced a bill that would extend hospital-based health care insurance coverage to those currently on Social Security.[19] The program, as proposed, would be funded by a 0.5 percent increase in both employer and employee contributions to Social Security. What made the plan so alarming to the AMA was not only that it was tagged on to an existing popular federal program, or that it targeted a population at ground zero in the explosion of chronic disease, but that the proposal had rapidly drawn very public endorsements from labor, the American Public Welfare Association, and the National Association of Social Workers, among others.[20] The ranks of the American Hospital Association had held, but its solidarity was deemed tenuous given that its members had begun to complain about having to absorb the cost of large numbers of ill elderly people who landed, unfunded, in hospital emergency rooms.

The AMA's reasoning was that payers make the rules, and that rule makers control not only the conversation but the price. Doctors had somewhat managed the growth of private insurers by expressing their preference for Blue Cross and Blue Shield plans that were controlled by medical societies and had boards with heavy physician representation. This kept a cap on the growth of potential private corporate insurance competitors and offered a defense against the growing public assertion that public government insurance was needed because no other options were available. Doctors viewed with skepticism the emergence of competing private plans, even as they had yielded to the rapid growth of employer-sponsored health insurance in the postwar period. But when it came to involving the government, they drew the line. The AMA launched a full-court attack on Forand and his bill, even appealing for help to Eisenhower's personal physician. Ultimately AMA prevailed, at least in the short term. On March 31, 1960, the House Ways and Means Committee voted down the measure. In August 1960, a Senate version of the bill also failed. But in the process, the issue of medical care for the elderly poor had come front and center.[21]

Congressman Wilbur Mills (D-AR), a veteran deal maker, then joined Senator Robert Kerr (D-OK) in providing Congress with what they believed would be an acceptable compromise. Termed the Kerr-Mills Bill, it dropped the notion of federal controls and funding through Social Security contributions and substituted a much more targeted approach.[20] To begin with, the program would support only those over age 65 who did not have the financial means to care for themselves. Second, while the program would be funded in part through federal contributions or grants to the states, it would be administered by the states. Finally, the program would be voluntary, available only to those states that actively chose to participate.

If all the states decided to participate, the numbers looked pretty good to advocates for the poor elderly. There were 14 million Social Security beneficiaries, with 2.4 million poor elderly people on state welfare rolls. But another 10 million were estimated to be potentially eligible for the new benefits. The extent of those benefits would ultimately be determined by each participating state. The federal government's contribution would be from 50 percent to 80 percent of the total projected cost of the program in each state. The AMA still felt it was a "foot in the door" for "socialized medicine," but eventually it bowed to reality, and Kerr-Mills became law in 1960.[22]

As was the case with Obamacare's Medicaid-expansion offering 50 years later, voluntary participation was spotty. One-third of the states never participated, and ultimately five large industrial states—California, Massachusetts, Michigan, New York, and Pennsylvania—with 32 percent of the poor elderly population nationally, drew 90 percent of the federal funds expended.[22] More important, those that supported a more comprehensive federal program, dubbed Medicare, didn't stop pushing when Kerr-Mills was enacted. In fact, they tried harder.

The AMA's shift in support of Kerr-Mills had been a defensive position, a means, the association felt, of blocking the progress of more comprehensive Medicare. But the election of John F. Kennedy brought the group's concerns back to the surface. Shortly after the election, Congressman Cecil King (D-CA) and Senator Clinton Anderson (D-NM) brought forward a new proposal that would cover the cost of hospital care and nursing home care for elders, but excluded reimbursement for surgeries and outpatient visits to physicians, as a way to control costs.[20] To the AMA, the King-Anderson Bill was a double insult. Not only did it move boldly toward socialized medicine, but it deliberately cut doctors out of the reimbursement scheme as well.

The AMA's concerns were both pragmatic and political. Job number one, as always, was to protect its physician members' financial interests.

In its capacity as a trade organization, the AMA responded by expanding its budgets for state and federal government relations, and by organizing and launching the AMA Political Action Committee (AMPAC) in 1961.[20] For the next two years, those advocating a large federal role and those opposing it fought to a stalemate.

The AMA quickly became one of the largest and, arguably, most successful lobbying forces in Washington. With government relations as an integrated element of a larger professional public affairs program and a vertically integrated network of national, state, and county organizations, as well as the ability to communicate directly to patients though member doctors' offices on a wide range of issues, it set out to make King-Anderson a line in the sand beyond which AMA members would not go.

In this it was not short on allies. Other provider organizations such as the American Hospital Association, the American Dental Association, and the American Nursing Home Association were equally nervous about allowing government to become their paymaster. Also lining up in opposition were the National Association of Manufacturers, the National Chamber of Commerce, the Pharmaceutical Manufacturers Association, and the Health Insurance Association of America.[20] Once again, prefiguring the battle to come against Obamacare, critics argued for more tailored and flexible benefit packages, more selective eligibility, and greater risk-bearing for those currently uninsured.

To defeat King-Anderson and stop Medicare in its tracks, the AMA set out to generate thousands of "spontaneous" letters—notably from nonphysicians—voicing opposition. Its stealth approach was to use doctors' spouses by tapping into the AMA's Woman's Auxiliary, a network of state and local chapter organizations focused on community service and advocacy for AMA members.[23] In 1961, the auxiliary members were almost all women, and the spouses were almost all home-based. To attract thousands of local audiences, and to motivate tens of thousands of volunteers to write letters, the AMA needed someone who could draw these women out of their homes to attend a "special event."

The "trusted spokesperson" recruited in 1961 was a B-movie actor who had already made the transition to corporate spokesman, and who was also the son-in-law of an archconservative physician and Chicago-based AMA bigwig named Loyal Davis.[24]

The man in question, Ronald Reagan, had gained some policy experience as president of the Screen Actors Guild, but his true education in these matters came from Lemuel Boulware, who had served as Roosevelt's operations vice chairman of the War Productions Board, then moved on to one of the military's largest suppliers, General Electric.[25] At the war's end, labor relations all over America had gone from bad to worse as a result of the rapid end of war contracts, conversions to peacetime production, the return of 12 million servicemen to the labor force, and the movement of many unionized women workers back into the home. In 1946, nearly 4 million American workers, including autoworkers, steelworkers, coal miners, electrical workers, railroad workers, meatpackers, and others, went out on strike.[26] During this period, the General Electric Company found itself tangled up in a nasty 17-week work stoppage. As the corporate leaders tried to develop a strategy, they noticed that 16,000 workers in seven of their unionized supplier shops had chosen not to strike. Those seven units, which had stayed on track, meeting their target revenue goal of $150 million in sales, were under the supervision of Lemuel Boulware.[27]

When GE's consultants analyzed this anomaly, they found that Boulware had a philosophy of "going over the heads" of union leaders. Instead of confrontation, he employed comprehensive, ongoing communications and economic education directed not only at workers at all levels in his organization but also at their spouses and families.[28]

Boulware had fostered newsletters, symposia, book clubs, and courses that included a heavy dose of basic conservative economics, but they also touched on entrepreneurship, management philosophy, investment, retirement, health, and family education. Sprinkled in reliably were messages reinforcing the idea that high taxes, government regulation, meddlesome bureaucracy, and outside agitation against free market practices were just not the American way.[29]

The top ranks at GE obviously liked what they saw, and in no time at all, Lemuel Boulware was corporate vice president in charge of public affairs and human resources. Within a short period of time, he had developed a full-blown public affairs training program focused on turning employees into instruments of GE's government-relations effort. With a new army of 3,000 employee-relations mangers and the attention of 12,000 supervisors whose performance evaluations were in part tied to active participation in his efforts, Boulware went about "winning the hearts and minds" of GE's own employees.[30] There were bowling leagues and book clubs, parties and brigades.

The new medium of television was becoming a factor in American life, and another of Boulware's bright ideas was to launch a new TV show called *General Electric Theater*. He turned to Ronald Reagan to host the weekly dramatic series and appear in some of the episodes, as well as to be a goodwill ambassador for the company. Reagan's movie career had stalled, and his adoring second wife, Nancy, thought the shift would take her husband in a promising new direction. The actor would spend a quarter of his time traveling with company executives, addressing and meeting employees and their families, answering their questions, educating them, and ever so gently guiding them into alignment with senior management. The goal was to have workers reject what management saw as negative union propaganda, while embracing the belief that the company was "fair but firm" and supported the "balanced best interests" of its workers.[25]

Over the next eight years, Reagan visited and addressed more than 250,000 GE employees and customers at 139 different GE sites. He read and absorbed the unique Boulware reading list, debated the various views of leading conservative economic thinkers, and observed the workings of senior management in one of the largest and most successful corporations in the world. He also consulted with hundreds of GE lobbyists and public relations professionals, and met most of the important political figures of the day.[30]

So when the AMA began to look for someone to help fight the scourge of socialized medicine, Ronald Reagan was the ideal public opinion operative. Prefiguring Pfizer's Viagra campaign of 30 years later, the AMA in 1961 began to plan a "military style" assault on proposed governmental health insurance. Operation Hometown, the first aspect of this assault, enlisted local medical societies and their physician members to write letters, but also to distribute a range of other print materials, study guides, and high school debate tool kits, throughout their communities to address the grave threat of socialized medicine.[31] Major radio, television, and print advertising would augment and energize these efforts.

The second arm of the campaign, which the AMA called Operation Coffee Cup, was even more devious.[23] It involved using the Woman's Auxiliary and its network to orchestrate thousands of home-based gatherings, or "coffee klatches," as they were called, to advance goals revealed only after the participants had been gathered. As for the question "How do we get them there?" the hook was self-evident: A package for each participant included an LP vinyl record whose cover featured the glamorous movie star, with the name Ronald Reagan in bold, red capital letters, followed in black script by "speaks out against SOCIALIZED MEDICINE."[32]

The record was an 11-minute condensed version of the pro-business, pro-American, anticommunist speech Reagan had been giving for GE for almost a decade, only now with a special focus on how Medicare would be the death knell for American civilization. It reviewed the Forand Bill and the Kerr-Mills Bill that the AMA had ultimately endorsed. And it disparaged the King-Anderson offering, suggesting that its proponents were simply trying to supplant Kerr-Mills before it had time to work. But following his mentor Boulware's methods, Reagan, in his primary call to action, spoke directly to the women's vested interests—the security and future of their husbands' careers, their families, and their status in their communities. Organizers and Woman's Auxiliary "hostesses," on hearing the recording, jumped on board. They were instructed to simply "Drop a note—just say 'Come for coffee at 10:00 a.m. on Wednesday. I want to play the Ronald Reagan record for you.'"[33]

On the record, in his most reassuring tones, Reagan said, "The doctor begins to lose freedom. . . . First you decide that the doctor can have so many patients. They are equally divided among the various doctors by the government. But then doctors aren't equally divided geographically. So a doctor decides he wants to practice in one town, and the government has to say to him, you can't live in that town. They already have enough doctors. You have to go someplace else. And from here it's only a short step to dictating where he will go. . . . All of us can see what happens once you establish the precedent that the government can determine a man's working place and his working methods, determine his employment. From here it's a short step to all the rest of socialism, to determining his pay. And pretty soon your son won't decide, when he's in school, where he will go or what he will do for a living. He will wait for the government to tell him where he will go to work and what he will do."

Then he asked: "What can we do about this? . . . We can write to our congressmen and to our senators. . . . And at the moment the key issue is, We do not want socialized medicine. . . . In Washington today 40,000 letters, less than 100 per congressman, are evidence of a trend in public thinking."

Along with the recording, each local sponsor also received a tool kit that included a cover letter with key messages like "The chips are down, in the next months Americans will decide whether or not this nation wants socialized medicine"; a list of members of Congress; a 10-point checklist on how to write effective letters to Congress; instructions to hosts that carefully detailed the steps to be taken, down to "Provide guests with stationery, pens and stamped envelopes. Don't accept an 'I'll do it tomorrow' reply—urge each woman to write her letters while she's in your house—and in the mood!"; and a report form listing the number of attendees, the number of times the accompanying record was played, and the number of letters written.

Unlike Operation Hometown, Operation Coffee Cup was intended to stay on the "down low." And with 3,000 kits distributed far and wide, and letters pouring into Congress, it would have remained just that if not for an article titled "Hollywood Star vs. JFK," written by Washington-based investigative reporter Drew Pearson, which was distributed nationwide by Bell Syndicates on June 17, 1961.[34] Pearson succinctly sized up the playing field:

Ronald Reagan of Hollywood has pitted his mellifluous voice against President Kennedy in the battle for medical aid for the elderly. As a result it looks as if the old folks will lose out. He has

caused such a deluge of mail to swamp Congress that congressmen want to postpone action on the medical bill until 1962.
What they don't know of course is that Ron Reagan is behind
the mail, also that the American Medical Association is paying
for it. Reagan is that handsome TV star for General Electric
who is frequently opening national political conventions with
the singing of the Star-Spangled Banner and who has starred
in *Hasty Heart*, *John Loves Mary* and *Voice of the Turtle*. He is
also a breeder of thoroughbred horses, trainers and jumpers.
Just how this background qualifies him as an expert on medical
care for the elderly remains a mystery. Nevertheless thanks to
the deal with the AMA and the acquiescence of GE, Ronald
may be able to out influence the president of the United States
with Congress.

Pearson went on to outline in detail the process map for the stealth
operation. Congressmen reading the report that day discounted the flood
of mail from energized doctors' wives. Yet the AMA campaign was enough
to slow down the congressional process.

The press-induced transparency continued to haunt the AMA in the
months ahead, but not more than its constant collision with the facts and
advancing demographics. Between 1950 and 1963, the number of Americans over 65 had grown from 12 million (8.1 percent of the population)
to 17.5 million (9.4 percent of the population). The cost of hospital care
in the early 1960s was accelerating at a 7 percent annual clip. Insurance
premiums were on the rise, with insurance brokers struggling to bring
on new enrollees. The proportion of covered individuals had stalled at
about 50 percent, and the coverage was anything but comprehensive.
Putting it all together, a Senate study committee in 1964 confronted the
reality that only 25 percent of the elderly had adequate health insurance.[20]
Something had to give.

As previously mentioned, at this same time just above our northern
border, Canada was completing a three-year process that would place universal coverage of hospital and physician health costs under the national

government with responsibility for delivering a uniform set of benefits placed in the hands of each province or territory. The name of the new program was Medicare.[35] In addition, reviews of positive results of the US military's making national health care a part of nation building in Germany and Japan under the Marshall Plan had already demonstrated that carefully orchestrated national approaches to health insurance yielded higher outcomes at lower cost.[36,37]

Still, the majority of physicians across America continued to oppose our own more modest version of Medicare, a universal plan for those over age 65. And physician members were willing to devote a portion of their limited time to the AMA causes, as were many of their spouses. Most saw nothing positive to be gained by further governmental intrusion into the health care space. More dramatically, most saw the AMA and their medical profession as under attack and needing their support. A few were militant. On May 5, 1962, the *New York Times* reported that 200 New Jersey doctors had signed a resolution proclaiming their intention to "refuse to participate in the care of patients under the provision of the King-Anderson Bill or similar legislation." As for charity care, they agreed to "continue to care for the medically indigent, young and old, as we have in the past."[38]

On May 20, at Madison Square Garden in New York City, President Kennedy delivered a major address on health care to a full house of 20,000 senior citizens. The speech was broadcast without advertising by all three major networks as a "news event," and it reached an estimated viewership of 20 million.[39] He directly challenged the AMA and its health care lobbyists, who were flooding the hallways and mailrooms of Congress. Kennedy said, "Some organizations have six, seven, and eight hundred people spreading mail across the country, asking doctors and others to write in and tell your congressman you're opposed to it. The mail pours into the White House, into the congress and senator's office. Congressmen and senators feel people are opposed to it. Then they read a Gallup poll, which says 75 percent of people are in favor of it, and they say, 'What has happened to my mail?' The point of the matter is that this meeting and the others indicate that the people of the United States recognize, one by one, thousand by thousand, million by million, that this is a problem whose solution is long overdue. And this year, I believe as certainly or as inevitably as the tide comes in next year, that this bill is going to pass."

The AMA was livid. It demanded equal time from the networks to give a formal response to what it saw as a Democratic Party political address, but it was refused. Undaunted, the AMA board members gave the go-ahead to rent Madison Square Garden and pay to televise their rebuttal.

As their voice, they chose a Tallahassee surgeon, Dr. Edward Annis, who had been a debater in high school and college. Part of the AMA speakers' bureau, Annis, like Ronald Reagan, had been put on the road the year before to develop his own version of "the speech." He had delivered it dozens of times over the past five months and along the way had publicly debated UAW officials and Senator Hubert Humphrey.[40]

When he got to Madison Square Garden on May 22 to deliver a very personal rebuke to the president, Annis had two advantages. President Kennedy's earlier address, as his staff would later admit, was not his best. It lacked strong focus and delivery; it was heavy in facts and figures; and it admonished both the AMA and physicians, suggesting they had not done their homework or even "read the bill." The AMA also had Kennedy's speech on film and was able to build a point-by-point reply. Dr. Annis, in 30 minutes, mined the weaknesses of Kennedy's address, referencing filmed portions of the president's speech, and challenged the absent president directly as he went along.[40]

At the end of the speech, Annis admonished Kennedy: "The people have a right to remind their first servant that his election, even his present popularity, does not authorize him to change fundamental institutions that have proved a lasting value through the generations. Nor should he tamper with fundamental human relationships that are sacred, in that they involve the creation of human life, or the preservation of human life. There are few such things that touch so close to God. And the relationship between a doctor and his patient is one of them."

Then, as the cameras panned the empty seats in the vast arena, Annis said, "All of you who occupied these 18,000 seats yesterday, you are at home now. You have time to think. You have time to ask your doctor. To the millions of Americans who may have a doubt, who may want to take a moment to hear the views of one they know and trust, I implore you, 'Ask your doctor. Ask your doctor.'"

And ask they did, in droves. The AMA's paid televised address on the same networks Kennedy had accessed two days earlier was said to have reached 30 million viewers.[41] On July 17, 1962, the King-Anderson Bill went down in defeat in the Senate by a vote of 52–48.[20] But progressive forces were not to be undone.

On September 24, 1963, Kennedy signed the Health Professions Educational Assistance Act, which for the first time provided direct federal grants, in the amount of $175 million, to be distributed over three years in support of constructing training facilities for the medical and health professions.[42] Kennedy used the signing that day to save face and to signal that he had not given up on universal health insurance for the aged. Putting the best face he could on his very public defeat at the hands of the AMA a year before, he said:

"It gives me great satisfaction to approve the Health Professions Educational Assistance Act of 1963, the culmination of 14 years of effort by many devoted and dedicated citizens. . . . The measures authorized by this act cannot accomplish all the goals we have envisioned. But it is a good beginning, a firm foundation on which to build in the future. The legislative history of the act makes it clear that the intent was to inaugurate a program of action that can be reevaluated after a suitable period of time. This will enable the Congress to consider further measures after some experience with the program has accumulated."[42]

Recalling the AMA speech and events that followed, one veteran health policy analyst commented years later that, on the evening of Edward Annis's speech in 1962, "They [the AMA] had won the battle, but lost the war."[43] The Kerr-Mills Bill, with its state controls and welfare focus, would continue to be ineffective in the states where it was needed most. The demographics and disease burdens of elderly Americans would ensure that, absent a true, comprehensive national effort, older Americans would continue to devolve into poverty and despair. At the same time, the absence of universal coverage and universal contributions through payroll deductions would prevent the healthy and wealthy from cross-subsidizing the poor and ill.

Most of all, though, the AMA-led resistance failed because of John F. Kennedy's assassination on November 22, 1963. Vice President Lyndon Johnson assumed the presidency with Medicare at the very top of his legislative agenda.[44] As Johnson would later recall, "I had to take the dead man's program and turn it into a martyr's cause."[45]

Johnson brought to the task an encyclopedic knowledge of the federal legislative system, an energy that knew no bounds, and a skill set and style of negotiation that colleagues referred to as the "Full Lyndon." As Hubert Humphrey said, "He'd come on just like a tidal wave. He went through the walls. He takes a whole room over just like that."[46] The Full Lyndon involved using the full scope of his six-foot-four, 250-pound frame to tower over people in such close quarters that they felt both physically overwhelmed and verbally intimidated. Various victims subjected to this unpleasant treatment over the years described clutches, patting, pushing, and bumping intermixed with threats, promises, and flattery.[47]

Johnson's unique voice, accent, and communication style also made full use of storytelling, jokes, and shock humor.[48] As down-home and folksy, as lumbering and crude as Johnson could appear at times, he was also brilliant in wielding power, a cunning and patient strategist, and relentlessly persistent.[49]

By May 1964, six months after Kennedy's death, Johnson had captured the moral high ground for his "Great Society," which would now include the commitments that had been made within the dead president's New Frontier. It was about the "quality of our American civilization."[50]

A few weeks later, on July 2, 1964, President Johnson signed the Civil Rights Act.[51] A month later, he launched the War on Poverty. The third leg of the "martyr's cause" was Medicare.

History has traditionally credited the passage of Medicare on July 30, 1965, to the actions of Congressman Wilbur Mills, the shrewd chairman of the Ways and Means Committee. But newer documents have established that the "legendary coup" Mills sprang on his committee on March 2,

1965, had been in the works for 14 months, and that his coconspirator was Lyndon Baines Johnson himself.[52]

When Johnson first took office, Mills was reluctant to rock the boat, favoring some expansion of the state-administered program directed at the needy, sweetened with reimbursement for physician services. Johnson sequentially pushed him toward a nationally administered solution that would be funded through Social Security and that would be available to all participants. Mills's primary concern was economic.[53] He saw the costs exploding and the federal government being swamped by the obligations.

Johnson's response was to purposefully understate the costs and gradually get Mills to the point where he accepted that paying for the program would be the president's problem. In addition to covering the economic worries, Johnson assured Mills that the congressman would get all the credit. With a healthy ego and presidential ambitions of his own, Mills knew that Johnson would be true to his word. Both he and the president were also aware that the pollster Lou Harris had confirmed beyond doubt, in both 1962 and 1964, that national insurance for the elderly was a winning issue.[54]

As the 1964 election drew near, the two reached an agreement.[55] The original Kerr-Mills Bill would become a more generous federal offering, administered by the states and directed at needy Americans of all ages. The defeated King-Anderson Bill would be folded in and provide new broader coverage of all hospital costs for those over 65. Finally, physicians' services would be generously reimbursed on a cost-plus basis, meaning that doctors would receive the actual cost plus an additional service fee. The program would be financed through the federal government and contributions from citizens who had enrolled for the coverage. On top of it all, Social Security payment levels would be increased.[56] How the bill would be passed Johnson confidently left up to the more than capable Mills.

The presidential contest of 1964 between Johnson and Barry Goldwater was a landslide for the Democrats. Johnson received 61 percent of the roughly 70 million votes cast, and 486 electoral votes to Goldwater's 52.[57] The AMA, which had very publicly run a "Doctors for Goldwater" PR campaign, had egg on its face. Postelection, it went on the offensive, attempting to move an alternative proposal, a Kerr-Mills on steroids paired with a voluntary physician payment scheme, and, as always, avoiding federally administered benefits.[58] But after the 1964 landslide, Mills needed no further encouragement to move the legislation ahead.[59]

On March 2, 1965, Chairman Mills took his Ways and Means Committee into a closed session to discuss a proposal by John Byrnes (R-WI), who had agreed to advance the AMA's alternative proposal to provide coverage for physician services to the elderly who voluntarily elected to enroll themselves. Mills surprised the committee with, "You know, John, I like that idea of yours."[55] He then proposed a "three-layer cake" that folded in the expanded Kerr-Mills and the rejuvenated King-Anderson layers. These would later become Medicare A, Medicare B, and Medicaid. Surprisingly, the committee members supported the program in principle, and when Mills came out of the closed session to announce what they had done, the news was met with thunderous applause.[60] The same thing happened when he soon afterward laid out the proposed legislation on the House floor.

Only 10 Republicans voted with the administration, and there were 63 Democratic defectors. The difference was the 1964 election that allowed the entry of an additional 44 supporters of the bill called H.R. 1, to signify its highest priority in the Johnson administration, and later called simply the Mills Bill.[61] On April 8, 1965, Mills presented all 296 pages of the bill to the House of Representatives, where it would pass 313–115.[61] Over the next few months, efforts were made by the bill's opponents to kill it by loading it up with additional benefits, including pharmaceutical coverage, catastrophic insurance, and an expansion of coverage to younger citizens. Johnson's team fought these off, knowing that the economics of the legislation were already tenuous.[62]

On July 30, 1965, Johnson flew to Independence, Missouri, to celebrate the passage of Medicare with Harry and Bess Truman at his side. In his remarks, he said, "It was really Harry Truman of Missouri who planted the seeds of compassion and duty which have today flowered into care for the sick and serenity for the fearful. . . . Many men can make many proposals. Many men can draft many laws. But few . . . have the courage to stake reputation, and position, and the effort of a lifetime upon a cause when there are so few that share it. . . . Perhaps you alone, President Truman—perhaps you alone can fully know how grateful I am for this day."[63]

However, as Johnson flew back to Washington, he knew that the success of Medicare was by no means ensured. He had given President Truman the first Medicare card, but now, 19 million other potential recipients needed to be enrolled. The administration had only 11 months before the program would go live, and the scope of the communications and public education challenge was unprecedented, with doctors threatening to boycott the program, and Southern states threatening to resist it.[64]

In the 1960s, hospitals throughout the South still maintained segregated restrooms and segregated floors and wards designed to separate black and white populations. The passage of the Civil Rights Act in July 1964 had sent a clear warning: Title VI of the bill stated, "No person in the United States shall, on the grounds of race, color, or national origin, be excluded from participation in, denied benefits of, or be subject to discrimination under any program receiving federal assistance."[65] After formal review by the Justice Department, HEW secretary Anthony Celebrezze informed the Senate that the new hospital insurance program would indeed be subject to the requirements of Title VI.[66] As a result, all hospitals, in order to qualify for federal Medicare certification, would have to prove that they were no longer segregating patients. Johnson took no chances, deploying 1,000 federal inspectors across the country to ensure that the letter of the law was being implemented. Even with this, 10 months after Medicare had been signed into law, and a month or two before the launch date, half the hospitals inspected in 12 Southern states were still noncompliant.

Johnson called a special cabinet meeting and leaned on Vice President Humphrey to head south and communicate directly with every mayor in the noncompliant Southern cities and simply, one way or another, get the job done.

By May 23, 1966, all hospitals were compliant except in Alabama, Louisiana, Mississippi, and South Carolina. By July, they were clearly heading in the right direction, though 320 hospitals had not yet completed the conversions. Though some would still lag behind on the day Medicare went live on July 1, 1966, all would soon comply.[67]

At the same time the administration was waging this war against segregation in health care, it was focused on herding in recalcitrant physicians. Johnson saw this challenge as one only he could address. As the Senate was closing in on final approval of Medicare, in early June 1965, AMA president James Appel called the White House to request a meeting.[68] It was scheduled on June 29, the day the Senate would vote its final approval of the bill. When the delegation arrived with Dr. Appel in the lead, Johnson began by reading to them verbatim from the proposed bill: "Nothing in this title shall be construed to authorize any Federal officer or employee to exercise any supervision or control over the practice of medicine or the manner in which medical services are provided." He then reviewed the use of Blue Cross and private insurance "intermediaries" to administer the program, thus keeping government at arm's length. He spent the next half of the meeting "hugging" the doctors, thanking them for their service, day and night, to patients "like his daddy." He expressed his respect and gratitude for their devoted and selfless service, then asked whether they would be able to help him round up some doctors to address the pressing needs of the war-ravaged Vietnamese people.[69]

The response from the doctors was unconditional—they were at the president's and the nation's service. Johnson then immediately pivoted, calling for "a couple of reporters," who arrived quickly on cue. Johnson praised the doctors and their leaders by name, and the reporters not surprisingly wanted to know whether the AMA intended to support Medicare. Johnson interrupted, visibly shocked by the question. "These men are going to get doctors to go to Vietnam where they might get killed. . . . Medicare is the law of the land. Of course they'll support the law of the land. Tell him, you tell him," he said, pointing directly at the AMA leader. Appel had no choice but to confirm their support, stating modestly, "We are, after all, law abiding citizens."[69]

Johnson then left the doctors with his ace health-policy leader, Wilbur Cohen, whom he instructed to work out the details.[69] With a pledge in hand that the government would not "interfere with the patient-physician relationship" and confirmation of cost-plus reimbursement for the doctors, inclusion of hospital doctors under Part B, some adjustments to disease-specific areas, and a role for private insurers, the AMA delegation left with what it needed—an explanation to the AMA's more conservative members for its willingness to cooperate with the administration on this heinous new law.

At the September AMA house of delegates meeting, the AMA top executive proclaimed, "I think it is fair to say that [we] . . . succeeded in bringing about at the White House level a series of 'improving amendments' which . . . should allay the fears of the profession."[70]

One week before the actual launch of the Medicare program, on July 1, 1966, Johnson sent a telegram to the AMA president, timed to arrive dramatically at the AMA's National Convention gathering in Chicago. The message read:

"ON JULY 1 THE MEDICARE PROGRAM WILL BECOME A REALITY. . . . PERHAPS NEVER—EXCEPT IN MOBILIZING FOR WAR—HAS THIS GOVERNMENT MADE SUCH EXTENSIVE PREPARATIONS FOR AN UNDERTAKING. . . . WE SHALL CONTINUE TO SEEK YOUR COUNSEL IN THE MONTHS AHEAD—AND WE SHALL BE AVAILABLE TO EVERY DOCTOR AND EVERY HOSPITAL OFFICER TO DEAL WITH ANY PROBLEM THAT ARISES."[71]

The implementation was not perfect, but considering the size of the challenge, it was amazingly smooth. There were no major organized doctor protests or significant holdouts. Physicians soon came to appreciate that Medicare delivered much better payment across the board than did private insurers. As they aged, retired, and moved from the provider to the consumer ranks, they found Medicare enrollment to be a great relief, highly responsive to their needs, and with none of the trickery of commercial insurers attempting to maximize their profits by limiting their outlays in response to legitimate claims of enrollees.

Rather than bringing on the collapse of American democracy—or perhaps of Western civilization—as the AMA had predicted, Medicare and Medicaid became two of the US government's most popular and effective programs. They also proved to be, along with Social Security, the most expensive.

A few years after they were enacted, underfunding of these programs led Richard Nixon to state in 1972: "We have made the mistake in
addressing issues such as the exploding costs of health care in ways that
removed market forces from the equation. We have erred by separating
health care consumers from concern about the costs of the care being
provided. We need to work out a system that includes a greater emphasis
on preventative care, sufficient public funding for health insurance for
those who cannot afford it in the private sector, competition among both
health care providers and health insurance providers to keep down the
costs of both, and decoupling the cost of health care from the cost of
adding workers to the payroll."[72]

Nixon supported a number of new cost-containment initiatives that
restricted patients' choice of doctors and hospitals under the banner of
health maintenance organizations (HMOs). As he said in 1972: "The
richest country in the world cannot tolerate the fact that we have the
highest per capita health care costs in the world and yet 38 million of
our people are unable to get adequate medical care because they cannot
afford it."[72] But these efforts were controversial, promoting the use of
primary physicians over high-cost specialists, and pitting doctors and
hospitals against insurers.

With Nixon's resignation, Gerald Ford initially signaled support
for a national health insurance bill, but high inflation and a persistent
recession made the politics untenable.[73] Inadvertently, President Ford
did have a lasting impact on health policy when he signed legislation to
protect pensioners, and a small attachment prevented employees from
suing their companies for health mishaps if the company self-financed
its own employee health plans. This innocent action led to a mass movement of large corporations to self-fund their employees' health insurance.
Employer self-funding transformed corporate human resource departments into a new and powerful lobby that would, though unsuccessfully,
try to contain and control health care costs through the turn of the century.

Nearly 20 years later, when Bill Clinton launched the next initiative
to create universal health care, his plan was rightly criticized as being too
bureaucratic, dogmatic, and complicated. As already noted, his proposal

led to open warfare, as the pharmaceutical industry, insurers, and the AMA launched the notorious "Harry and Louise" ad campaign, which suggested that the government plan would direct patient choices in the future and force Americans to leave their own doctors and hospitals.[74]

Fifteen years later, the political climate had changed, and President Obama elected to use the majority of his political capital to pass the Patient Protection and Affordable Care Act. More and more voters had begun to see the provision of health coverage as a right of citizenship and a powerful economic equalizer. In the past four decades, as more and more low-wage Americans have faced medical bankruptcies and middle-class wages have been largely frozen, the earnings of the top 1 percent have tripled.[75]

The provisions of the Affordable Care Act had a major impact on health insurers nationwide. Over the next eight years, roughly 24 million additional uninsured Americans received coverage, half from the expansion of Medicaid programs and half from the creation of subsidized individual insurance markets. Insurers were mandated to accept all comers regardless of preexisting conditions and to provide a uniform generous benefit package with the same premium pricing to all, regardless of a citizen's prior medical history. Insurers also had to provide up to 85 percent of their premium revenue to direct clinical care of their enrollees. To pay for these programs, as we'll see in chapters ahead, the MIC pillars in the hospital, insurance, pharmaceutical, and medical fields made specific concessions in return for the opportunity to serve more insured patients. In addition, under the new law all citizens not already insured were mandated to purchase health insurance or pay a federal penalty or fine. This mandate was designed to share the financial risk of caring for all Americans across the population, so that the high costs of treating those who are sick would be subsidized by the low cost of caring for those who remain well.[75]

In the years that have followed, the Trump administration and the Republican-controlled Congress have continued to wage a pitched battle to undermine President Obama's signature legislation at every turn. By and large the legislation has survived in the courts of law and public opinion. The price Americans have paid in the interim has been a lost opportunity to refine and expand the national movement toward universality and solidarity when it comes to embracing health care as a right of citizenship.

While expanding health insurance to an additional 24 million citizens, the Affordable Care Act was not designed to address either the quality issues or the cost issues that have chronically plagued American health care since World War II. As costs consume roughly 20 percent of our economy, too many members of the Medical Industrial Complex continue to conflate and confuse scientific progress with human progress, and too much of corporate America continues to favor profit-seeking entrepreneurship over collective social health planning.

And yet, as US health care costs continue to rise and US health outcomes decline compared with outcomes in nations whose rational health care systems we helped design, there are signals everywhere that fundamental change is under way. Consider, for example, the shifting fortunes of stand-alone health insurers like industry giant Aetna. In 2017 it agreed to be purchased outright for $69 billion by a retailer that had been launched with a single location in Lowell, Massachusetts, in 1963. Today, the company owns pharmacies nationwide, is one of the largest pharmacy benefit managers (PBMs), has integrated several thousand patient-friendly MinuteClinics, and has annual revenues in the vicinity of $200 billion. A half century ago, it was called Consumer Value Stores. Today we know it as CVS.[76]

There is no mystery to how CVS became so powerful in such a short period of time. The company inserted itself into the middle of the Medical Industrial Complex and extended its profit-seeking tentacles from the center outward. Beginning with the simple sale of pharmaceuticals and related retail products, it became an active marketing partner with pharmaceutical companies that were willing to pay for strategies to enhance their product choices over competitors' at the point of sale. When the public outcry demanded strategies to control costs, it entered the PBM business, making the case that its ever-enlarging database could be leveraged to support cost-control initiatives like tiered drug choices, co-pays, and hidden financial kickbacks to compliant drug companies and insurers, all for a fee. Completing the loop, with its move to acquire Aetna, CVS has made a bid to become the insurer itself, acquiring not only a wealth of new clients but, perhaps more important in the long run, the clients' medical profiles and health data as well.

In the arena of crass modern capitalism, the highest compliment is imitation. Recognizing that data control and efficient movement of money and product are the power levers of the MIC syndicate operation, Jeff Bezos (Amazon), Warren Buffett (Berkshire Hathaway), and Jamie Dimon (JPMorgan Chase) announced in March 2018 that they had entered a cooperative venture initially focused on the public-spirited goal of bringing down the health care costs for their combined 1.2 million workers.[77] A few months later, they announced the hiring of a highly respected voice in health care, Atul Gawande, MD, to lead their effort.[78] But financial analysts, reading between the lines, were quick to identify profit seeking as the titans' ultimate destination point. They noted a recent rash of hiring at Amazon, including "experts from biopharma, primary care, health insurance, and other sectors." They also placed a spotlight on existing partnerships with large wholesale drug distributors like Cardinal Health; investments in electronic-medical-record firms; state-by-state procurement of pharmacy licenses; an alliance with Merck to explore the use of its voice-technology platform, Alexis, for assisted home management of chronic disease; and logistics dominance and mastery as evidence of a multifront assault on the hugely profitable health care sector.[77] Disruptors like Amazon and CVS shift the locus of control, but they do not resolve the fundamental issue. If capitalistic exploitation of health care following World War II is what has led to the dismantling of appropriate checks and balances, unconscionable variability in quality and access, and profiteering complexity on a vast scale, it is unreasonable to believe that the solution lies in injecting more capitalism.

Consolidation, simplification, and nationalizing of our health insurance payment system alone will save our nation an estimated 15 percent on an annual expenditure of $4 trillion.[79] But to wisely reapply that $600 million in savings will require national health planning, setting and funding of priorities, reestablishing appropriate checks and balances to curtail schemers and profiteers, and addressing the basic question we ignored in 1945: "How do we make America and Americans healthy?"

Chapter 8

Masters of Manipulation

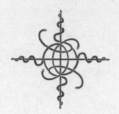

The Temple of Dendur, one of the world's most prized antiquities, sits in the Sackler Wing of New York's Metropolitan Museum of Art.[1] That name is also attached to the Sackler Gallery at the Smithsonian's Freer Gallery of Art in Washington, the Sackler Museum at Harvard, and the Arthur M. Sackler Museum of Art and Archaeology at Beijing University.[2] The same Arthur M. Sackler who gave so generously to the art world and was rewarded with naming rights also endowed numerous medical institutions, but exactly how he made his fortune was never well known. In fact, Sackler himself was remarkably obscure until fall 2017, when two profiles appeared almost simultaneously in two different publications, *Esquire* and the *New Yorker*.

What those magazine pieces made clear is that the more one knows about Sackler's career as the ultimate manipulative marketer, and the careers of his brothers, and the more one understands his family's contribution to drug addiction in the US, the more one is forced to view his philanthropic legacy in a different light. His impact on the infrastructure of American health care is comparable to the influence on New York City of Robert Moses, the infamous urban planner who destroyed neighborhoods to build freeways instead of mass transit.

As Allen Frances, former chair of psychiatry at Duke University Medical Center, told the *New Yorker*, "Most of the questionable practices that propelled the pharmaceutical industry into the scourge it is today can be attributed to Arthur Sackler. His activities, along with those of his younger brothers, helped the family amass a collective net worth of $13 billion, more than the Rockefellers or the Mellons."[3] Sackler was trained as a physician, but he made his mark as a businessman. He brought direct-to-consumer advertising into medicine, created industry-funded (and industry-manipulated) continuing medical education programs, and invented the medical infomercial and (at least in the biomedical context) fake news, while unleashing armies of detail men to ingratiate themselves with compliant doctors. Within the world of Sackler's spin, the job category he invented existed not to push pills but merely to provide professionals with the details of drug actions and applications.

When Americans first bet the nation's health on an entrepreneurial system of care, we grossly underestimated just how far certain individuals and institutions would go in pursuing financial incentives, how benefits might be overstated and risks downplayed, and how side effects including drug addiction and lost productivity could bring a large portion of society to its knees. We also grossly underestimated just how much such a system could be gamed and, in that gaming of the system, how pivotal a player one highly determined individual could be. In a market-driven system, Arthur Sackler showed how to both create and drive the market.

Sackler's biography is somewhat murky, especially the story of his early years, in which he passed through various guises and settings like a medical-industrial version of Woody Allen's Zelig, the human chameleon who showed up everywhere.

Born in Brooklyn in 1913, Arthur Mitchell Sackler was the son of immigrants from the Ukraine and Poland.[4] He had two younger brothers, Mortimer and Raymond, each of whom followed his lead into the medical business. Over his lifetime, Sackler actively presented a rags-to-riches narrative, but by the time he was 24, he had completed college and medical school; had married his beautiful and sophisticated first wife, Else Finnich Jorgensen; and was already collecting art.[5] After a year of general medical training, he jumped into pharmaceuticals. Within just three years, young Sackler somehow became head of the medical research division at Schering Corporation, an American subsidiary of the German parent company Schering AG.[6,7]

With the wartime US government seizing the assets of German companies, Sackler's term at Schering was short-lived, but he recovered quickly, joining the William Douglas McAdams advertising agency in sales and marketing rather than the Army, and within five short years, while most doctors his age were overseas serving their country in war zones, he somehow gained a controlling interest in the firm.[8,9] The source of his good fortune and funding remains a mystery. Clearly he was an opportunist. As thousands of shell-shocked veterans streamed into US mental hospitals during and after the war, he enrolled in a psychiatric residency at New York's Creedmoor Psychiatric Center.[10]

By the time he completed his psychiatric training in 1947, Sackler had divorced his first wife; two years later, he married his second, Marietta Lutze, the third-generation manager of yet another German pharmaceutical firm, and likely a rich source of business contacts for his growing advertising firm.[11] By 1952, this son of an immigrant grocer in Flatbush, now a successful medical advertising man and twice divorced, was able to begin exercising in earnest his penchant for art collecting and for philanthropy, for which he would be best remembered.

The period of Arthur Sackler's rise was the same period in which other nations were choosing to more directly address the well-being of their citizens. During that same era, the US made critical decisions that would enshrine health care as just another business opportunity, and Sackler was the man for the moment. At the beginning of his career, traditional infectious diseases and childhood epidemics were declining as a cause of early death, but longer life spans prefigured an increased incidence of chronic diseases such as congestive heart failure and arthritis. Cigarette use, alcohol consumption, heavily marketed and easily prepared processed foods, anxiety, and depression, as well as the overuse of prescription medications, made heart disease and cancer the number one and number two killers, creating heavy demand for the blockbuster drugs that Sackler would prove so adept at selling.[12] First, though, came a midcentury gold rush in new antibiotics, which made the top pharmaceutical companies a fortune, with Pfizer in the lead, and Sackler as its lead advertiser.[13]

In 1952, Sackler put a multipage insert in the *Journal of the American Medical Association* to push Pfizer's new antibiotic, Terramycin, but here, too, the consummate spin doctor avoided using such a vulgar term as "advertising," claiming instead that the drug company's investment was purely for informational and educational purposes.[13] Between 1950 and 1957, the revenue from the "informational" ads Sackler produced for *JAMA* for broad-spectrum antibiotics increased sevenfold. Terramycin was marketed as a breakthrough, but it wasn't unique. It was built by adding one oxygen atom onto Pfizer's original tetracycline, Tetracyn.[14]

During this period, nearly every *JAMA* issue also included, bound right in, an in-house magazine from Pfizer called *Spectrum*, developed by Sackler.[15,16] In 1953, Pfizer followed Sackler's advice and purchased the marketing juggernaut Roerig, a nutritional–vitamin supplement company, in order to make use of its direct-to-consumer product profile and as a seed for what would become the greatest pharmaceutical sales force of the 20th century.[17]

This is when the detail man began to flex his full marketing muscle. The drug company sales rep, typically a conservatively dressed, middle-aged white man who matched up well with the typical physician of the time, would visit doctors' offices to distribute glossy color publications extolling the virtues of the latest discoveries, along with a variety of branded giveaways such as pens, notepads, and coffee mugs. The most important giveaways, though, were small samples of the latest drugs the detail man represented.

Not surprisingly, pushing drugs to the medical profession led to a sharp rise in drug dependency. The first wave was barbiturates, popular throughout the 1950s as sedatives, hypnotics, sleep aids, anticonvulsants, and anesthetics.[18] By the end of the decade, as postwar America struggled to accommodate its new, more frenzied pace, one in seven adults would be using tranquilizers.

In 1957, Pfizer wanted to launch its new solution for anxiety, Atarax, and once again the marketing maven the company turned to was Sackler.[19] Tranquilizers at the time were described as "ataractic," a term which refers to a "mental and physical state of bliss." On behalf of Pfizer, Sackler created a 13-minute "public service presentation" called "The Relaxed Wife."[20] It featured an anxious husband dressed in pajamas and a silk bathrobe being comforted by his loving spouse. As the couple sat on twin beds suitable for Rock Hudson and Doris Day, the wife explained what she had learned about "tension" and "relaxation," which was that "relaxation techniques don't work for everyone." Ten minutes in, the voice-over introduced the audience to the ancient Greek word *ataraxia* and went on to explain in terms that a guru from the sixties might appreciate that "doctors are now prescribing an ataraxic medicine" that offers the "calming peace of a cloudless sky." Then the announcer gave a simpler directive that would become a mantra in the pharmaceutical business: "If you have tension problems, discuss them with your doctor." Pfizer's new drug, Atarax, was never named—and it didn't need to be.

During the same era, Sackler, as head of the William Douglas McAdams agency, persuaded a number of drug companies to amplify their already lavish funding of continuing medical education by creating allegedly scientific journals, like the *Journal of Clinical and Experimental Psychobiology*, that published allegedly scholarly articles primarily devoted to experimenting with new drug therapies. These articles were, in fact, lightly veiled advertisements for drugs developed by Sackler's clients. Sackler hired ghostwriters for articles and attached the names of compliant physicians and scientists who were more than happy to become "authors" and "thought leaders," designations which in turn led to handsome fees for giving speeches (arranged by Sackler) at medical meetings. But Sackler was hardly alone in his willingness to doctor science in pursuit of commerce.

The heyday of Arthur Sackler was a period of crossover in the methods used for the marketing of prescription drugs and the marketing of the drug delivery system known as the cigarette. Sackler's counterpart in the tobacco industry, and fellow master of manipulation, was John Hill of the public relations giant Hill & Knowlton.[21] Sackler and Hill shared authorship of such techniques as third-party advocacy, subliminal message reinforcement, junk science, phony front groups, advocacy advertising, and using advertising dollars to buy favorable "news" to report. Thus the Medical Industrial Complex created an amazingly unlikely odd-couple alliance with the industry representing the very antithesis of health—tobacco.

Between the world wars, smoking became as American as mom and apple pie. Not only a majority of Americans but also a majority of their physicians smoked, a trend that would continue into the 1950s.[22] In the *Mad Men* television series, a doctor memorably performs a gynecological exam with a cigarette hanging out of his mouth. A great period detail for the series, this was not an over-the-top joke but an accurate reflection of just how ubiquitous cigarettes were even into the 1970s.

In the 1930s, when money was tightest during the Depression, the tobacco industry sponsored medical meetings and supplied advertising revenue that kept alive the two top medical journals in the country, *JAMA* and the *New England Journal of Medicine*.[23] In midcentury, during the American Medical Association's annual convention, the tobacco giant Philip Morris placed special ads in *JAMA* inviting doctors to visit the company's smoking lounge on the convention floor, where they could "drop in, rest . . . read . . . smoke . . . or just chat." At the associated exhibit, doctors were invited "to be amazed by the dramatic visualization of nicotine absorption from cigarette smoke in the human respiratory tract," as well as "giant photo-murals of Camel laboratory research experiments."[24]

When consumers began to express anxiety in the 1940s about the rising rates of lung cancer and respiratory distress and the apparent link between these afflictions and smoking, Big Tobacco tried to create an even deeper partnership with members of the medical profession, and the profession not only played along but also seemed to enjoy the attention. Tobacco companies fielded sales forces to visit doctors' offices with free cigarettes and glossy reprints of the companies' non-peer-reviewed "scientific" publications.[25] One memorable ad appearing in *Life*, *Look*, and the *Saturday Evening Post* proclaimed, "L&M Filters Are Just What the Doctor Ordered!" For validation, the ad included a copy of a letter endorsing L&Ms, written by a Dr. F. R. Darkis, who was actually a PhD chemist, not an MD. He was also the director of research for Liggett and Myers Tobacco.[26]

Philip Morris couldn't do much about the carcinogens embedded in its product, but the company did try to ameliorate throat irritants, at least to the extent of underwriting the research of two Columbia scientists— Michael Mulinos, a pharmacologist; and Frederick Flinn, a physiologist— who demonstrated that injecting diethyleneglycol rather than glycerin into tobacco leaves as a moistener made the eyes of rabbits less subject to irritation.[27] In a *Saturday Evening Post* ad in 1937, the company stated that in "a report on the findings of a group of doctors . . . when smokers changed to Philip Morris, every case of irritation cleared completely and definitely improved." The company went a step further in ads in medical journals, encouraging doctors to request copies of the "scientific" articles—the ones created, of course, by the tobacco company.[28]

In 1942, RJ Reynolds upped the ante by creating its Medical Relations Division to carry out experiments and to publish results claiming that its Camels were the "slowest burning" cigarettes, and thus had the least nicotine absorption. The public couldn't know that the division was directed by A. Grant Clarke, an advertising executive with no medical or scientific background whatsoever, or that all mailings, in and out, were being processed by an ad agency.[29]

In 1946, RJ Reynolds launched its "More Doctors" campaign in *Ladies' Home Journal* and *Time*, claiming that doctors far and wide, GPs and specialists, had "named their choice" of cigarette and that their choice was Camel.[30] In the same year, eager to ingratiate itself with its best ally against the rising tide of alarming health news, RJ Reynolds launched an unsolicited PR campaign on behalf of American doctors, extolling their service in the war while excoriating President Truman for his attempts to undermine them with a national system of health insurance, which the company called "socialized medicine."[31]

In 1951, though, the Federal Trade Commission broke up the alliance between doctors and cigarette makers by forcing the American Tobacco Company to drop health claims related to acid levels, throat irritation, and nicotine levels in its ads for Lucky Strike.[32] The RJ Reynolds brand Camels had to reverse its own claims that the popular cigarettes "aided digestion," "calmed the nerves," and "increased energy levels." A second round of regulations in 1954 specifically barred all tobacco industry advertising or claims related to the "throat, larynx, lungs, nose, parts of the body, digestion, nerves or doctors."[33]

The real challenge to Big Tobacco came in 1952, when *Reader's Digest* ran a piece by Roy Norr, originally published in the *Christian Herald* and titled "Cancer by the Carton."[34] In it, Norr wrote, "What gives grave concern to public health leaders is that the increase in lung cancer mortality shows a suspicious parallel in the enormous increase in cigarette consumption (now 2500 cigarettes per year for every human being in the United States)." The industry's survival required either denying the facts or manipulating the public's perception of those facts. Almost immediately, tobacco companies began to pump up their advertising budgets, which rose from $76 million in 1953 to $122 million four years later.[21]

With the *Reader's Digest* piece, the cozy relationship between tobacco and the medical profession seemed over. In 1953, *JAMA* stopped accepting cigarette ads for its journals, and the AMA prohibited cigarette companies from exhibiting at its conventions. A *JAMA* editorial one year later went so far as to condemn the "unauthorized and medically unethical use of the prestige and reputation of the American Medical Association."[35]

But Big Tobacco was not easily bowed, and along the way, Big Pharma would watch and learn from the cigarette makers' gutsy and totally unscrupulous techniques. Deprived of the protective cover that had been provided by the AMA, the tobacco companies once more enlisted Hill & Knowlton, which proposed mirroring the professional education approach by the Pharmaceutical Manufacturers Association (PMA) in forming what it called the Tobacco Industry Research Committee (TIRC), an entity that could have been more accurately described as the Tobacco Industry Office of Disinformation and Propaganda.[36] The TIRC's Scientific Advisory Body did not include anyone who acknowledged the direct connection between cigarette smoking and disease. Instead, the advisers called the cancer link an "inconclusive theory" and—anticipating

coal company statements a half century later about global warming—
determined that "there is no agreement among the authorities regarding
what the cause is."[37,38]

The manipulation then became more subtle and more sinister,
spreading into the surprisingly corruptible branch of the Medical Industrial Complex known as academic medicine. To continue selling cigarettes
in the face of devastating scientific evidence of tobacco's link to both lung
cancer and cardiovascular disease, the companies had to come up with an
alternative explanation for the rise in cardiac deaths that clearly tracked
alongside the rise of cigarette smoking. Their savior was a Hungarian-
born endocrinologist named Hans Selye, a man nominated multiple times
for the Nobel Prize.[39]

Selye was famous for his formulation of the concept of stress as the
source of microscopic injuries to the cell.[40] But he was also known for
his ability to attract research funding, an ability that was enhanced by his
willingness to tailor the evidence to suit the highest bidder.

In numerous court cases during the 1960s and 1970s, the Tobacco
Industry Research Committee relied on Selye as an expert witness to
make the argument that smoking, rather than being a health hazard,
might actually provide a measurable benefit in the form of stress relief.
Meanwhile, Dr. Selye was turning to the tobacco industry for major grants
to support his growing research enterprise and to enrich himself. Years
later, as part of document disclosure during litigation by state attorneys
general against the tobacco industry, communications between Selye
and industry representatives proved that he had conspired to hold back
supportive testimony and publications suggesting a link between tobacco
use and stress reduction until he received his cash.[41]

In the mid-1950s, two New York cardiologists, Meyer Friedman
and Ray Rosenman, had observed 3,000 men and speculated that those
who developed heart disease were more likely to be what they labeled
"type A." They postulated that certain people were genetically hardwired
to experience and magnify stress, and that these hard-charging type A
personalities were sitting ducks for heart disease, cancer, and early death,
as they explained in their 1974 book, *Type A Behavior and Your Heart*.[42,43]

For the leadership at the Tobacco Industry Research Committee, here were findings that offered beautifully plausible deniability. When a 45-year-old man dropped dead during a Saturday-afternoon softball game, it wasn't cigarettes; it was stress. In fact, if anything, he should have smoked more—it might have relieved some of his tension.

Tobacco litigation documents released in 1998 as part of the Master Settlement Agreement between 46 state attorneys general and the five largest cigarette manufacturers in America demonstrated that both Selye's research and that of the creators of type A was subsidized by large grants from the Tobacco Industry Research Committee.[44] Selye's research and papers were even vetted by the TIRC, and their content and wording were adjusted by his tobacco patrons. As for the type A research, repeated studies over subsequent decades could never replicate the level of speculative association Friedman and Rosenman found between stress and heart disease. Only four papers out of hundreds claimed a link, and three of those four were underwritten by the tobacco industry. Yet, in a tribute to the enduring power of branding, the label "type A" endures as a cultural artifact and Google search favorite.[45]

When Hans Selye died in 1982, he was regarded as a venerable scientist, but the tobacco industry's funding of his work, and Selye's willingness to recruit additional scientists to present tobacco's messages in meetings and publications, would later be cited by the US Department of Justice as a clear example of racketeering.[46]

Selye's transgressions were not unique, nor even unusual. For decades, academic researchers throughout the country had been doing the same thing—leveraging their expert status to obtain funding—only from drug companies rather than cigarette makers. Selye was following a well-worn path whereby companies selling drugs, tobacco, automobiles, paints, chemicals, agricultural products (even milk), and packaged foods used otherwise legitimate researchers to lend credibility to their claims in order to boost profits, while the researchers used a portion of those profits to fund their laboratories and their lifestyles.[47] Unsurprisingly, in 1967, when the Tobacco Industry Research Committee was looking for a vice president for public relations, it hired William Kloepfer, former director of public relations for the Pharmaceutical Manufacturers Association, the man who had led Big Pharma's effort to capture, integrate, and underwrite physicians and scientists who would toe the PMA line.[48]

In 1960, Arthur Sackler launched *Medical Tribune*, a publication that, in time, reached more than a million physicians each week in 20 countries, publishing editorials that supported free enterprise and the unified political agenda of the American Medical Association and the Pharmaceutical Manufacturers Association.[49] These columns promoted the drug industry's friends and hammered its foes, castigated both regulators and the makers of generic drugs, and extolled unbridled research—all points of view perfectly aligned with those of the drugmakers.

Two years later, Sackler was brought before the Senate Judiciary Committee, where Senator Estes Kefauver questioned him about misleading and deceptive drug advertising. In his appearance before Congress, Sackler portrayed himself as a highly respected New York academician, a cutting-edge research psychiatrist, and a compassionate physician dedicated first and foremost to his patients' welfare and to the ethical standards of the profession of medicine. But in reality, he was already the top medical marketer in the United States; the 1952 purchaser of the fledgling drug company Purdue Frederick and its star laxative, Senekot; a human experimenter in the use of unproven psychotropic drugs on hospitalized mental patients in his own branded research institute at the New York Creedmoor Mental Institution; a secret collaborator and partner with his supposed PR arch-competitor; and the secret owner of MD Publications and Medical and Science Communications Associates, which had FDA leaders on the payroll to ensure their support of pharmaceutical clients' products.[50]

At least one Senate staffer understood at the time who Sackler really was. He prepared a memo that summed up the Sackler approach: "The Sackler empire is a completely integrated operation in that it can devise a new drug in its drug development enterprise, have the drug clinically tested and secure favorable reports on the drug from the various hospitals with which they have connections, conceive the advertising approach and prepare the actual advertising copy with which to promote the drug, have the clinical articles as well as advertising copy published in their own medical journals, (and) prepare and plant articles in newspapers and magazines."[50]

But Sackler was as slippery as the proverbial eel, even when confronting basic facts. Senator Kefauver asked him specifically about a small company called Medical and Science Communications Associates that was known for disseminating "fake news."[51] Even though the company shared the same Lexington Avenue address as the MacAdams Advertising Agency headed by Sackler, the doctor testified that he held no stock in MSC Associates and that he had never been an officer of it. This claim proved to be true, so Senator Kefauver moved on. What Sackler failed to mention was that the company's sole shareholder was his former wife, Else Sackler.[52]

But the ne plus ultra of Sackler's chutzpah may have been his recommendation to prescribe Valium, an addictive benzodiazepine, to people with no symptoms whatsoever, relying on the line: "For this kind of patient—with no demonstrable pathology—consider the usefulness of Valium." One editorialist in the journal *Psychosomatics* responded, "When do we *not* use this drug?" Sackler went to nearly equal depths of chicanery in parsing the difference between Librium, launched in 1959, and its chemical cousin Valium, released in 1963, drugs both made by Hoffman–La Roche that worked in a very similar fashion to calm the nerves. Sackler managed to convince the world that these two products were entirely different medications for entirely different purposes. Librium was for "anxiety," while Valium was for the quite different problem of "psychic tension."[53] Thus clearly partitioned, the two medications would not cannibalize each other's markets, and Hoffman–La Roche would get two bites at the apple of emotional distress among medical consumers. By 1964, Valium had become the first $100 million drug, a then staggering sales figure.[54]

Roche Labs, the American subsidiary of Hoffman–La Roche, spent somewhere in the vicinity of $200 million, in 1960s dollars, in the US alone to promote sales of the drugs, with Sackler receiving a bonus tied to each dollar spent. Roche even gave him interest-free loans as advances against future advertising work, largesse that he was able to invest in a bull market to amass an even greater fortune to buy even more art, which he could later donate to burnish his legacy within the Medical Industrial Complex as a benefactor of premier academic medical centers and the Foundation of the NIH.[55]

The talented Dr. Sackler not only created daylight between two nearly identical drugs; he also contrived new medical conditions for which new medications could be marketed.

For Upjohn, he helped promote the "happy baby vitamin," B6, which could be administered through a product called Zymbasic drops. Dr. Charles B. May, editor of the *Journal of the American Academy of Pediatrics*, became alarmed by the surge in supplements with B6 and consulted with some of the experts whose work Sackler had misrepresented in product promotions. One of these, Arild E. Hansen of the University of Texas, made it clear: "Never by any stretch of the imagination have we implied that there is such a thing as a 'happy baby vitamin.'"[56]

Sackler also sat on the editorial board of an antibiotics journal, *Antibiotics and Chemistry*, for which he created ads for Sigmamycin, a drug that would later be shown to cause jaundice and liver damage. After his death in 1987, it was discovered that he secretly owned MD Publications, a company that had funneled $287,000 to Henry Welch, the FDA regulator who headed the agency's division of antibiotics.[57,58]

Following Sackler's death, his third wife, Jillian, whom he had met when she was a secretary at his publication the *Medical Tribune*, engaged in a nasty, decade-long battle with his children for control of his estate. One of the revelations coming out of the legal battle was that, while he had always portrayed himself as being in fierce competition with the other most dominant drug advertising agency of the time, L.W. Frohlich, he and Frohlich had in fact been partners all along.[59] One of their joint ventures, in which Sackler enjoyed a hidden ownership stake, was IMS Health, originally Intercontinental Marketing Statistics, which aggregated prescription data. Sackler realized by 1960 that merging the database with purchased AMA Physician Masterfiles would allow the creation and subsequent sale of physicians' prescription profiling data used to microtarget compliant physicians and direct detail reps to soft targets, a process that would critically enable the progression of the opioid epidemic decades later.[59]

Today, Sackler's band of detail men, which he launched in 1952, is an army of more than 60,000 pharmaceutical sales representatives, servicing some 900,000 prescribers, and representing an industry investment of around $5 billion.[60] Most are employed by the top 20 companies with combined 2016 US-based revenues of $316 billion.[61] These new drug reps are 52 percent female; they are younger than the prior generation; one-third are former military people; and they are evaluated more on their discipline and aggressiveness than their congeniality. Now they come armed with exact monthly statistics of how many prescriptions each of the doctors they "detail" has written in the past month for each of their company's drugs, thanks to Sackler's arrangement with the IMS-laced Physician Masterfile data from the AMA.

But Sackler's legacy is actually far deeper, more pervasive, and pernicious. Ultimately, he helped condition us to look for the quick fix in the form of a pill, and he helped create an environment in which physicians oblige that patient reflex with sloppy prescribing and where overconsumption of drugs is stoked by enormous budgets for direct-to-consumer advertising. The idea that there should be a quick and seemingly efficient fix distracts us from the fact that we are the only nation in the world that spends more on health care than on social services—the kinds of services like good nutrition, safe air and water, and affordable housing that reduce the need to "fix" disorders after health has been compromised. It also sustains the illusion that scientific progress, in and of itself, equates with human progress, and that we don't need to pay equal attention to the effect of the social fabric on long-term health outcomes.

During the decade I spent at Pfizer, beginning in 1997, I accommodated the worldview that there is always a pharmaceutical fix with benefits that outweigh the risks, that advertising is consumer education, and that professional collusion is merely collaboration. But I never anticipated just how far the masters of manipulation would be willing to go in pursuit of profit and/or professional prestige until I witnessed Sackler's devotees place a large portion of our very young children on psychotropic drugs for reasons that are not at all clear.

According to the American Psychological Association, attention deficit hyperactivity disorder (ADHD) affects 5 percent of America's youngsters, though nearly 15 percent of high-school-age boys have been labeled with the condition.[62,63] Yet no blood test or imaging study is available to confirm the diagnosis; there's just a weakly validated 39-question yes-or-no survey that's distributed far and wide in pediatricians' offices, through the media, and through public and private schools nationwide. When the diagnosis is broken down by gender, demographics, and geography, the distribution of ADHD becomes even more mystifying and disturbing. Rates can double and triple in areas, most notably Arkansas, Kentucky, Louisiana, and Tennessee, where schools promote the diagnosis and local physicians are willing to play along and prescribe.[64] Meanwhile, the Centers for Disease Control and Prevention reports that among poor and disadvantaged two- to five-year-olds who carry the diagnosis of ADHD, more than 75 percent are placed on drugs, while only half ever receive "any form of psychological services."[65]

New York Times investigative reporter Alan Schwarz calls ADHD the "most misdiagnosed condition in American medicine."[62,66] It is also the logical extension of the promotional methods pioneered by Arthur Sackler: Pay and promote the careers of compliant physician "thought leaders," send sham patient-education materials into enabling institutions (in this case public schools), create quasi-medical associations and bogus pro-industry publications to liberalize diagnostic criteria for conditions, and expand drug use in treatment, ultimately relying on acquiescence from professional organizations—in this case the American Psychiatric Association (APA)—to support a disease category and the monetizing of it rather than find less intrusive and more effective ways to promote children's health and well-being.

Clearly some children benefit from drugs like Ritalin and Adderall, but in the world of pharmaceuticals I inhabited, marketers never settle for "some," even when only some might legitimately benefit. As I came to understand all too clearly, the Medical Industrial Complex creates markets, often by inventing a disease to be "treated" by a compound already in the works. One need only cite one of the latest market entries—opioid-induced constipation (OIC)—to illustrate how far pharmaceutical companies will go to medicalize conditions, including those that their own products have created. The next step is broadening the definition of the malady, then overstating and overpromoting benefits while minimizing risks. In the case of ADHD, this kind of "mission creep" has led to the astonishing belief, in many quarters, that the medicated youngster is actually better than he or she would be nonmedicated. And patient advocacy groups are fully on board with the mission.

Encouraged by a million-dollar grant from CIBA pharmaceuticals (originally Chemical Industries Basel) in 1989, Children and Adults with Attention Deficit Hyperactivity Disorder (CHADD), with 34,000 members in 640 chapters, currently trumpets, on its website, the "12 amazing superpowers" associated with hyperactivity.[67] According to CHADD, medicated juveniles multitask with a "laser focus" and score high on tests, a result no parent or teacher would object to. In 2012 comedian Stephen Colbert critically labeled the behavior "meducation."[68] The problem is that even when these pills deliver short-term, positive results, they short-circuit the child's development of strategies that can provide long-term solutions and success in adulthood. And as one might predict, anything in our culture that promises a quicker route to academic success is an invitation for illicit use.

Ironically, the ADHD pandemic began with the search for a profitable solution to a problem created by the medical profession itself. In the 1930s, Charles Bradley was a pediatrician responsible for troubled youth at the Emma Pendleton Bradley Hospital in Rhode Island.[69] His search to find the cause of varied psychiatric afflictions led him to routinely perform spinal taps for spinal fluid analysis on the children in his care, procedures that led to widespread spinal headaches among his patients. This occurred around the time that Philadelphia-based Smith, Kline & French came across a new remedy for nasal congestion, Benzedrine sulfate, which constricted nasal blood vessels and decreased nasal mucosal swelling.[70]

Dr. Bradley decided to try Benzedrine on 30 of his headache-afflicted charges, ages 5 to 14, in the hope that he could relieve the problems he had created with the spinal taps.[71] The drug failed miserably as a pain reliever, but suddenly the kids taking the stimulant embraced their studies. They began to perform better in school, and follow-up measurement confirmed that they appeared calmer as well. In November 1937, Bradley published his findings in the *American Journal of Psychiatry*.[72]

Most adults don't have to cope with exams, piano recitals, and homework assignments, but they, too, welcomed the boost Benzedrine provided. Popularity led to blowback, including a 1937 article in *Time* magazine called "Pep Pill Poisoning."[73] When college students from the Universities of Minnesota, Wisconsin, and Chicago collapsed from overdoses while cramming for exams, Smith, Kline & French began to retreat from marketing Benzedrine for use by children and focused instead on selling it for the treatment of depressed women, and this remained Benzedrine's market for the next two decades.

To ameliorate the drug's side effects, the company made minor changes to the formulation and rechristened the stimulant Dexedrine in late 1937.[74] It was used by soldiers in World War II to promote alertness. But the new version still maintained the overriding drawback of its precursor—addiction. Winston Churchill personally authorized its use by British soldiers until the soldiers' abuse of the drugs induced hallucinations that had tank drivers spinning in circles.[75] Combining the drug with the barbiturate amobarbital to form Dexamyl, including an extended-release version in the 1950s, only made matters worse. That's when Pfizer entered the market in 1956 with Atarax and hired Arthur Sackler to promote it by way of his infomercial, "The Relaxed Wife." It wasn't just for stressed-out women though. The company also targeted the youth market with ads claiming that the drug was capable of lengthening "the child's attention span for better schoolwork and easing his relations with teachers, classmates, and parents."[75] The question of Atarax's potential for causing addiction remained unresolved.

At about the same time, Harvard-trained psychologist Keith Conners, working at Johns Hopkins Medical School, went back to Dr. Bradley's

1937 Benzedrine paper.[76] He examined the research in detail and suggested to his boss, Leon Eisenberg, that they repeat the study. Soon they had a grant from the relatively new National Institute of Mental Health (NIMH) created with a healthy behind-the-scenes push from Mary Lasker.

Conners and Eisenberg did their experiment in 1961 with the updated formulation Dexedrine, giving it to a group of African American boys who were said to be hyperkinetic and impulsive—descriptions that could apply to just about any kid at one time or another. Their experiment was done at a reformatory called the Boys Village of Maryland. Despite side effects, most notably loss of appetite and weight loss, the drug seemed to work, making the boys calmer and more compliant.[77]

One year later, a replacement called methylphenidate hydrochloride was introduced that was supposed to be free of side effects. It had been created in 1956 by a CIBA company chemist, Leandro Panizzon, whose wife, Marguerite, was a tennis enthusiast looking for that extra oomph. Her nickname, Rita, provided the brand name—Ritalin. Although the company initially marketed the drug—with a 5,000 percent markup—for the treatment of depression and fatigue, in time it pivoted to a novel marketing pitch to therapists and counselors. These clinicians, CIBA said, should give the drug to their patients before a session because it could "help psychiatric patients talk in as little as 5 minutes."[78]

Thus did ADHD and Ritalin come of age together, coevolving along with renewed grants from the NIMH and cashable checks from a very supportive CIBA. Conners was recruited back to Harvard Medical School, where he began work on a measurement scale for the now fully endorsed "disease" of ADHD. In 1969, only one year after the most recent *Diagnostic and Statistical Manual*, the bible of psychiatry, had coined the term "hyperkinetic reaction of childhood," he published his original 28-question "Teacher Rating Scale" for ADHD in the *American Journal of Psychiatry*.[79] He would receive royalties for this testing instrument for the rest of his life.

With a deft touch that would have made Sackler, Hill, and even Selye proud, Conners described his study results this way: "The drug has energized the children, apathetic and discouraged by previous school failure, into making use of abilities available to them." CIBA's Ritalin ad stated simply, "Ritalin helps the problem child become lovable again."[80]

Of course, Conners's scale was not only a lever for manipulation; it was an invitation for abuse. On June 29, 1970, the *Washington Post* introduced the nation to Byron B. Oberst, an Omaha, Nebraska, pediatrician whose office treated approximately 6,000 kids referred by a school administration instituting what it called a behavior modification program. The kids being "modified" attended the mostly black North Side public schools. The district head of health services justified the program by saying, "It makes them happier." Dr. Oberst's comment was that he was in the prevention business, as in preventing "vandalism, riots, and anarchy against society."[81]

In September 1970, congressional hearings revealed that Conners was on the receiving end of $450,000 in grants from the drug industry to explore minimal brain dysfunction. A particularly generous benefactor was Abbott Labs, whose new product Cyclert promised greater effectiveness and safety for hyperkinetic kids.[82]

By 1975, portions of the medical establishment began to show concern that "minimal brain dysfunction" had become a catchall diagnosis for any child with even mildly nonconforming behavior.[83] But a number of influential psychiatrists simply doubled down, saying the issue requiring their immediate attention was a brain-related disorder that interfered with "attention span." By the time the 1980 *DSM* was printed, the condition had a new name, attention deficit disorder, accompanied by 16 definable traits that, once again, could describe just about any child having a bad day.[84,85]

Supplementing CIBA's $1 million under-the-table 1989 payment to CHADD, in 1995, a cooperative and compliant Department of Education provided another $750,000 to help the organization produce two ADHD information videos, one for parents and the other for schools. It also produced "A Child's Call for Help," a public service announcement that reached 19 million viewers and generated more than 100,000 follow-up calls to CHADD's headquarters.[85,86,87]

Harvard child psychiatrist Edward Hallowell's influential and bestselling 1994 book, *Driven to Distraction*, advocated psychotherapy and coaching, in addition to medications.[88] In 1996, writing in the Sunday supplement *Parade*, he referred to ADHD as "a good-news diagnosis."[89] And so it arguably was for some desperate parents who were at their wit's end. On the other side of the issue were critics such as Dr. Peter Breggin, a Harvard-trained psychiatrist and consultant to the National Institute of Mental Health, who raised suspicion of ulterior motives on the part of educators: "Who's suffering? These drugs alleviate the suffering of teachers in over-crowded classrooms."[90]

Public debate continued for another two years before the NIH decided in 1998 to hold a consensus conference on the topic headlined by Keith Conners, who had recently left Harvard for Duke. But Massachusetts pediatrician Mark Vonnegut offered the most succinct assessment: "The diagnosis is a mess."[91]

The 1948 patent on Ritalin that had allowed the 5,000 percent markup had long since expired. The market continued to grow, however, and so did the search for new patentable pharmaceuticals that could be used to "treat" ADHD-labeled children. Ironically, the race was won not by an eminent scientist but by a former Lederle Laboratories detail man named Roger Griggs.[92]

In the early 1990s, Griggs had started his own firm, Richwood Pharmaceutical, with the strategy of acquiring the rights to sell already patented drugs. Initially, he focused on Rexar's Obetrol, a weight-loss product that in 1991 earned a meager $40,000.[93] Its side effects in adults included anxiety, tension, and sleeplessness, but its effects in children had not been studied. What salesman extraordinaire Griggs noticed that others missed was the unusual number of scripts being written by a Utah pediatrician named Ron Jones. When Griggs investigated, he discovered that Jones was prescribing Obetrol to children off-label for ADHD. More than that—the pediatrician claimed a 70 percent success rate with the drug when it was used on kids who had failed a trial of Ritalin.[94]

Griggs bought Rexar and with it control of the drug Obetrol, which he renamed Adderall (as in "ADD for all"). Then, without even asking the FDA's permission, he launched the compound as a "unique alternative" for ADHD. The FDA was not amused and aggressively moved to shut down his company, but in 1995, according to *New York Times* columnist Schwarz, the child of an unidentified but influential senator did well on Adderall after failing on Ritalin, and that was all it took for the FDA to approve the drug a year later.[95]

However, by now, the claims of successful ADHD drug treatment had become more explicitly focused on academic achievement and the return to normalcy. In 1993, Larry B. Silver, MD, wrote an informational pamphlet, sponsored by the British pharmaceutical company Shire, stating, "Parents should be aware that these medicines do not 'drug' or 'alter' the brain of the child. They make the child 'normal.'"[96] In a culture ever more accepting of the idea that test results determine future placement in college, and that the name recognition of the college attended could determine the quality of life, this was a powerful argument, well amplified in the popular press. Company-funded, doctor-fronted ADHD information pamphlets added legitimacy to the idea that the administration of drugs was the only responsible thing to do.

Domestic Adderall sales by 1997 were $18 million. That year, Griggs was approached by Shire with an offer to buy Richwood for $186 million, and he took the money and ran.[97] Others saw more staying power, even growth, buoyed by the results of an NIMH trial headed by none other than Keith Conners. This study, published in the *Archives of General Psychiatry* in 1999, compared Ritalin with cognitive behavioral therapy for ADHD and gave the edge to drugs, even though nearly half of those on medication alone showed no benefit.[98]

And then the spiritual heirs of Arthur Sackler began to imagine the profit potential if only ADHD could be defined as a *lifelong* condition. Companies that targeted children with ADHD saw an upper limit of school-age patients at about 3 million, but if sales could be projected into adulthood, a universe of 10 million was entirely possible. Shire and its drug Adderall took the lead in advancing the cause of adult ADHD, but soon Novartis, having purchased CIBA's Ritalin, and Johnson & Johnson, with its new once-a-day Ritalin-like drug called Concerta, joined the pack.

On June 18, 1994, the cover of *Time* magazine proclaimed, "Disorganized? Distracted? Discombobulated? Doctors Say You May Have

ATTENTION DEFICIT DISORDER. It's not just kids who suffer from it."[99] By the end of the decade, Shire was selling $250 million worth of Adderall each year. More contenders would soon arrive, and they would all pass through the Duke lab of Conners, whose construct of ADHD was so well established at this point that he had his own medical journal, the *Journal of Attention Disorders*.[100] But Conners was aging, and the market was attracting new champions—at the top of the list was a Czechoslovakia-born, Argentina- and Israel-schooled Harvard child psychiatrist named Joe Biederman.

Known for an overly aggressive personality, Biederman also had an uncanny ability to churn out papers on ADHD—nearly 300 in the decade between 1995 and 2005.[101] As a result, he became the go-to guy for activities in continuing medical education by any and all companies with ADHD products to sell. That lucrative business was curtailed in 2008 when Senator Chuck Grassley (R-IA) investigated and found that, between 2000 and 2007, Biederman and his two top subordinates at Harvard had collected $4.2 million in fees, much of it from Johnson & Johnson, which, in addition to Concerta, owned the psychotropic Risperdal and pushed for treatment not only of ADHD but also of another Biederman-marketed concoction, "childhood bi-polar disease."[102]

By 2002, Adderall sales exceeded $1 billion; five years later the drug crossed the $3 billion threshold.[103] Along the way, Shire and Johnson & Johnson received help from yet another corner of the Medical Industrial Complex that had become an ever more reliable partner in manipulation—academic medical centers trolling for clinical subjects to participate in NIH-supported studies. In 2007, an alarming print ad created by the advertising firm BBDO for New York University's Child Study Center ran for two weeks in the New York City market. It stated: "We are in possession of your son. We are making him squirm + fidget until he is a detriment to himself + those around him. Ignore this + your kid will pay. ADHD." But this copy was not written to sell a movie; it was written to enlist study subjects for medical research. After 3,000 email messages, 70 percent negative, were sent to the center's director, Dr. Harold Koplewitz, he pulled the ad.[104]

Since the 1970s, entrepreneurial psychiatrists like Dr. Paul Wender had been pushing the American Psychiatric Association to include the adult form of ADHD in the *Diagnostic and Statistical Manual*. The APA resisted, but by 2007 the barriers had been worn down by 40 years of relentless persuasion.[105] The latest industry-created vehicle was called the National Alliance for the Advancement of ADHD Care and was funded by Lilly—not surprisingly, a company whose own ADHD entry, Strattera, had joined the fray in 2002 and promised fewer side effects.[106] A familiar barrage of simulcast conferences, continuing medical education boondoggles, pamphlets, and papers followed.

Not to be outdone, Shire commissioned a loosely referenced booklet for doctors' offices, fronted by Denver psychiatrist Dr. William Dodson, who stated, "We know now that about 10 percent of adults have ADHD, which means you're probably already treating patients with ADHD even though you don't know it." The 10 percent figure was unsubstantiated, and Dodson at the time was collecting speaker fees from three different manufacturers.[107,108] Shire also commissioned a survey designed to prove that people with untreated ADHD were far more likely to drop out, get divorced, or become addicted. The company then underwrote a scientific version that was published in May 2004 by the *Journal of Clinical Psychiatry*. The Shire press release read, "Survey of Adults Reveals Life-Long Consequences of Attention-Deficit-Hyperactivity Disorder."[109]

Eli Lilly's Strattera had failed as an antidepressant but gained FDA approval for use in ADHD. In 2004, Biederman spearheaded a study, funded by Lilly, to create a diagnostic survey for adult ADHD. His original 18-question survey was tested on 1,001 adults and glowingly portrayed in a press release. He subsequently whittled the survey down to six open-ended questions that were laughably nonscientific.[110]

1. How often do you have trouble wrapping up the fine details of a project, once the challenging parts have been done?
2. How often do you have difficulty getting things in order when you have to do a task that requires organization?

3. When you have a task that requires a lot of thought, how often do you avoid or delay getting started?
4. How often do you have problems remembering appointments or obligations?
5. How often do you fidget or squirm with your hands or feet when you have to sit down for a long period of time?
6. How often do you feel overly active and compelled to do things, like you were driven by a motor?

Using this measurement tool, the team soon declared that 4.4 percent of American adults were afflicted with this dread disorder, and thus they were in need of the products the drug industry was eager to sell. In 2007, adult scripts for ADHD numbered 5.6 million. By 2012, they topped 16 million, most of them written for folks in their 20s and 30s. Student health offices on college campuses noted a huge uptick of students requesting Adderall for their chronic ADHD.

The Centers for Disease Control and Prevention was remarkably compliant with ever-escalating estimates of the number of kids affected by ADHD. In 2010, it accepted a range between 7.8 percent and 9.5 percent. By 2016, it had approached 11 percent.[111] But estimates like these, and new industry ads suggesting, "Drug Therapy for Parents' ADHD Improves Kid's Behavior," had become too much even for Keith Conners. North Carolina, the home state of his treatment center at Duke, now had the highest proportion of kids on ADHD drugs in the nation—16 percent.[112]

Ultimately, what brought Conners around was not criticism from professional colleagues but rather the plight of a family member. Conners began to express a different point of view after a May 2014 meeting with a local school superintendent, attended and recorded by the *New York Times'* Schwarz.[113] Conners's grandson had been receiving a hard push by school officials to get diagnosed and treated for ADHD, and at last Connors, writing in the *Huffington Post* on March 28, 2016, admitted the obvious. "A vast proportion of [kids] on medication received an incorrect diagnosis," he said. "Testing and funding is at stake and nobody wants these kids dragging down the numbers. School systems have developed some secret process—teachers have a way of talking to parents. And it's not just teachers either; it's school personnel. There's a roundabout system because the incentives are for the school system to deliver better test scores, more end-of-school graduation rates."[114]

His grandson's school superintendent dispassionately shifted the blame: "That sounds like a question for physicians. Because they write the prescriptions." When asked how the kids got in to see those doctors, she said, "That's a question for the parents."[113,114] Conners apparently didn't press the issue further, perhaps in part because he was still collecting royalties for the use of his diagnostic scale.

Just as troubling as knowing that schoolchildren and young adults are being heavily medicated based on dubious criteria is the news that, as CDC epidemiologist Susanna Visser recently confirmed, more than 10,000 American infants two and three years old are already receiving physician-prescribed psychotropic medication for ADHD.[115]

As one might expect from the spiraling feedback loops seen within the Medical Industrial Complex, admissions for Adderall drug *rehabilitation* began to rise. Doctors focused on the opioid epidemic have been slow to acknowledge that their sloppy prescribing has created another front in the health professions' war on drugs.[115] But as British imperialists learned with opium in China long ago, nothing succeeds quite like addiction when you're looking to develop a customer base.

Since 1966, the annual consumption of stimulants by Americans has expanded fourfold; for Adderall, Ritalin, Concerta, Strattera, and their generic offspring, consumption has grown 10-fold. We are just over 4 percent of the global population, and yet we consume close to 90 percent of the world's prescription-level stimulants. An estimated 16 million American adults use prescription stimulants.[116,117]

In the US, any physician, physician's assistant, or nurse practitioner can prescribe one of these drugs.[118] In marked contrast, countries like France and Canada look first at what can be accomplished through social services and behavioral adjustments. To get the diagnosis of ADHD in France you must be evaluated by a psychiatrist or neurologist. If you are among that small 0.5 percent believed to actually have ADHD in France, psychotherapy or family counseling is the treatment of choice. Children and their parents leave the office with lifelong strategies rather than pills. Schools contribute as well, not by encouraging medical treatment but by expanding access to the outdoors, eliminating sugary processed foods, and adjusting classroom design and rules to make them less confining.[119]

The widespread and growing expansion in the US of the ADHD diagnosis, and the explosive abuse of Adderall and growth of treatment programs to rescue the addicted, reflects more than just sloppy physician prescribing, pharmaceutical greed, or a consumer over-appetite for pharmaceuticals, fed by direct-to-consumer advertising. It is rather a tangible expression of the perverse outcomes that one might expect when health care is considered a business opportunity rather than a public good, when health planning is conflated with health profiteering, and when complexity and obfuscation are deployed with the intent to monetize, in situations where simplicity and transparency are essential.

In all of this, Arthur Sackler, the master of manipulation, had shown the way. Sadly, the most dramatic legacy of the strategies he devised is in the domain of highly profitable addiction. Early on, in 1952, when he was still developing his playbook for capturing hearts and minds, he and his brothers acquired a small company called Purdue Frederick.[120] Little more than a shell with annual revenues of only $22,000, it had been founded in 1892 to produce patent medicines. One of its big sellers was Gray's Glycerine Tonic Compound, which consisted mostly of sherry.

In 1955, Purdue expanded to sell a brand of laxatives, and then an earwax remover. During this period, the Sackler brothers continued to actively experiment with the use of psychotropic drugs to address the symptoms of mental illness, and then they began to investigate what seemed to be an overlooked area—the treatment of pain. In 1964 Purdue acquired a British counterpart called Napp Pharmaceuticals, which in turn acquired a Scottish drug producer, Bard Pharmaceuticals.[120] The Sacklers' primary interest in Napp and Bard was not a specific drug but rather their prolonged-release technology called Continus which was suitable for administering morphine. At the time, highly addictive morphine sulfate was the mainstay of pain relief for surgical and cancer patients. The Sackler brothers felt that a slow release might be less addictive. In 1972, they patented a system called Contin in the US and began to sell a new slow-release morphine sulfate drug called MST in England. In 1987, they released a new and improved version called MS Contin in the US, and a decade later they modified the chemical formula to create OxyContin.[121]

Arthur Sackler died in 1987 at the age of 73. But Purdue remained very much a family business, run by his brother Raymond and a nephew, and operating very much in the Sackler tradition.

When the FDA approved OxyContin in 1996, no clinical studies to determine the risk of addiction had been performed, yet the FDA-approved package insert said that the drug was safer than rival painkillers because its delayed-absorption mechanism was "believed" to reduce the likelihood of abuse.[122] That same insert was an invitation to an epidemic in its warning against ingesting the drug in any way other than the pre-scribed capsule form. People quickly discovered that if you ground up the pills and snorted them, or dissolved them in solution and injected them, you could get the punch of heroin.

The opioid epidemic was built on three big lies, each of which was relentlessly exploited by Purdue.[123]

1. There was an epidemic of untreated pain throughout America—it was the neglected "fifth vital sign."
2. OxyContin was less potent than morphine.
3. OxyContin provided relief for a full 12 hours—thus two pills a day would do the trick.

This third claim, central to OxyContin's basic selling proposition, was made despite the fact that in Purdue's first study, conducted in 1989 and focused on 90 women recuperating from abdominal or gynecologic sur-gery, over one-third complained of pain at the 8-hour mark. That study was never published.[123]

Instead, Purdue became even more aggressive, increasing the number of its sales reps from 318 in 1996 to 671 in 2000.[124] The reps traveled far and wide, spreading the message that this miraculous, no-risk opioid should be prescribed not just for severe postsurgical pain but for arthritis and sports injuries and C-sections—the kind of use that gets people hooked. These sales reps were given special training in overcoming objections and in understating the potency of the drug. The party line was that less than 1 percent of patients who took the drug became addicted—a statistic pulled from thin air. In 1999, when Purdue funded a study of the drug as used for headaches, investigators found an addiction rate of 13 percent.[125] Purdue supported a speakers' bureau that paid thousands of clinicians to deliver presentations about the glories of OxyContin at "pain seminars" in appealing vacation spots. Purdue's AMA-provided tracking system showed that doctors who attended these seminars in 1996 wrote scripts for OxyContin at more than twice the rate of those who didn't attend.[126]

In 2001, a year in which Purdue would pay $40 million in sales bonuses, Michael Friedman, a Purdue executive vice president, claimed in testimony before Congress that Purdue's marketing of the drug had been "conservative by any standard."[127] As for the epidemic of opioid abuse sweeping the nation, he said, "Virtually all of these reports involve people who are abusing the medication, not patients with legitimate medical needs." When a crackdown seemed imminent anyway, Purdue hired former New York mayor and lawyer Rudolph Giuliani, who successfully warded off government intervention.[128]

In fact, Purdue was following the Arthur Sackler playbook in every detail. First, help create the American Academy of Pain Management, a quasi-medical organization, housed within the AMA Federation for legitimacy. Then provide funding to the organization to sponsor quasi-academic vehicles (journals and continuing medical education programs) to publish supportive articles and reeducate practitioners toward the medicalization of the target condition and the need for treatment of this condition with its therapy. Integrate these programs with the mainstream intelligentsia by ample funding in high-end medical journals and generous philanthropic support of high-end academic institutions and medical organizations, so that, by simple name association, the brand's integrity is reinforced. Then sell, sell, sell, using AMA-enabled physician prescription profiling to identify the soft physician targets. Finally, when overprescribing causes a backlash, generously and magnanimously participate in the corrective steps made necessary by one's actions.

In 2003, the Drug Enforcement Administration found that the opioid epidemic was far more attributable to these Purdue marketing techniques than to a sudden upsurge in the number of would-be thrill seekers. The agency also concluded that the company had deliberately minimized the drug's risks. At the same time, the FDA was sending Purdue warning letters about ads that "grossly overstate the safety profile of OxyContin." Purdue responded to government concern by airing a public service announcement showing a teenager raiding his parents' medicine cabinet.[129] (In 2017, Purdue began running full-page image ads in the *New York Times* saying, in effect, "Of course we're concerned.")

Purdue also distributed a pamphlet in which it introduced the concept of "pseudo-addiction." In Purdue corporate-speak, when patients crave another hit of a drug because they continue to be in pain, that's not really addiction. And yet selling a product that promises 12 hours of relief with one pill, when you know full well that the effect will wear off after 8 hours, is an engraved invitation to abuse.[127]

Under pressure from attorneys general to change its tactics, Purdue was forced to reveal internal documents showing that it knew all about the bait and switch it was selling, and that the company was indeed concerned, but not because its lies were getting people hooked. Executives were worried that the truth would undercut the sales rationale for the drug and that the drug's niche would be overtaken by immensely cheaper generic morphine.[127]

Between 2006 and 2015, Purdue spent nearly $900 million on lobbying and political contributions and paid more than $600 million in fines. The company is also currently fighting more than 100 state and city lawsuits claiming damages for the immense social costs attributable to OxyContin.[130,131] Leading the effort against Purdue Pharma is former Mississippi attorney general Mike Moore, the legendary figure behind the exposure of Big Tobacco's true intent and its costly multistate settlement two decades ago. With approximately 100 Americans dying each day from opioid overdoses, the potential liability could exceed the settlement faced by tobacco companies: $200 billion over 25 years. According to legal experts, conviction for violating consumer protection standards could carry a $10,000 fine per occurrence for each prescription written. That could add up to trillions in penalties. An unapologetic Purdue spokesman in 2017 rejected the tobacco comparison while hiding behind a familiar MIC shield, stating, "Unlike tobacco companies, our products are medicines approved by FDA, prescribed by doctors, and dispensed by pharmacists, as treatments for patients suffering pain."[131]

In August 2010, Purdue replaced the original drug with a reformulated version that when crushed yielded not a fine powder but rather a gummy mess.[132] But again, the motive was more to block competition from generic morphine that to cure a social ill. Also, the patent on the original formulation was due to expire in 2013. The net result was that many of those already addicted moved from OxyContin to heroin.[127]

The reformulation meant a 50 percent drop in prescriptions for OxyContin, but Purdue, following yet another strategy borrowed from the tobacco industry playbook, had already responded to domestic health concerns by moving its marketing focus overseas, where it now uses the same unscrupulous techniques in places like Mexico, China, and Brazil.[127]

Even more astoundingly, in August 2015, Purdue received FDA approval to market OxyContin to children age 11 to 16, justifying its action as an important option for teens with cancer who need daily, round-the-clock, long-term pain relief. But studies now show that 1 in 25 high school seniors has abused OxyContin. The FDA approval came without the FDA ever convening an advisory committee to assess the risks and benefits of its controversial decision.[133]

Chapter 9

Equal Parts Politics and Science

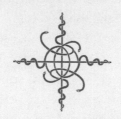

The Saint Regis Mohawk Tribe, a community of nearly 3,000 Native Americans, occupies a remote area along the south bank of the St. Lawrence River in upstate New York. In 2017, the tribe, best known for a gambling casino and allegations of smuggling across the Canadian border, became the owner of the patent for a bestselling dry-eye drug, Restasis.[1] Not that the tribe members were tearless or had suddenly gone into drug development. They had simply joined in a scheme to take the drug's patent out of contention in a lawsuit.

Under the terms of the deal, Allergan, the drug's manufacturer, transferred patent ownership to the Mohawk and paid the tribe $13.75 million for accepting it. In exchange, the tribe—a nation of indigenous people unto itself—claimed "sovereign immunity" as grounds for dismissing a patent challenge by Teva Pharmaceuticals, a company seeking to produce a generic version of the drug. Given that Restasis brought in $336.4 million in revenues in the second quarter of 2017, and that it's Allergen's second-biggest-selling product, behind the wrinkle treatment Botox, the company is not eager to have a lower-cost alternative on the market. The courts have cried foul, but the company is appealing a ruling to invalidate the patent transfer. If the transfer is allowed, the tribe will lease the patent back to the drugmaker and will receive $15 million in annual royalties until the year 2024, when the patent expires.[2]

This odd-couple alliance is only one of many strategies used by members of the Medical Industrial Complex to circumvent regulations and maximize profitability. The extreme cynicism it exposes reflects the success of nearly a half century of a deliberate and slowly progressive erosion of checks and balances restraining corporate greed.

Initially few and far between, episodes of MIC collusion are now more the rule than the exception, and victims one day become offenders the next. Which is why, in 2016, 20 states, tired of federal inaction, joined in a civil suit against the very same Teva Pharmaceuticals, and against Mylan and four smaller firms, for brazen price-fixing.[3] It is also why, one year later, five other state attorneys general initiated a civil action against Lilly, Novo Nordisk, Sanofi, and CVS and its pharmacy benefits management firm, charging that they had colluded in an insulin price-fixing scheme that led patients to ration their own insulin, with deadly consequences.[4]

If the first two decades following World War II were the years when Vannevar Bush and George Merck launched the integrated Medical Industrial Complex, supported by Arthur Sackler's bag of marketing tricks, the following three decades represented a proof of concept.

As early as 1980, Arnold Relman, MD, editor of the *New England Journal of Medicine*, was drawing unwelcome comparisons between the MIC and the military-industrial complex and its penchant for embracing competition and collusion in equal measures. He said:

A final concern is the one first emphasized by President Eisenhower in his warning about the "military-industrial complex": "We must guard against the acquisition of unwarranted influence." A private health-care industry of huge proportions could be a powerful political force in the country and could exert considerable influence on national health policy. A broad national health-insurance program, with the inevitable federal regulation of costs, would be anathema to the medical-industrial complex, just as a national disarmament policy is to the military-industrial complex. I do not wish to imply that only vested interests oppose the expansion of federal health-insurance programs (or treaties to limit armaments), but I do suggest that the political involvement of the medical-industrial complex will probably hinder rather than facilitate rational debate on national health-care.[5]

As Arthur Sackler worked inventively to parse the difference between Valium and Librium, and with one in seven Americans in 1960 taking tranquilizers, a subtle power shift was emerging that would in time reshape institutional relations within the Medical Industrial Complex.

In 1963, Stanley and Sidney Goldstein opened their first store in Lowell, Massachusetts, to sell health and beauty products. Restless and aggressive businessmen, they expanded to 17 Consumer Value Stores throughout Massachusetts and Rhode Island within the year, and by 1967, when their new red-and-white logo simply read "CVS," they had pharmacies in several of the stores. By 1975, the chain had 300 locations in the Northeast and the Midwest, sales in excess of $100 million, and standardized inventory and ordering systems that made it a powerhouse.[6] Four decades later, it is the dominant player in America's complex and opaque pharmaceutical and insurance supply chain, a major employer of health professionals and provider of direct health care services. In 2017, CVS made a $67 billion offer to purchase the health insurance giant Aetna.[7]

In 1940, few would have predicted the appearance of CVS on the market, let alone its stratospheric rise. In that year there were 80,000 druggists in the US, 3,000 of them hospital-based, and their prestige was probably at a low ebb.[8] With war on the horizon and the official Medical Corps and Nursing Corps in place, the American Pharmaceutical Association lobbied the Surgeon General's Office for a commissioned Pharmacy Corps, but the official response merely added insult to injury. After stating that the Army's three-month pharmacy-technician course seemed sufficient, the surgeon general summed up the work of a military pharmacist by saying that "any intelligent boy can read the label."[9]

Pharmacists never received the bump up in status that other health care professionals did during the war. No accurate census of the number of pharmacists who served was ever taken, but that number is estimated to be somewhere between 10,000 and 14,000.[8] Because of the lack of pharmacists and the impact of war rationing, 15 percent of America's drugstores closed during the war. As a result, those that remained open filled 13 percent more prescriptions and realized an 80 percent increase in overall sales.[10]

The American Pharmaceutical Association's modest attempts to support an expansion of its members' professional privileges in 1950 were aggressively opposed by the American Medical Association and by the Pharmaceutical Manufacturers Association. A major source of contention for the pharmacists was the growing list of branded me-too drugs that exploded onto the market in the 1950s and added to the clutter of generic products on drugstore shelves. Pharmacists were required to follow the physician's prescription orders to the letter, and no substitutions were allowed. As a result, they were forced to absorb the expense and inconvenience of carrying an enormous inventory of products.[10]

The right to substitute generic drugs for branded varieties became the proxy in a battle between doctors, pharmacists, hospitals, pharmaceutical manufacturers, and insurers for control during the next two decades. The AMA's and APA's unwillingness to compromise on this issue and share turf and profitability with pharmacists, and their preference for conspiring and colluding with each other, helped create the Medical Industrial Complex. The arrival of pharmacy corporations like CVS created new dynamics, and the MIC adjusted to this new reality. To evolve and survive, competing sectors collaborated behind the scenes, utilizing shared patient databases and an army of cross-sector leaders able to pass seamlessly between academia, government, and the various branches of industry to effect cooperation.

By 2018, cross-sector leaders in the health industry were ubiquitous. That year 340 former congressional staffers worked for MIC firms they had once regulated, and more than a dozen former MIC industry execs had jobs on Capitol Hill, including the former Eli Lilly executive Alex Azar, who replaced the disgraced Dr. Tom Price as head of the Department of Health and Human Services. All were experts in the inner workings of both government and industry, and also on a first-name basis with scores of academicians, hospital leaders, industry lobbyists, and insurance executives.[11]

The role model for many of them was the physician and pharmacologist Louis Lasagna, who had trained at Johns Hopkins. In 1956, he lobbied the FDA to develop a separate metric beyond "safety" to assess the effectiveness of new drugs coming to market.[12] As a contrarian, he was an equal-opportunity offender, often sought after for media commentary. He had challenged the pharmaceutical industry's over-the-top marketing claims, outrageous prices, and deceptive relationships with doctors nationwide, but also was not shy about criticizing his fellow physicians' dismal lack of expertise in all things pharmacologic.

The AMA in 1960 had already acknowledged that physicians' familiarity with new drug developments was sketchy, and that the instructions dealing with dosage, indications, side effects, and routes of administration that the industry put into pill packages were seldom read. So the organization created a yearly book, *The Physicians' Desk Reference*, which presented all the information contained in the package inserts in an orderly, indexed format available free to all AMA members each year.[13] It also created a subscription serial pamphlet for practicing physicians called *The Medical Letter*, with Lasagna as one of its advisers, which provided monthly updates of new discoveries and controversial issues in pharmacology.[14]

In 1962, Lasagna's knowledge and outspokenness led to an invitation to join the government team evaluating FDA policy. When he appeared before Estes Kefauver's congressional committee, he made headlines in Arthur Sackler's hometown by lamenting the fact that money was corrupting doctors' professional decision-making choices, or as he put it, "Madison Avenue" had discovered "Medicine Avenue."[15] He also labeled the science involving the "equivalency" of generic products "abysmally ignorant" and the standards for quality "inadequate."[16]

The committee to which Lasagna said all these things went on to craft the Kefauver-Harris Amendment, or the Drug Efficacy Amendment, to the Federal Food, Drug, and Cosmetic Act. Adopted in 1962, the amendment introduced a requirement for drug manufacturers to provide proof of the effectiveness and safety of their drugs before approval, required drug advertising to disclose accurate information about side effects, and prevented cheap generic drugs from being marketed under new trade names as "breakthrough" medications.[17]

These requirements were retroactive, meaning that more than 4,000 drugs that had appeared on the market between 1938 and 1962 needed to be critically evaluated. To determine these drugs' effectiveness, the government created the Drug Efficacy Study (DES), which involved multiple panels of experts drawn from the National Academy of Science and the National Research Council.[18]

The lead voice on the DES was the outspoken Louis Lasagna. He had acknowledged industry support of his fellowship programs in clinical pharmacology at Johns Hopkins,[19] and, with the support of the American Enterprise Institute, he had endorsed collaboration between "universities and the pharmaceutical industry . . . to join forces in providing reasonable advice to government . . . to prevent unwise participation of the government in drug development."[20] If Lasagna occasionally slammed the drug industry as well, that was just Lou being Lou.

Not shy in promoting himself or his ideas, Lasagna had a knack for deleting embarrassing details from his ever-expanding professional narrative. Few knew that he had unsuccessfully pressured the FDA to approve thalidomide on behalf of its US manufacturer, Richardson-Merrell. Fewer still remembered his publicly quoted remark following the barbiturate-overdose death of Marilyn Monroe in 1962: "If Marilyn Monroe's physician had been able to prescribe that drug [thalidomide] instead of barbiturates she might still be alive."[21] But remarks such as these eventually drove a wedge between him and his academic colleagues, and fueled his desire to create a new and independent leadership platform that he alone would direct.

Between 1965 and 1970, with the advent of Medicare and Medicaid, health care costs had moved front and center. Congress had realized from the start that the presence of health care coverage for those over age 65 and the poor would drive up utilization of services. Total costs had risen by more than 6 percent a year during the first five years of the program. By the mid-1970s, the steep rise continued, with about 40 percent attributed to hospital expenses and 25 percent attributed to physicians. Drug costs accounted for about 10 percent, and that price tag made the industry a favorite target for legislative reform.[22]

When the Subcommittee on Monopoly of the Select Committee on Small Business convened in 1967 to examine the effect of competition on drug pricing, it focused on lower-cost generics as a solution.[23] The pharmaceutical industry and the AMA said that forcing generic substitution would be an assault on physician autonomy as well as a health risk inasmuch as there was no proof that generic copies were as safe and effective as the parent compounds.[24] Even though a compound's active ingredients appeared equivalent, they argued, this was no guarantee that the two drugs were actually "therapeutically equivalent."

In his testimony, Pharmaceutical Manufacturers Association president C. Joseph Stetler referred to the case of a powerful antibiotic, chloramphenicol. A head-to-head study of the parent drug and a generic copy had just revealed that the absorption rates of the two varied widely in humans. In a commentary in *JAMA*, a physician had added: "The pharmaceuticals manufactured in some of these loft factories are sometimes a combination of dust, ground-up cockroaches, and drug."[25] The FDA shortly thereafter pulled nine different generic "chloramphenicols" off the market.[26]

In many instances, however, no therapeutic differences between the branded drug and the generic substitute could be established, and Senator Gaylord Nelson (D-WI) labeled Stetler's line of defense "gobbledygook," as well as "propaganda."[27] In May 1968, Senator Ted Kennedy (D-MA) and Nelson, who had taken over the antitrust watch from Estes Kefauver, launched a decade-long struggle to bring the drug giants to heel.[23] The industry's rather grandiose line of defense was expressed in a Pfizer annual report that described pharmaceutical innovation as being "not only a scientific process, but also a socio-political one," a variation on its earlier portrayal of the business of selling drugs as a bulwark against Soviet communism.[28]

Senator Kennedy, as chair of the Senate Subcommittee on Health, opened hearings in 1973 and 1974 focused on physicians' dependency on brand-name drugs and the army of pharmaceutical detail men they relied on for their prescribing information.[29] This was at a time when employers were seeing the inflation of medical costs eating into their profitability, and when escalating oil prices were tipping the economy into a deep trough. Thus, Kennedy had a rather broad mandate to explore "legislative solutions to the problems surrounding the way drugs are developed, marketed and used in this country."[30]

Members of the pharmaceutical industry clearly felt heat at their back and went looking for allies. They turned to Lou Lasagna, in whom they had seen the qualities of a future cross-sector leader a decade earlier. Dr. Lasagna's outspoken nature and public overexposure had led to a break with his professional colleagues over the Drug Efficacy Study deliberations on the safety of combination drugs in the 1960s. But he made a smooth landing thanks to the patronage of Allen Wallis, the conservative chancellor of the University of Rochester, New York, and a corporate darling whose views related to free enterprise, entrepreneurship, and cross-sector leadership were well aligned with Lasagna's.[31]

In 1970, Lasagna became chairman of the Department of Pharmacology and Toxicology at the University of Rochester's School of Medicine,[32] where he founded the Center for the Study of Drug Development (CSDD), a common meeting ground for free market–minded academics, government officials, and corporate leaders.[33] By 1976, he had moved his center to Boston's Tufts University. He was now a renegade scholar, a successful entrepreneur, and a lightning rod for controversy. But within the business community, he was a sought-after speaker, much as Reagan had been.

From the start, Lasagna's CSDD was a multifaceted and highly productive platform, providing professional development courses in clinical pharmacology, drug development, research processes, and pharmaceutical regulations.[34] It generated influential white papers and reports on everything from clinical research design to the growing trend of outsourcing work to contract (or clinical) research organizations (CROs). It also provided customized reports helping individual clients design their government-relations strategies in pursuit of favorable policies.

The 1962 FDA legislation had left much to be desired in the area of drug development. It had created complex regulations without adequate staffing or funding. In the early years following the thalidomide disaster, the American people and their government were willing to accept the new rules and the delays in drug development these rules fostered. However, they became less tolerant a decade later when a deep recession, accompanied by high interest rates and extraordinarily thin pipelines for new discoveries, stubbornly resisted corrective steps.

Lasagna was all about free enterprise and eliminating what he viewed as excessive government regulation. That worldview was well capsulized in remarks he made in 1976. Quoting Rochester chancellor Wallis, Lasagna said, "The remedy . . . is obvious and simple, but implausible. Return the power to the people. Give each doctor and each patient the right and responsibility for making his own decisions freely in light of his own best knowledge (or ignorance) and judgment (or folly). Inevitably, some doctors and some patients will make some unwise decisions, perhaps even some that harm other people. But there is no possibility that the greatest harm these errors could do would even approximate the least harm that the government can do."[35]

Throughout the 1970s, the pharmaceutical-industry-funded CSDD under Lasagna laid the statistical groundwork to "prove" that the pharmaceutical industry was "high risk/high gain," that government-induced delays eroded patent life and profitability, and that inadequate protection of intellectual property rights discouraged investment, discovery, and innovation.[36] Lou pegged the cost of bringing a new drug to market at $800 million and the losses associated with a one-month delay in a product review by the FDA at $10 million for the sponsoring company. Multiplied by the average approval time required for a new drug application—31 months—that amounted to real money.

New drug launches in the US had dropped to around 40 per year, and for nearly all of these, the drug's appearance in Europe preceded its US debut by approximately two years. Not surprisingly, multinational pharmaceutical companies were choosing to launch their new products in Europe rather than in the United States in 80 percent of cases.

In the early 1970s, physicians were relatively unconcerned about what Lasagna labeled the "drug lag." Their earnings, which had ratcheted up for decades, surged with Medicare approval. A 2014 *Wall Street Journal* analysis found that in 1940, the 2010 inflation-adjusted mean income of all doctors on average was $40,000. By 1970, it was closing in on $250,000—six times the median American household income at the time.[37] This was good news for the ability of doctors to join country clubs, but not good for their image, and neither the government nor private insurers were amused by the way physicians could, and often did, bump up earnings simply by ordering another test or doing another procedure. Some medical leaders went so far as to implore their colleagues to practice restraint or, as the president of the New Haven Medical Society in Connecticut put it, "to quit strangling the goose that can lay those golden eggs."[37]

The doctors received a partial wake-up call in 1971, when consumer advocate Ralph Nader, in partnership with physician Sidney Wolfe, created the Health Research Group, which put rising health care costs squarely in the crosshairs.[38] Their initial goals were to reverse the state anti-substitution laws that restricted generic use in the marketplace and to get rid of the detail men, whom they saw as being largely responsible for the tripling of per capita US prescription rates since 1950.[39]

But in testimony before Congress, Nader also made it clear to physicians that their open-ended support of the pharmaceutical industry came at their own peril. He appealed to their almost priestly image of themselves, pointing out the irony that doctors were "fighting all attempts to encroach on their professionalism, and yet, in prescribing drugs, they take the words of highly articulate, persuasive pitchmen called detail men, who have nothing . . . beyond the mission of maximizing sales for the company. In other words, here you have professional people relying on rank amateurs to advise them as to what drugs to prescribe for what ailments. If it was not so absurd, one could almost describe the process as having tens of thousands of physicians belonging to a 'Drug of the Month Club.'"[40]

Still, physicians remained relatively content and oblivious to the way their world was about to be turned upside down. In 1973, only 15 percent of doctors surveyed said they might forgo a career in medicine if they had to choose again. By 1981, that number would exceed 50 percent.[37] Between those two dates, cost containment became the number one issue in health care, the rates for malpractice insurance soared, and corporate benefits managers were coming up with new "managed care" strategies, including the health maintenance organization (HMO), to curtail the cost of doctors and hospitals.

In 1975, energized by Nader's dramatic testimony before the Senate, with public opinion coalescing, and with corporations increasingly concerned about health care costs, Senator Kennedy sponsored the Drug Utilization Improvement Act.[41] Among other provisions, it proposed a National Center for Clinical Pharmacology "to improve the education of each member of the health care team." The new body, as proposed, would control the creation and dispersal of new drug information and "prohibit the giving of any gift product, premium, prize or other thing of value to a physician or pharmacist by the drug companies." The bill failed in 1977 and again in 1978 as a result of solid opposition from the pharmaceutical manufacturers and the AMA, which feared government intervention would lead to socialized medicine, price controls, and a loss of professional autonomy.[42]

Lou Lasagna's CSDD had now been connecting leaders in medicine, industry, academia, and government for nearly a decade, with a special emphasis on managing health policy outcomes. He had been propagating his view of the medical world, its major trends, and his vision of what was possible through a series of negotiated compromises and changes with his corporate clients. The facts were clear. The country was in a stubborn recession, the cost of innovation was way too high, a gold mine of government science patents derived from NIH grants were locked away and inaccessible for private exploration, and the cost of health care was increasing at an alarming rate with insurers and employers in full revolt. But as a brilliant strategist, Lasagna could see a number of these issues breaking his way. The stubborn recession combined with the escalating cost of employer-based health benefits was beginning to fuel the demand for innovative solutions. Lasagna was skilled at converting concern about cost into demands for efficiency and for less regulation of industry. And he already had the right messaging in hand.

The phrase "drug lag" had first appeared in a 1973 paper written by Lasagna's colleague Dr. William Wardell, a University of Rochester pharmacologist, who found that Britain had approved four times the number of new drugs approved by the United States during the previous decade.[43] Not only that, but for individual drugs, Britain beat the US to the market, on average, by two years. This competitive disadvantage in medicines played poorly in the midst of a countrywide recession, and the drug industry made the most of the findings, blaming its lack of "new medical miracles" on government inefficiency. Conquering the drug lag became Lasagna's rallying cry with FDA reform still a decade away.

The focus on cost had also received an unexpected boost in 1974 from a little-appreciated add-on to a pension bill. A one-hour NBC prime-time documentary in 1972 titled *Pensions: The Broken Promise* told the scandalous story of unprotected workers at the automaker Studebaker in South Bend, Indiana, who had lost everything when the company went belly-up.[44] The resultant pension reform bill, titled the Employment Retirement and Security Income Act, or ERISA, remedied the situation.

A small provision in the bill, Section 514—the ERISA preemption—allowed employers who decided to fund their own employee health plans, rather than outsource the funding to insurance companies, to be shielded from any employee lawsuits connected to the company plans. The bill was signed by President Gerald Ford eight days after President Nixon's resignation. This seemingly insignificant fragment of legislation started a wave of employer conversions to self-funded health plans. Within 30 years, 89 percent of employers with 5,000 or more workers would self-insure their employees. The practical impact was a new focus by business leaders on the cost of health care.[45]

During this same time period, the growth of CVS emboldened the American Pharmacists Association to push for its pharmacists to be seen as "bona fide members of the health care team," and to renew the battle to eliminate the state anti-substitution laws that had tied the hands of state licensed pharmacists for decades.[46] By February 1977, New Jersey approved generic substitution.[47] Pharmacists could now substitute a less expensive copy for the prescribed brand-name drug unless specifically directed not to by a physician. Within two years, 40 states had adopted similar laws.[48] The CSDD followed these changes and realized that CVS, which in 1994 would launch one of the first pharmacy benefit management (PBM) firms, was fast evolving into a data management company. It promised greater quality at lower cost, and would soon change the MIC balance of power. CVS was already cross-linking doctors, hospitals, and insurers, and had a long lead in the creation of electronic medical records, plus a national network of retail outlets that would reach 10,000 in a few decades.

Lasagna and the CSDD were also tracking the issue of intellectual property. Ever since the birth of the NIH, there had been a prohibition against private ownership of patents that had emerged from research supported by federal grant dollars.[49] As the thinking went, discoveries supported by public dollars were a public trust and should benefit the public at large, not private individuals. The downside of such idealism was that private investors shied away from trying to commercialize intellectual property that they couldn't own and control. As a result, by 1978, a backlog of 28,000 scientific patents for federally funded discoveries sat in government vaults, largely unused and undeveloped. At a time when the economy was still lagging, fewer than 5 percent of these innovations had been commercialized.[50]

Indiana's Purdue University was one of many institutions sitting on new health-related discoveries that had been supported by NIH grants. In the face of the country's "economic doldrums," the university decided to hire some lobbyists to try to gain control of its NIH-grant-supported patents and their future profitability. They approached Senator Birch Bayh (D-IN) and were delighted by his enthusiastic response.[51]

At about this time, Senator Bob Dole (R-KS) was exploring the same legislative territory, and Purdue encouraged the two senators to fashion a bipartisan bill to liberalize patent restrictions, not only as a way of eliminating "bureaucratic regulatory waste" but also as a means of stimulating moribund local economies within their two states. The technology-transfer legislation swept through the Senate Judiciary Committee with unanimous support, and passed the Senate in a 91–4 vote on April 23, 1980.[51]

While the House and Senate negotiated the final version of the bill, the 1980 elections showed Democratic president Jimmy Carter to the door, along with 12 Democratic senators, including Bayh. Even so, after considerable horse trading, the bill was unanimously approved and sent to the White House. Lame-duck Carter dragged his feet, but on December 12, 1980, he signed the bill.[52]

In 1980, such soon-to-be biotech behemoths as Biogen and Genentech were still obscure start-ups launching a shift away from "small chemical" therapies to "large biologic" cures. The change in patent law that resulted from the Bayh-Dole Act helped spur the rise of genetic engineering and the biotech industry as a whole.[53] While 380 patents were granted to health care institutions in 1980, by 2009 that number had soared to 3,088.[51] Those patents, now under the control of individual scientists and the universities where they worked, could be licensed to corporations for the codevelopment of a range of products and applications.

The CSDD and other organizations carefully tracked the economic benefits of the bill. According to one estimate, the resultant impact on the nation's gross domestic product reached $47 billion in 1996 and soared to $187 billion a decade later.[51] In three decades, 4,000 new companies appeared, giving rise to a vibrant new sector of the American economy. The act created thousands of new jobs and the complete reshaping of such academic-industrial tech capitals as San Francisco and CSDD's hometown, Boston.[51,54]

A less visible measure of the Bayh-Dole Act's impact is the fact that all major research universities today have a formal office of technology management to oversee issues related to intellectual property. In 1979, their trade association, the Association of University Technology Managers, had 113 members nationwide.[54] By the dawn of the new millennium, that number had swelled to 2,178.[55]

But as we saw in the case of Jesse Gelsinger's death during that University of Pennsylvania clinical trial, there has been a downside as well to this bonanza for academic health systems, their physicians, and the Medical Industrial Complex. In 2005, the *Economist* published "Bayhing for Blood or Doling Out Cash?"[56] Reviewing the impact of the legislation and the moral crisis that has followed, the article stated: "Many scientists, economists and lawyers believe the act distorts the mission of universities, diverting them from the pursuit of basic knowledge, which is freely disseminated, to a focused search for results that have practical and industrial purposes. Whether that is a bad thing is a matter of debate. What is not in dispute is that it makes American academic institutions behave more like businesses than neutral arbiters of truth. . . . Researchers (and particularly their minders in university patent-licensing offices) are increasingly reluctant to share materials and knowledge with others unless such sharing is accompanied by legal agreements about 'reach-through' royalties on potential findings and the right to restrict publication of results."

For Lou Lasagna, access to government patents was helpful, but it would have had limited economic impact unless the drug lag he had helped identify was addressed through legislative reform. As luck would have it, Carter's successor, President Ronald Reagan, had identified the dismantling of government regulations as one of the major principles of his trickle-down economic theory designed to address a stubborn recession.

The battle between research pharmaceutical companies and their generic competitors was now decades old. The research companies relied on patents to compensate them for their costly investment in the risky process of discovery. Patents, a form of intellectual property, are exclusive rights granted by the government for a specific period of time in exchange for detailed public disclosure of an invention. As a result of the 1962 Kefauver-Harris Amendment, the FDA required research companies to submit a new drug application to begin the approval process of a new discovery. The patent clock began to tick the day the file was submitted. To unravel what he perceived as overregulation of government-funded science, President Reagan had established an Office of Technology Assessment in 1981, and the office shone a critical light on the fact that it took an average of 7 to 10 years to develop and launch a new medicine.[57] Studies supported by the CSDD noted that most of the patent protection provided to companies, an average of 14 years at the time, was being eaten away during the time the therapy was still seeking FDA approval. Recouping an investment, let alone showing profitability, was problematic.[58] These studies further argued that current incentives were not adequate to drive investment in drugs that sold in smaller quantities, because they were designed to treat rare conditions called "orphan diseases." The final grievance was that generic companies had an unfair advantage in that they could simply copy the hard work of research companies and provide cheap products without any front-end investment in discovery.

During this period, Senator Kennedy remained focused on pharmaceutical prices and the range of tactics used by brand-name manufacturers to slow down and suppress the use of generic drugs. Where others saw an impasse, Lou Lasagna saw the makings of a compromise and shared profit for all. Until now, the forces of change for policy on generics at the federal level had been beaten back not just by claims of quality deficiency, but also by accusations that the proponents of change were intruding on the sacred territory of the patient-physician relationship. However, that resistance rapidly melted away once the possibility of patent extensions was dangled in front of the major pharmaceutical companies and their new academic medical-center partners. By the time the compromise reached a vote, the negotiations had been going on for more than two years.

In the summer of 1984, Representative Henry Waxman (D-CA) and Senator Orrin Hatch (R-UT) worked out a compromise.[59] Generic manufacturers would be allowed to bring their products to market without having to repeat expensive tests that had already been conducted by the originating company. All they had to do was to demonstrate "biologic equivalency," meaning that their pill delivered the same biologic blood levels on absorption as the parent compound. This streamlining of process ensured that the new generics, available when the brand-name parent went off patent, should theoretically be far less expensive to produce than their predecessors.

In return for this concession, brand-name pharmaceutical companies were granted an additional 5 years of patent protection, as well as additional patent time based on regulatory delay. The net effect was to expand the patent-protection time on average for new drug discoveries to approximately 20 years.

The compromise benefited both sides, and very rapidly prescriptions for generics exceeded scripts for brand-name drugs.[59] Before Hatch-Waxman, fewer than 15 percent of prescriptions were filled by generics. Today that number approaches 90 percent. As for pricing, consumers initially benefited by reductions averaging close to 80 percent off the original brand drug's price.[60,61] But in recent years, generic prices have skyrocketed, driven by speculators and unscrupulous companies that have skirted the law.

In 2015, the prices of more than 60 drugs doubled.[62] Public outrage was triggered by the brash hedge fund manager and owner of generic manufacturer Turing Pharmaceuticals, Martin Shkreli, who had purchased a 62-year-old generic antiparasitic drug and bumped its price up from $18 to $750 overnight, and with no apology.[63] When he called a CBS reporter a "moron" on September 22, 2015, the Pharmaceutical Research and Manufacturers of America (PhRMA) was quick to tweet, "@TuringPharma does not represent the values of @PhRMA member companies." A year later, Shkreli was sentenced to seven years in prison for conspiracy and securities fraud.[64]

Slightly less outrageous brand-name manufacturers, believing that 20 years wasn't quite enough payback time, developed a variety of delay tactics to protect or extend aging patents, including making minor revisions in a drug's chemical structure or mode of action or administration, or colluding with Native American tribes, while also paying off generic producers not to proceed with plans to offer lower-priced copies.

In the early years that followed passage of the Hatch-Waxman Act, the pharmaceutical industry remained ultra-focused on the patent issue. During the Reagan administration, all members of the MIC worked more cooperatively among themselves in a domestic environment that celebrated innovation and profitability and detested what they viewed as overregulation and high taxation. But what Lou Lasagna recognized at the CSSD, and at the multinational pharmaceutical companies he served, was that patents for his multinational clients were a global issue that affected long-term growth. Many emerging economies had no patent laws, and others had laws that were laughably enforced. Brazil and India were notorious for brazen pharmaceutical pirating—creating copies of a branded product atom for atom, and mimicking the physical pill they were copying and its packaging so accurately that it became nearly impossible to distinguish counterfeits from real products. Patent-protecting countries like the US were an easy mark. Their investigative and enforcement efforts were weak and ineffectual, and the companies' registrations were often incomplete; for example, they might choose to protect the process of creating the product but not the product itself, rendering the patent meaningless.[65]

Without protections for intellectual property, global expansion was out of the picture. For drug company CEOs, this meant that lobbying, which had already morphed into "governmental affairs," needed to expand its reach around the world. In the 1980s Pfizer was a CSDD client and its CEO, Ed Pratt, an admirer of Lou Lasagna, was ideally positioned to lead the global charge for intellectual property (IP) protections. Pratt was chairman of the powerful US Business Roundtable and also the formal adviser to Reagan's US trade representative, Bill Brock.[66] Pratt's first move was to form a task force on intellectual property with his chief ally, IBM CEO John Opel. Their recommendation to Brock that a position be created within the Office of the US Trade Representative for a director of international investment and intellectual property sailed through.[67,68]

The challenge remained in linking intellectual property protections to ongoing multilateral-trade negotiations that currently involved 123 nations. This was a leap, because trade agreements normally helped prevent monopolies, while intellectual property protections were viewed by many nations as supporting monopolistic companies. Rather than fight the battle head-on, Pratt and his followers finessed the whole discussion by advocating for the creation of a collection of regulatory policies to prohibit product piracy, under the title Trade-Related Aspects of Intellectual Property (TRIPS), which would become an add-on to the multilateral general trade negotiations.[67]

At the helm of this sophisticated public affairs assault, Pratt placed Constantine "Lou" Clemente, a young lawyer with IP expertise, who was appointed chairman of the new Intellectual Property Committee (IPC) of the powerful US Council on Business. This provided a platform for the next step in organizing a global effort. In 1983, Pratt and Opel approached the leaders of 10 other large US-based multinationals, including General Electric, General Motors, DuPont, Johnson & Johnson, and Monsanto, requesting their participation on the Intellectual Property Committee and creating a united front across industries.[67,68,69]

Trade representative Brock knew that they would not carry the day with a US-centric campaign, and he made it clear that the support of Europe and Japan was a must. With the IPC in the lead, Clemente helped orchestrate the support for TRIPS by the European Employers Association and the Japanese Federation of Economic Organizations, which carried with it the endorsement of corporations like Toyota, Mitsubishi, Nissan, and Sony. At the same time, IPC let the involved governmental bodies know that unless TRIPS was included it would work to scuttle the entire 123-nation multilateral trade agreement that had taken more than a decade to negotiate.[66,67,68,69]

At Bill Brock's request, Pratt, leaning heavily on Clemente, worked tirelessly to build a multisector global coalition of major corporations to engage the United Nations and World Trade Organization. Domestically, he worked with the chambers of commerce, business councils, business committees, and trade associations. Pfizer executives, who occupied key positions in strategic business organizations, were directed to engage with their cross-sector colleagues and gather the support of leaders in manufacturing, entertainment, technology, and consumer goods for the attachment of TRIPS intellectual property protections to the new trade agreement. As one analyst recounted, "With every such enrollment, the business power behind the case for such an approach became harder and harder for governments to resist."[68]

During Reagan's first term as president, and with the input of Lasagna and the CSDD, the term "piracy" became popularized and connected to American ideas that were being stolen by greedy foreign nations, denying companies like Pfizer and IBM their "rightful rewards." The messaging was reinforced by generous underwriting of well-funded think tanks across the political spectrum, from the American Enterprise Institute to the Brookings Institution. Pfizer supported a comprehensive public affairs strategy with press releases, speeches, white papers, conferences, op-eds, and special briefings, all reflecting the CSDD's own views and designed to strengthen the connection between free trade and intellectual property.[69]

It took more than a decade to accomplish the goal, but when the eighth round of the General Agreement on Tariff and Trade was signed in 1994, it had 123 signatories, and established the World Trade Organization with intellectual property protections for multinational corporations.[70] During the years when the battle was engaged, Pfizer developed resources in government relations, investor relations, media relations, public affairs, and shareholder relations that would facilitate the same kind of coordinated, global-strategy support for its product line of ever-emerging blockbuster drugs.

In this way, the battles of the 1970s and 1980s, supported by a new brand of MIC cross-sector leaders like Lou Lasagna, helped solidify the pervasive structure of the Medical Industrial Complex that exists today. The dismantling of regulatory checks and balances to speed drug approval, the release of government patents, the formation of academic health system/industry centers of innovation, the negotiation of an MIC truce on generics and the extension of patent life for brand-name corporations, the accommodation of new pharmacy corporations like CVS and its pharmacy benefit manager subsidiaries, and the forging of global agreements on intellectual property protections—all had given the MIC unparalleled clout. The MIC policy wars supported by the CSDD had been waged in a deliberate fashion over decades, not merely months or years. Leaders were battle-hardened and well funded. And the forces in opposition, led by politicians like Ted Kennedy and social warriors like Ralph Nader, routinely underestimated the Medical Industrial Complex's determination and strength.

The MIC was now equal parts politics and science. At Pfizer, Pratt and his successor as CEO, Bill Steere, moved Lou Clemente from his corporate counsel position and reassigned him as executive vice president of a new department, Corporate Affairs, reporting directly to the chief executive. At his disposal was the same sophisticated and integrated public affairs machinery he had directed in the global IP fight. In his new post, Clemente would drive the success of Viagra, soon to be Pfizer's most famous product, and engineer the successful hostile takeover of Warner-Lambert in 2000, a move that delivered Lipitor, Pfizer's most profitable product ever, to its doorstep. I would be his final major hire.

Chapter 10

Strange Bedfellows:
Health Care, Politics,
and the Christian Right

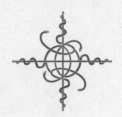

In the immediate aftermath of World War II, Canada to our north, and
Germany and Japan under the American-taxpayer-funded Marshall
Plan, carefully developed and budgeted national health care systems.
These structured approaches not only defined other nations' priorities
but also reinforced the integrity and ethical boundaries of these systems.

In choosing to fight disease through individual enterprise, rather
than to promote the nation's health as a matter of public policy, the
United States invited aggressive partnering and profit seeking, as well as
an endless stream of supporters and beneficiaries promoting unhealthful agendas. As the tobacco industry well illustrated, those seeking the
support of physicians or their associated health care institutions became
part of the Kevlar fabric of the MIC, which helps explain the durability
of our health care system's many failings.

The politics of health care in the United States involve strange bedfellows and often lead to unintended consequences, but no matter how
tangled the lines, one might hope that the debates would stay within the
boundaries of scientific fact and genuine concern for the well-being of

all Americans. The potential threats of the tobacco industry or climate-change deniers or the beverage companies funding research to dissociate sugar from rising obesity rates are easy to recognize. Yet religious institutions have intruded into health care for many decades under the radar. More insidiously, they have pursued distinctly unhealthful objectives like maintaining racial segregation in hospitals, severely limiting women's health services, placing embargoes on promising medical research, tolerating the forced separation of illegal immigrant mothers from their babies, and promoting health policies that actively discriminated against poor and vulnerable citizens.

Politicians now routinely justify their core beliefs about health care issues based on religious orthodoxy, while the religious coalitions that helped place them in office demand allegiance with all the subtlety of the National Rifle Association.

The case of Representative Tom Price of Georgia, the devoutly Presbyterian orthopedic surgeon who was President Trump's first, very short-lived secretary of the Department of Health and Human Services, is a striking example of just how far religious ideology, conveniently aligned with economic and/or political self-interest, can distort the health care mission.

In his rhetoric, Tom Price emphasized the noble cause of making our health care system "more responsive and affordable to meet the needs of America's patients and those who care for them."[1] Yet when he was a congressman, patients' needs did not appear to be high on his list of priorities. For example, he supported expanding private insurers' control over Medicare, converting federal support of Medicaid programs into "block grants" that would no longer require states to provide a basic medical benefit package, allowing hospitals to turn away Medicaid and Medicare patients seeking nonemergency care if they could not afford co-payments, permitting doctors to bill Medicare patients for amounts above those covered within the agreed-upon fee schedule, and allowing doctors to negotiate with insurance carriers en masse without violating antitrust statutes. Price also ignored public health priorities when he opposed regulating tobacco as a drug; expanding mental health services; funding global programs to prevent malaria, AIDS, and tuberculosis; financing stem cell research; expanding funding of the State Children's Health Insurance Program (S-CHIP) and the National Institutes of Health; and expanding insurance coverage within the Affordable Care Act.

Yet this was the man chosen to head the federal department overseeing the programs that provide health care for roughly half of all Americans. More shockingly, Price was heartily endorsed by both the American Medical Association[2] and the Association of American Medical Colleges[3] as one of their own, which is to say, as a reliable advocate for their narrow economic interests.

Price was undone not by his extreme policy positions—grounded, he said, in a conservative, Christian worldview—but because of his penchant for wasting $341,000 worth of taxpayer money on private jets.[4,5] However, he was only the most visible fundamentalist with peculiar ideas about how to translate the message of Christ ("Inasmuch as ye have done it unto one of the least of these my brethren, ye have done it unto me") into health care policy.

Modern-day politicians go to great lengths to signal their appreciation to their religious backers through health policy messaging and appointments. Valerie Huber, the woman President Trump appointed to be chief of staff for the Office of the Assistant Secretary for Health at HHS, a position with direct influence over policy affecting HIV/AIDS, women's health, and adolescents' health, had been head of the National Abstinence Education Association.[6] For assistant secretary of public affairs in HHS, Trump appointed Charmaine Yoest, former president of Americans United for Life, where her focus was on restricting access to abortion state by state. (Along the way, she labeled transgender people "crazy.")[7] With the encouragement of these two women, the Trump administration abruptly eliminated the final two years of funding for the Teen Pregnancy Prevention Program, ignoring the fact that this comprehensive federal effort, which provides $89 million a year to 81 organizations, had helped drive teen birthrates down significantly.[8]

The encroachment of "faith based" health policy in the US has a long history. Since the beginning of the 20th century, the Catholic Church has been waging a pitched battle against "artificial contraception," which it views as not only interfering with God's plan but also challenging priestly authority. Birth-controllers were lumped with "adulterers, fornicators, prostitutes, drunkards, Mass Skippers" who had given way to "madness of the senses."[9] In the immediate post-WWII period, faced with a cascade of worldly returning soldiers and hormonal science pointing toward a future contraceptive pill, the Church borrowed tactics employed at the time by the tobacco industry to undermine science. Its Madison Avenue–styled Cana Conferences for couples about to be married relied on Catholic physicians to hard-sell a unique brand of medical quackery in the form of the "rhythm method" of contraception, which unreliably predicted those days each month when a woman was fertile on the theory that by avoiding intercourse on those days couples could avoid pregnancy as well.[10]

The physicians' value in selling "natural" birth control as instructors in the program was laid out without apology in the 1957 *Basic Cana Manual*.[10] The Catholic training manual drew its title from the New Testament account (John 2:1–11) of the wedding at Cana where Jesus changes water to wine. In the updated version, it was the doctor, not Jesus, who performed the miracles. On page 94 the manual states, "The doctor's role is to add his authority, personal and professional, to the teachings of the Church. Speaking with warmth and concern, and yet with a degree of clinical detachment, he can properly take up some areas that priests or laymen can avoid. His prestige, though often overrated, can be used to advantage."

The issues of birth control and women's health not only defined the boundaries of priestly authority; they were the fundamental differentiating features separating Catholic hospitals from their competitors. These Catholic institutions, which today make up more than 12 percent of US hospitals, prohibited instruction in the use of contraceptives and procedures like vasectomies and tubal ligations. Most important, they outlawed the performance of abortions and aggressively campaigned against the legalization of the procedure and have remained in the lead in attempts to overturn *Roe v. Wade*, which legalized abortions in the US in 1973. Once run by nuns "in the service of God," these hospitals are predominantly under secular management these days, with their boards tightly supervised by Catholic bishops.[11]

Evangelical Christians, for their part, came late to the struggle against legalized abortion. As recently as 1968, the membership of the Christian Medical Society refused to endorse a proclamation that labeled abortion as sinful.[12] In 1971, America's leading conservative religious organization, the Southern Baptist Convention, went on record as encouraging its members "to work for legislation that would allow the possibility of abortion under such conditions as rape, incest, clear evidence of severe fetal deformity, and carefully ascertained evidence of the likelihood of damage to the emotional, mental, and physical health of the mother." In 1973, both the Southern Baptist Convention and the Christian Medical Society chose not to actively oppose the Supreme Court ruling known as *Roe v. Wade*, against a Texas law prohibiting abortion, and they reaffirmed that position in 1974 and 1976.[12]

The Southern Baptist Convention's views on abortion were part of its long-standing support for the separation of church and state, and Baptist medical communities largely opposed the idea of churches and their pastors wading into delicate health care issues.[12] After all, the basics of *Roe v. Wade* were reasonable. As most doctors saw it, what possible good could come from putting politicians in the middle of such complicated, emotion-ridden, and highly personal patient-physician decisions?

In addition, abortion was an issue long associated with "the other team," namely Roman Catholics.[12] To take up abortion as a moral (and political) issue would require cooperation with the very group that Protestantism had long ago risen up in protest against.

But in 1970, a Nixon-era journalist named Paul Michael Weyrich arrived on the political scene.[13] A staffer at the *Milwaukee Sentinel* who served as a weekend anchor at the local ABC affiliate WISN-TV, Weyrich went on to serve as press secretary to Colorado senator Gordon Allott. From there it was a short walk to the offices of conservative beer mogul Joseph Coors, who was funding the creation of a new right-wing think tank called the Heritage Foundation. Weyrich became its first director, and he summed up his mission this way: "The New Right is looking for issues that people care about. Social issues, at the present, fit the bill."[14]

This new "Christian" movement, however, espoused conservative politics first, social issues second, and fundamentalist religious fervor a distant third. What was truly best in terms of health in the early days of the movement was not even part of the discussion.

The 1960s and early 1970s had been socially disruptive, creating a firm sentiment in certain circles for the need to "stand up for God and country," with both defined in staunchly conservative terms. An event that helped the movement coalesce took place in 1977 in Dade County, Florida. At issue was a county ordinance that banned discrimination based on sexual orientation, which Anita Bryant—former Miss Oklahoma, former recording star, and a devout Christian—tried in vain to defeat.[15] Undaunted, Bryant and other social conservatives began collecting signatures to demand a referendum.[16] Lending a hand was a Christian broadcaster named Jerry Falwell, who would ultimately take credit for the record-breaking Dade County turnout that approved the antigay referendum in June 1977 by a margin of more than two to one.[17] Campaigns in other states to reverse gay rights ordinances soon followed, with operatives faithfully gathering names and addresses that would be instrumental in creating an effective conservative Christian political movement. In 1978, change was in the air. For the first time, pro-life candidates took both Senate seats in Wisconsin, and a pro-life Senate candidate in Iowa, who was expected to be badly defeated, won his seat after pro-life advocates leafleted churches, branding his opponent as pro-abortion, the weekend before the election.

Falwell's battle cry was, "Number one, get people converted to Christ; number two, get them baptized; number three, get them registered to vote."[15] But not until 1979 did he decide to focus on abortion as the ultimate wedge issue. Feeling the political winds at his back, Falwell suddenly declared, "The Roman Catholic Church for many years has stood virtually alone against abortion. I think it's an indictment against the rest of us that we've allowed them to stand alone."[18]

Aligned with him in newfound antagonism to this health care service for women was Pat Robertson, who had inherited his conservative bona fides from his father, A. Willis Robertson, a senator from Virginia; and his religious zeal from his mother, Gladys.[19] While enrolled in law school, he impregnated his future wife, a Catholic nursing student named Dede Elmer, who was six and a half months along when they married on August 27, 1954.[20] In 1955, he failed the New York bar exam, a failure which caused him to contemplate suicide. Instead, he followed his mother's recommendation and was "born again."[21]

A managerial job with an electronics firm followed, and during this stint he became obsessed with the Bible, announcing his plan to temporarily abandon his young family to attend a protracted summer religious retreat in Canada in 1956. At this point, as reported in the *New York Times*, his wife tried to reason with him, saying, "I'm a nurse. I recognize schizoid tendencies when I see them, and I think you're sick."[22]

Robertson went to Canada anyway, and on his return, he enrolled in the Biblical Seminary of New York. There he immersed himself in all things evangelical, speaking in tongues, exorcising demons, selling household possessions, and moving his family to the Bedford-Stuyvesant section of Brooklyn to serve the people.[22]

In 1959, he moved again, to Portsmouth, Virginia, where, according to his own account, "the Lord" led him to a bankrupt UHF TV station, then helped him arrive at the purchase price for the facility: $37,000.[23] He bought the station and changed the call letters to WYAH for the Hebrew "Yahweh," which set the tone for the broadcasts that would follow.[24] In its first two years of broadcasting, it was failing financially, unable to attract sponsorship. But in 1962, Robertson announced a special telethon broadcast and appealed to his audience to be among 700 viewers who would donate $10 per month to support his television mission. The appeal was successful, and the program was renamed *The 700 Club*, which by 1966 had grown into a two-hour nightly Christian variety show. By 1976, the year that President Ford went up against a Baptist peanut farmer from Georgia, Pat Robertson and his new Christian Broadcasting Network, supported by state-of-the-art direct-mail solicitations, were going all out on mixing religion, politics, and entertainment.

That November, 55 percent of Baptists voted for Jimmy Carter, a gain of 22 percent on the previous Democratic presidential nominee.[25] But the new activist breed of fundamentalists like Robertson didn't appreciate Carter's belief in what they called the "archaic Baptist tradition of a wall of separation between church and state." Carter made no effort to pack his cabinet with evangelicals, and Billy Graham never even got the call to come and pray in the Oval Office. Moreover, while Carter didn't like abortion, he refused to support a constitutional amendment to override *Roe v. Wade*, and he didn't think homosexuals threatened the moral fabric of America. He also got along with Catholics.[14,25]

For those and other reasons, operatives like Weyrich, Falwell, and Robertson listened intently to then candidate Ronald Reagan in the summer of 1980 address the Christian Coalition's annual policy meeting and say, "I know you can't endorse me, but I want you to know that I endorse you and what you are doing." This new Moral Majority got "their man" (a divorced, completely secular product of Hollywood and corporate America) into the White House. Whereas 61 percent of conservative Christians had voted in the 1972 presidential election, 66 percent voted in both 1976 and 1980, and they voted overwhelmingly Republican.[26] That was enough for Jerry Falwell to confidently claim that the Moral Majority had elected Jimmy Carter and, when Carter had displeased them, replaced him with Ronald Reagan.

But another three years would pass before the real tidal wave of evangelicals in politics would hit, and the seismic force that created the wave was the financial survival of Christian nonprofit schools that promoted racial purity. In 1983, the Supreme Court ruled that Bob Jones University, often called "the buckle on the Bible Belt," could not receive federal funds so long as it continued to discriminate on the basis of race.[12] The university's namesake and founder had been an early-20th-century evangelist with such Bible-pounding zeal that he was said to have at least once shattered a pulpit. What really engaged his fervor, though, was the trend of children raised in the church going off to college and losing their faith. So in 1927, shortly after the Scopes "monkey" trial, in which William Jennings Bryan defended the "literal truth" of the Bible against Clarence Darrow's defense of Darwin and science, Jones founded the institution of higher learning that bears his name.[27]

Twenty years on, he bequeathed to Bob Jones Jr., his son, the Greenville, South Carolina, school, which, until 1971, would continue to exclude black students.[28] When at last it relented under federal pressure, it still required that black students be married to attend the school. After 1975, it opened the door to single blacks as well, but still prohibited interracial marriage and dating. This relative "enlightenment" was still not enough for the IRS, which on January 19, 1976, rescinded the university's tax-exempt status for failure to comply with federal civil rights regulations.[29]

In the hands of Paul Weyrich, this dispute over taxes and compliance with laws banning racial and gender discrimination became not only a David-versus-Goliath battle but a direct attack on Christian teachings. The Supreme Court ruled against Bob Jones and its racial policies on May 24, 1983.[29] By then, lily-white "Christian academies" had proliferated throughout the former Confederacy, and all of them now felt threatened. Their health curricula were already infused with abstinence-only values education and bans on contraceptive information. The merger of health and education conservative priorities gave Weyrich confidence that he now had an explosive and powerful force that could rally the Southern electorate and ensure Reagan's success.[30]

Within this highly charged environment, Ronald Reagan, the newly elected president and former AMA crusader against Medicare, faced the customary decision of whom to nominate to become the "nation's doctor." In considering his options, Reagan leaned heavily on the powerful conservative senator Jesse Helms (R-NC) for his pick for surgeon general. Senator Helms's nominee, one intended to express gratitude to the Christian Coalition, which had helped elect Reagan, was C. Everett Koop, the born-again doctor who had labored long and hard to save the lives of children with a range of congenital deformities, a career focus that for him did not rest comfortably with the reality of legalized abortion. He had expressed his thoughts on this and related issues of medical ethics in a 1976 book called *The Right to Live, the Right to Die.*[31] In his view, the nation risked moving inexorably from abortion to infanticide to the destruction of children who were merely inconvenient or socially embarrassing.[32] He developed a five-part film series called *Whatever Happened to the Human Race?* which contained an image of dolls splayed out on the beaches of the Dead Sea to illustrate the human carnage of *Roe v. Wade*'s "abortion on demand."[33] In the early months of 1979, he took the show on the road, signaling to doctors and their organizations that it was acceptable, even necessary for Christian physicians, to oppose *Roe v. Wade.*[34]

Carl Anderson, a Catholic aide to Senator Helms, had informally approached Koop about making a play to become surgeon general well before the 1980 election. When Reagan won, conservatives fell in line to support Koop, but the American Public Health Association (APHA) came out in full-throated opposition—something it hadn't done in 100 years.[35] The American Medical Association, which saw Koop as unpredictable, was already on record as supporting the University of Texas vice chancellor of health affairs Edward Brandt Jr.

But these slaps in the face were nothing compared with the *New York Times*' assessment. On April 9, 1981, the lead editorial declared, "Dr. Unqualified."[36] The editorial acknowledged in the first line that Koop had a "fine reputation as a pediatric surgeon" but found him "not deserving" of the role of surgeon general. The charge that he had no "significant experience in the field of public health" was no surprise, especially given that the APHA had torched him. But the editorial struck a deeper vein in declaring that his "attractiveness to the Administration must lie elsewhere." Addressing the implication, the editors observed, "That 'elsewhere' may be his anti-abortion crusade. Two years ago he toured 20 cities with a film whose message was that abortion led inexorably to euthanasia for the elderly. And he has described amniocentesis, a procedure used to detect congenital disorders like Down's syndrome and Tay-Sachs disease in fetuses, as 'a search-and destroy mission.'"

In January 1981 former Pennsylvania governor Richard Schweiker was appointed secretary of Health and Human Services, the department then responsible for appointing the surgeon general. Schweiker then decided to split the difference between the AMA and Senator Helms, and made Brandt the assistant secretary of HHS and nominated Koop for surgeon general. To shore up the candidate while the Senate deliberated, Schweiker put Koop on the payroll as an assistant to Brandt.[37] The months dragged on, and Koop, encouraged by Schweiker to stay under the radar, focused on establishing as many relationships as possible.[38]

Coincidentally, Koop took a number of positions that caused legislators on both sides of the aisle to question their assumptions. Most notably, his opposition to the Reagan administration's promotion of baby formula over breastfeeding in the developing world angered baby food manufacturers. Then in October, while testifying before Congress, he stated clearly, "It is not my intent to use any government post as a pulpit for theology."[39] Apparently, Koop's Christian conservative backers thought this was nothing more than the "tell 'em what they want to hear" customary for job seekers in Washington. But for Democratic leaders like Henry Waxman and Ted Kennedy, it was enough to soften their opposition. In November, the Senate confirmed him with a vote of 68–24, and on January 21, 1982, more than a year after the battle had been engaged, C. Everett Koop was sworn in as the 13th surgeon general of the United States.[40]

Koop's focus at the time was on the nation's chronic disease burden, especially cardiovascular disease and cancer, which had been fed by the postwar explosion of tobacco use. One month after his swearing-in, he appeared on a panel to release what had become rather routine by then—another surgeon general report on smoking.[41] But when Koop rose to deliver what all thought would be brief, inconsequential remarks, he wasted no time before attacking the Tobacco Institute for lies and deceit in daring to suggest that there was anything less than overwhelming evidence that tobacco caused cancer. The *New York Times* report that day led with Koop's saying, "Cigarette smoking is clearly identified as the chief preventable cause of death in our society."[42]

In his candor, Koop offended many of the business leaders who were part of the Southern conservative cabal. Not least among these was his old patron Senator Jesse Helms, from the Big Tobacco state of North

Carolina, who had been so thrilled with Koop's original nomination that he had called President Reagan to thank him personally.

But now RJ Reynolds CEO Edward Horrigan complained in a letter to Reagan about Koop's "increasingly shrill preachments."[43] Cigarette consumption in the US was already in free fall, and by 1987, 40 states would have laws banning lighting up in public places; 33 states had bans in public transportation; and 17 already had eliminated smoking in the workplace.[44]

Undaunted, Koop kept pressing to see how far he could push the industry. In public speeches and in testimony before Congress, he railed against the industry's advertising approaches, its marketing to children, its bogus research operation, and its unwillingness to come clean on nicotine addiction. He said its product was more addictive than heroin, then called its leadership "morally corrupt." He informed the public about the dangers of secondhand smoke, smoking while pregnant, and smoking in public places, including hospitals. He was relentlessly provocative, and he used tobacco to field-test his approach to hands-on public health campaigning. Everything from public schools to medical groups to women's associations to civic enterprises wanted him to come and speak. Beginning in late 1982, he would arrive in full regalia as a vice admiral in the US Public Health Service, ribbons and epaulets against a backdrop of navy blue. His aide, also in uniform, always carried along for distribution a bag of buttons that read, "The Surgeon General personally asked me to quit smoking."[45]

Koop's campaign readiness was well timed, because a new health crisis, first recognized one year earlier, was rapidly gaining momentum. The disease would soon pit conservative Christian biases squarely against medical necessity—as well as against common sense. Dr. Michael Gottlieb and Dr. Joel Weisman, infectious disease experts whose patients included many members of the gay population in Los Angeles, had first raised the alarm after noting five cases of *Pneumocystis carinii* pneumonia associated with a strange immune deficiency disorder in California men. Inside the Centers for Disease Control, a debate ensued about how best to keep physicians and the public informed without offending the gay population or inflaming homophobes.[44]

On June 5, 1981, the CDC issued its first account in the *Morbidity and Mortality Weekly Report* but posted it on page 2, with no mention of homosexuality in the title. The header read simply: "Pneumocystis pneumonia—Los Angeles."[46] But the editorial note at the bottom of the entry issued a clear warning: "*Pneumocystis* pneumonia in the United States is almost exclusively limited to severely immunosuppressed patients. The occurrence of pneumocystosis in these 5 previously healthy individuals without a clinically apparent underlying immunodeficiency is unusual. The fact that these patients were all homosexuals suggests an association between some aspect of a homosexual lifestyle or disease acquired through sexual contact and *Pneumocystis* pneumonia in this population."

On April 13, 1982, three months into the new surgeon general's tenure, Senator Henry Waxman held the first congressional hearings on the implications of this new disease. The CDC testified that very likely tens of thousands were already infected. On September 24, 1982, the condition was for the first time identified as acquired immune deficiency syndrome, or AIDS.[47]

As surgeon general, Koop had been successful in his first months on the job in raising the esprit de corps of the 5,600-person Public Health Corps, who were now required to wear uniforms to enhance their visibility and ideally contribute to the long-term funding viability of the institution.[48] But in the most pressing public health challenge of the day, HIV/AIDS, the Public Health Corps was absent. Edward Brandt and his boss, the new HHS secretary Margaret Heckler, closely attended by Reagan's domestic policy adviser and "family values" enforcer Gary Bauer, had given themselves the duty of addressing all questions on the topic while making it explicitly off-limits to the outspoken C. Everett Koop.[49]

Not surprisingly, the situation deteriorated rapidly. Heckler at one point suggested that AIDS was Reagan's "number one priority," even though the president had never uttered the term "HIV" or "AIDS" in public.[50] She also told the public—in 1984—to expect a curative vaccine within two years.[51] When Brandt tried to align with the increasingly vocal and activist gay community that was pressing for increased funding for research and treatments for the disease, and then agreed to attend their fund-raising event, conservatives made such a fuss about it that Heckler forced him to back down.[52] Soon after, Brandt resigned. Everyone felt the heat, including the CDC, which, after being accused by conservatives of promoting sodomy, removed funding for AIDS education.[53]

As more and more people died—not only gays but recipients of blood transfusions, intravenous drug users, newborns of infected mothers, and a surprising number of Haitians—Reagan's silence became deafening.

Inside his administration, Reagan empowered people like Secretary of Education Bill Bennett, who discouraged providing AIDS information in schools, and Bauer, whom Koop later described as his "nemesis," saying that Bauer "believed that anybody who had AIDS ought to die with it. That was God's punishment for them."[54] Even William F. Buckley, the voice of a more genteel, old-school conservatism, suggested in a *New York Times* article that HIV-positive gay men have their disease status forcibly tattooed on their buttocks.[55]

By October 1986, when Reagan first uttered the term "AIDS,"[56] more than 16,000 Americans had died. Jerry Falwell had declared the disease "the wrath of God upon homosexuals." Former Nixon speechwriter and conservative firebrand Pat Buchanan cruelly labeled the disease "nature's revenge on gay men."[54]

On April 10, 1987, with a federal budget calling for an 11 percent cut in AIDS spending from the prior year, actress Elizabeth Taylor had had enough. She went beyond Washington game-playing and gained access to political power based on Hollywood star power and a long-standing friendship.[57] She invited Ronald and Nancy Reagan to a dinner given by the American Foundation for AIDS Research.[58] The Reagans accepted, and on the evening of May 31, 1987, with 21,000 Americans dead and 36,000 more living with a diagnosis of HIV/AIDS, Reagan delivered his first major address on the topic—six years late.[47]

His prior behavior, unlike that of his Christian Right supporters, could not be blamed on ignorance or lack of exposure. Nor is it possible to say that his bias against gays was in any way "principled." In fact, he had defeated Jimmy Carter in 1980 with active gay support, especially in

California, where he himself had actively opposed Jerry Falwell and Anita Bryant when they had attempted to pass an antigay measure in 1978.[54]

Until this time, C. Everett Koop, the self-proclaimed "nation's doctor," had been forced by President Reagan to stand by idly and watch the epidemic explode.[59] From 1983 to 1985, he had been excluded from the Executive Task Force on AIDS established by his own boss, then HHS assistant secretary Edward Brandt. Now Brandt was gone, and Heckler, who had been burned twice by controversy, was more than willing to push the increasingly popular Koop out front. As the numbers of the dead and infected rapidly rose, the public was becoming more and more fearful. Since a test had been developed to detect the virus in blood, politicians, and some hospitals and physicians, were calling for testing to become mandatory in the interest of protecting health care workers.[57] This followed heavily publicized cases of death from HIV-tainted blood and fears that the entire US blood supply might be at risk.

On December 17, 1984, a 14-year-old hemophiliac from Kokomo, Indiana, named Ryan White had undergone a partial lung removal for severe consolidated pneumonia, after which he was diagnosed with HIV/AIDS.[60] He had been infected while receiving an infusion of a blood derivative, factor VIII. When he was cleared to return to school, 50 teachers and more than a third of the parents of students from his school signed a petition asking that his attendance be barred. After the state's health commissioner and the *New England Journal of Medicine* confirmed that Ryan White's disease could not be spread by casual contact, he was readmitted in April 1985.[61]

Koop clearly understood that continued inaction on his part would be unacceptable. He went far and wide collecting data without exposing his own bias. He interviewed AIDS activists, representatives from medical and hospital associations, Christian fundamentalists, and politicians from both sides of the aisle, but he held his cards close to his chest, and few knew exactly what he thought or planned.

In the fall of 1986, Koop carefully walked the administration through a draft statement tailored for approval, but to make it more difficult for his detractors to organize a blocking effort, he collected all print copies as participants left the room.

On October 22, the report was officially released, and it was, at least to conservative Christian tastes, shockingly explicit.[58] The surgeon general challenged parents and schools to discuss AIDS, and urged the public schools to offer sex education and to promote the use of condoms for prevention. The report drew immediate criticism from conservatives, but this was nothing compared with the furor that arose 19 months later.

After releasing the report, Koop hired the public relations firm Ogilvy and Mather to make certain he had the messaging, language, and imaging right. He then procured funding from private sources and from various branches of government to support the mass mailing (107 million copies, enough to fill 38 boxcars) of an eight-page pamphlet to every household in America. The huge print run required government printing presses to operate 24 hours a day for several weeks.[58]

Understanding AIDS was frank and factual, covering anal and vaginal intercourse, injectable drug transmission, and the proper use of condoms. The pamphlet promoted sex education beginning in elementary school and challenged the current messaging of the televangelists with this comment: "Who you are has nothing to do with whether you are in danger of being infected with the AIDS virus. What matters is what you do."[58]

When the pamphlets began to arrive in America's mailboxes, the phones in the Senate offices of conservatives like Jesse Helms started to ring. Falwell and Robertson were apoplectic, but there was no going back. The surgeon general's mailing was a fait accompli.

The medical community applauded loudly, as did the press and the majority of the public. When Koop's original patrons and their captive senators went after him, he responded, "I'm the nation's doctor, not the nation's chaplain."[58] The mountains of hate mail he received seemed merely to embolden him.

But then President Reagan was replaced on January 20, 1989, by another Republican beholden to the Christian Right, George H.W. Bush, who fired the embattled surgeon general. The vulnerable AIDS community had lost an unlikely champion, but as has occurred repeatedly within the Medical Industrial Complex, no public health crisis is so grim that it can't redound to someone's economic benefit—that someone being, more often than not, the major pharmaceutical companies.

To cash in on the AIDS crisis, Big Pharma had joined hands in 1988 with an unlikely partner, an AIDS activist group that had come together under the banner ACT UP (AIDS Coalition to Unleash Power).[51] ACT UP members were largely HIV-positive and were tired of being given the cold shoulder by government health officials in Washington. They decided that if they were going to die, they would go down fighting, by making in-your-face assaults on the individuals and institutions they felt had neglected the issue, a list that by 1989 included President Bush, Vice President Dan Quayle, the NIH, and the FDA.[52]

ACT UP consciously followed the tactics of the women's rights movement, the civil rights movement, and the antiwar movement.[51] At protests, the activists were well armed with press kits and a broad understanding of the FDA, its policies, and the range of issues that compromised the advancement of desperately needed cures. Scientists were making progress in understanding the viral disease, and in the early testing of a number of antiviral therapies that might be lifesaving. But activists believed that fast-track approval of these new therapies was being held up by excessive regulations and red tape. The pharmaceutical industry couldn't have agreed more. In assisting the AIDS activists in their fight for survival, it saw the potential to trigger legislation that would speed up drug approval overall and remove what it viewed as excessive FDA regulatory bottlenecks.

On October 11, 1988, at the end of a Columbus Day weekend of protests, including a march on the Health and Human Services offices in Washington, DC, 1,500 AIDS activists descended on the FDA campus, in a demonstration that drew broad national media coverage and led to 180 arrests. The activists gathered under a banner that read "Seize Control of the FDA," and their elaborate outfits and placards delivered a simple message: "You are either with us or against us." The wording that made it to the front pages of the nation's newspapers the next day was a bit more dramatic: "We recognize every AIDS death as an act of racist, sexist and homophobic violence." Also, "The government has blood on its hands. One AIDS death every half hour."[47,62]

ACT UP's list of demands was clear and focused:

1. Drugs must receive quicker approvals, with patients receiving access to any new discovery as soon as basic safety and toxicity studies had cleared phase I.
2. No placebos or double-blind studies should be used. Using them with this deadly disease is unethical.
3. Studies must include a diverse population of patients including young and old, male and female, and all races and sexual orientations.
4. The experimental drugs must be covered by Medicaid and private insurers.
5. The FDA must support community outreach and involve those with AIDS directly in the process.

According to ACT UP, the Department of Health and Human Services vacillated between being uninformed and being ineffectual. And all the while, people were dying. Nearly 83,000 by now had been infected and 46,000 were dead, 3 percent under the age of 18.[63] The only drug available was AZT, approved in 1987, but its developer, Burroughs Wellcome, had set the price at an unaffordable $10,000 a year, then under pressure reduced it to a still staggering $6,400.[64] Other experimental treatments were being studied, but they were locked up in an approval process that leaders of the pharmaceutical manufacturers had always viewed as antiquated and cumbersome.[65]

The response to the "Seize Control of the FDA" demonstration was almost immediate. Tony Fauci, director of the National Institute of Allergy and Infectious Diseases at the NIH, who in June 1988 had been described by ACT UP leader Larry Kramer as an "incompetent idiot," arranged meetings with leaders of the group to discuss their objectives.[66] Fauci was well respected within government and had been instrumental in directing NIH resources to investigators searching for a cure for AIDS. After meeting with Kramer in June 1989, Fauci endorsed a parallel track at the FDA for HIV drug approval.[66] This alternative approach would eliminate some of the regulatory steps to create a faster pathway for approval. The FDA was not thrilled with Fauci's going "off the reservation," but it still approved ACT UP's proposal for a fast-track process to make new AIDS treatments available immediately after they cleared phase I studies.[67] This helped to bring a second AIDS drug, dideoxyinosine, on line.[68]

Before leaving office, President Reagan had already approved the creation of the National Committee to Review Current Procedures for Approval of New Drugs for Cancer and AIDS. The task force included the top AIDS scientists and FDA and NIH staff, as well as leading HIV activists. Chairing the influential advisory committee, under both Reagan and Bush, was Big Pharma's friend, clinical pharmacology pioneer and head of the CSDD, Louis Lasagna, who had been favoring a streamlined approach to drug approval for more than a decade.[69]

When the committee released its final report on August 1, 1990, it pointed the nation toward a broader set of FDA reforms that, not surprisingly, would also achieve one of Big Pharma's most eagerly sought goals. The industry had been laying the groundwork for this moment for 30 years, connecting with a wide range of loyal academic researchers through a complex and nontransparent support system that included fellowships, lectureships, ghost journal articles, expert advisory boards, and other inducements.[70] Now, on the back of the HIV/AIDS crisis, and with support of AIDS activists, who had effectively neutralized Ralph Nader and other critics, the drug industry had achieved victory with its defensible argument that fewer regulatory hurdles and more flexibility would lead to more discoveries more quickly, and to more lives saved.

With each budget proposal since 1985, the Reagan and Bush administrations had promoted the idea of funding FDA service improvements by collecting user fees from pharmaceutical companies seeking new drug approvals.[71] In that same year, the Pharmaceutical Manufacturers Association, which had been staunchly opposed, had for the first time signaled that it might go along if the fees were tied to concrete performance goals.

The FDA itself was losing its resolve. Since thalidomide and the heroic stand of Frances Kelsey, the agency had become much more cautious about approval. But its caution had been blamed by Lou Lasagna and others for the drug lag, and now, by extension, was being blamed for the deaths of thousands of Americans from cancer and AIDS.

The new PMA president, Gerald Mossinghoff, had come from the Government Patent Office, where user fees were a part of everyday life.[72] He was quickly able to convince pharmaceutical CEOs that user fees tied to faster drug approval would actually save money. He also worked closely with FDA commissioner David Kessler, who had taken top FDA managers over to the Patent Office to learn how to structure such a user fee program.

At this point, even Ted Kennedy's objections, based on legitimate concerns that the agency might become captive to industry, dissolved in the face of heavy lobbying by AIDS activists and others. In the years ahead, Kennedy would point to 1989 as the year when his "provisions expanded home and community care of victims, made for easier access to experimental drugs, and created a new national commission to establish AIDS policy."[73,74]

A year later, Kennedy would team up with Senator Orrin Hatch and successfully pass the "groundbreaking Ryan White Comprehensive AIDS Resources Emergency Act, which created the single largest federal program for people with HIV/AIDS in the US."[74]

What emerged in 1991 was a plan to cover roughly 25 percent of the FDA's annual budget needs through three sets of fees.[73] If the fees were paid only at the time of each new drug submission, the FDA would be unable to budget effectively. So to even out cash flow, two other types of fees were included in the scheme: these would be paid by every company, whether or not it submitted a new drug application. One was an annual fee charged for each product currently on the market. The other would be attached to each manufacturing facility managed by each company. Each of the three types of fees would cover roughly one-third of the total industry contribution, in return for which the FDA agreed to a series of efficiency standards designed to speed up the decision-making process.

For the FDA, this meant a new culture of openness, collaboration, and transparency, with a management structure that was completely redesigned, simplified, and flattened. But most important, the FDA process would now be computerized.[73] One FDA director reflected years later that before the bill was passed, he had 66 staff members and two Wang computers. With the new financial support and management overall, desktop computers arrived, and specialized typists disappeared, leaving some to claim that credit for the elimination of the drug lag and the boost in productivity should go to the agency's sudden technological leap forward.[72] Over the next decade, new drug launches in the US would more than triple.[73]

The only casualty of the innovation may have been George H.W. Bush. He had won the White House in 1988 based on his dramatic proclamation: "Read my lips: no new taxes."[75] However, faced with a stubborn recession, Bush had increased the maximum individual income tax rate from 28 percent to 31 percent. Payroll and excise taxes had been increased as well, and allowances for itemized deductions had been decreased. Then on October 29, 1992, several days before the presidential election, Bush quietly signed the Prescription Drug User Fee Act (PDUFA), mandating user fees as law. It did not go unnoticed. Apparently one man's user fee was another man's tax, and in the eyes of conservatives, he had once again violated his "no new taxes" pledge and would be made to pay the price.[72]

President Bush's firing of Dr. Koop further emboldened the Christian Right. In choosing to be "the nation's doctor" and not "the nation's chaplain," Koop had sided with science over religion and thus committed an offense that his detractors would never forget. Today, it remains the dividing line for their support. In 2000, President George Bush, in his tortured ban on stem cell research, tacitly approved a scientific lie to maintain his conservative base.[76] A decade after Bush's departure, we are held hostage by many of the same voters and a Trump administration that lumps together global warming, sexual abuse, gun violence, discouragement of the breastfeeding of infants, and immigrant families' forced separations as "fake news."

Our health system rewards profit, not care. Its ever-growing MIC syndicate, reinforced by innocent-appearing collaborators and deeply infiltrated by special interests, shows no signs of backing down in its endless quest for profits. Yet its overreach is becoming obvious, and it appears to be loosening its grip on a public that now supports universal health care by a wide margin and is increasingly realizing that the creation of a real health care system will require that we actually care enough to start anew.

Chapter 11

Nigeria, CROs, and Research Biases

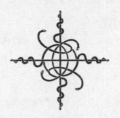

One major impact of World War II on the Medical Industrial Complex should have been a moral reckoning. In sorting through the legacy of Hitler's regime in Germany, one of the series of tribunals in Nuremberg delved into egregious examples of medical criminality, including Nazi experimentation on human subjects. Of 23 defendants, 7 were hanged, 7 acquitted, and the rest given sentences of from 10 years to life in prison.[1]

In making these judgments, the tribunal offered directives leaving no doubt that medical experimentation in humans could be justified only within certain well-defined boundaries:[2]

1. The voluntary consent of the human subject is absolutely essential. . . .
2. The experiment should be such as to yield fruitful results for the good of society. . . .
3. The experiment should be so designed and based on the results of animal experimentation. . . .
4. The experiment should be so conducted as to avoid all unnecessary physical and mental suffering and injury. . . .

5. No experiment should be conducted when there is an a priori reason to believe that death or disabling injury will occur. . . .

6. The degree of risk to be taken should never exceed that determined by the humanitarian importance of the problem to be solved by the experiment. . . .

7. Proper preparations should be made and adequate facilities provided to protect the experimental subject against even remote possibilities of injury, disability, or death. . . .

8. The experiment should be conducted only by scientifically qualified persons. . . .

9. During the course of the experiment the human subject should be at liberty to bring the experiment to an end. . . .

10. During the course of the experiment the scientist in charge must be prepared to terminate the experiment at any stage, if he . . . believes the experiment is likely to result in injury, disability, or death to the experimental subject.

This assessment was made by a worldwide Allied tribunal conducted under the direction of US judges and prosecutors and fully compliant with US standards of criminal procedure. Yet another 25 years would pass before any of the 10 agreed-upon standards were cited and recognized in a US court.[2]

Legal scholars such as Michelle Miller at Cornell Law School attribute this lapse to the self-regarding biases of leaders within the Medical Industrial Complex. As Jay Katz, a physician and professor of law at Yale, wrote in 1992 of the Nuremberg directives, "It was a good code for barbarians, but an unnecessary code for ordinary physician-scientists." In other words, it was assumed that American medicine's noble professionalism was adequate to ensure appropriate ethical standards. In fact, only after the war did the AMA fashion guidelines for the conduct of medical research.[2]

But the most significant influence on the direction of medical research in the post-WWII period was money. Over a short two decades, funding of medical research, flowing primarily through the federal government, exploded. Advances by 1950 to a total expenditure of $161 million seemed significant, but they were nothing compared with the $2.3 billion in federal funding that existed by 1968.[3] By then, financial incentives had solidified a deep and enduring bond forged by medical research leaders who traveled unimpeded from government to academia to corporate offices and back again as part of the ever-growing medical aristocracy.

A notable example is heart surgeon Michael DeBakey, who helped develop the mobile army surgical hospital (MASH) during the war, went on to develop the standard research systems for Veterans Administration hospitals, then became a prominent professor at Baylor College of Medicine.[4] At the same time, he chaired Mary Lasker's foundation while also serving a three-year stint on the National Advisory Heart and Lung Council of the NIH—and maintaining a close friendship with Arthur Sackler while serving as a close adviser for Sackler's advertorial magazine the *Medical Tribune*.

As we have seen, advances in regulatory oversight of health care in the United States have been hard fought. For the FDA, milestones occurred in 1906, 1938, and 1960, but only after the needless sacrifice of American children. In those years, legislators struggled to add protective labeling, demand testing for the safety and efficacy of products, and rein in false advertising and promotion. But at the same time, the government promoted easing access to government-funded patents and collaboration between MIC partners that used to provide checks and balances against each other's unethical practices.

In medical schools and academic hospitals a great deal of discussion about ethics has centered on clinical research since the Massengill tragedy in 1937, followed by the 1938 Food, Drug, and Cosmetic Act, which demanded safety data for drug approval, while also demanding presubmission of a company's research plans before it could proceed with human experimentation. But in reality, the pharmaceutical industry and its academic research partners within the MIC have often adjusted to the new regulations by skirting the boundaries of accepted ethical behavior or manipulating research findings to suit their needs.

Probably the lowest point in US medicine was discovered in 1964, when a young physician from Detroit, Irwin Schatz, came across an article in a medical journal titled "The Tuskegee Study of Untreated Syphilis: 30 Years of Observation."[5] Incredulous, he shot off a letter to the editor: "I am utterly astounded by the fact that physicians allow patients with a potentially fatal disease to remain untreated when effective therapy is available." The study he was referring to had begun in 1932 and, for experimental purposes, allowed the withholding of treatment from African American men with syphilis. When penicillin became standard therapy for the disease in 1947, it was deliberately withheld from the 399 African American patients in the study. It was later revealed that Dr. Schatz's message was read by Anne R. Yobs, one of the US Public Health Service employees who designed the Tuskegee Study, and who wrote to her superior, "This is the first letter of this type we have received. I do not plan to answer this letter."

Even with this first red flag, the study continued for another seven years.

On June 16, 1966, the *New England Journal of Medicine* published an article titled "Ethics and Clinical Research."[6] Written by a highly respected Harvard physician, Henry K. Beecher, the head of anesthesiology at Massachusetts General Hospital, the article referred to "troubling charges" that had grown out of "troubling practices" at "leading medical schools, university hospitals, private hospitals, governmental military departments (the Army, the Navy and the Air Force), governmental institutes (the National Institutes of Health), Veterans Administration hospitals and industry.

"Since World War II," Beecher continued, "the annual expenditure for research . . . in the Massachusetts General Hospital has increased a remarkable 17-fold. At the National Institutes of Health, the increase has been a gigantic 624-fold. This 'national' rate of increase is over 36 times that of the Massachusetts General Hospital. . . . Taking into account the sound and increasing emphasis of recent years that experimentation in man must precede general application of new procedures in therapy, plus the great sums of money available, there is reason to fear that these requirements and these resources may be greater than the supply of responsible investigators. All this heightens the problems under discussion. . . . Medical schools and university hospitals are increasingly dominated by investigators. Every young man knows that he will never be promoted to a tenure post, to a professorship in a major medical school, unless he has proved himself as an investigator. If the ready availability of money for conducting research is added to this fact, one can see how great the pressures are on ambitious young physicians."[6]

Beecher then reviewed 50 distinct contemporary American clinical studies with ethical violations judged by standards at Beecher's own Massachusetts General Hospital. These studies were performed in 1964 by academic clinicians in major institutions and published in peer-reviewed journals. In only 2 of the 50 was there any evidence of informed consent by the participants. In one of these studies, 109 servicemen with streptococcus infection—known to lead to rheumatic fever—had treatment with penicillin withheld because they were part of a placebo control group. In another study, 408 "charity patients" with typhoid were split into two groups. One group was given chloramphenicol, known to be effective against typhoid, while the other group received no treatment. Mortality rates in the two groups were 8 percent and 23 percent, respectively.

In yet another study, 50 patients, ages 13 to 39 and drawn from mental institutions and juvenile delinquency facilities, were given an experimental drug, TriA, known to cause liver damage. Significant liver dysfunction occurred in 54 percent of them, and 8 underwent invasive liver biopsies. Even worse, 31 patients were anesthetized and given carbon dioxide through their breathing tubes to create toxic levels that would lead to cardiac arrhythmias, including deadly ventricular fibrillation. Almost incredibly, 68 patients had their abdominal cavities entered through small incisions. Various organs were then retracted or pushed with instruments to gauge the effects on blood pressure levels. Mentally defective children were purposefully given live hepatitis virus to assess the infectiveness of the agent. Live cancer cells were injected into 22 human subjects to test immunity to cancer. A mother of a child dying from metastatic melanoma agreed to have the child's melanoma cells injected into her to gain understanding of the disease and possibly help the child. The child died the next day, and the mother died a year and a half later—of metastatic melanoma.[6] This is one of the two cases in which consent was documented.

Six years after Beecher's publication, Peter Buxtan, an epidemiologist for the US Public Health Service, finally and officially blew the whistle on the study of African American men being denied treatment. This led to a July 26, 1972, *New York Times* report titled "Syphilis Victims in U.S. Study Went Untreated for 40 Years."[7] Buxtan later said, "I didn't want to believe it. This was the Public Health Service. We didn't do things like that."[8]

But in fact, the US Public Health Service very much did things like that. And at long last, the grotesque breach of ethics was revealed.

This most grievous episode in the history of American medical research began in 1932, when the US Public Health Service, operating in Macon County, Alabama, home of Tuskegee University, launched a study of 399 African American men with syphilis, as well as 201 uninfected men who would serve as control subjects in the experiment. The goal of the study was eventually to gauge the effectiveness of antibiotic treatment and define the dosage and extent of treatment required to cure the disease. But when supplies of penicillin became limited, the researchers decided to provide selected infected men with placebos, and told them they were being treated with penicillin when in fact they were not. Local physicians participating in the study were asked to similarly withhold treatment for these patients, even after adequate supplies of penicillin later became available. After Irwin Schatz first raised the issue, the AMA still endorsed continuation of the study. Not until 1972, when the glare of publicity reached what was known as the "Tuskegee Experiment," was the study finally shut down. It led to a $10 million out-of-court settlement to cover the lifetime health needs and burial expenses of participants.[9]

Tuskegee also led to the 1974 National Research Act, which finally incorporated some of the protections recommended at Nuremberg. Voluntary consent was now required for all participants in US medical research funded by federal dollars. A study's design had to be reviewed and preapproved on ethical grounds by an institutional review board, a body of local professionals who would critique each proposed study and attest that it met ethical standards. Finally, the act established the National Commission for the Protection of Human Subjects of Biomedical Research, which was charged with identifying "the basic ethical principles which should underlie the conduct of biomedical and behavioral research involving human subjects."[2]

Even so, the official apology for the violations of the Nuremberg Code (also known as crimes against humanity) at Tuskegee would have to wait another quarter century, when President Bill Clinton at last acknowledged, "The United States government did something that was wrong— deeply, profoundly, morally wrong."[10]

But perhaps the most troubling legacy of this dark chapter was detailed in a 2016 assessment by the National Bureau of Economic Research. This report showed that the egregious breach of ethics in Macon County, publicized in 1972, created such a distrust of doctors and of the medical system on the part of African American men over age 45 nationwide that the Tuskegee Experiment alone, along with the subsequent avoidance of care it caused, accounted for a 1.5-year decline in life expectancy in these men in 1980.[11]

New standards imposed by the National Research Act of 1974 ensured that studies had institutional review board approval and were preceded by informed consent from patients who had not been coerced and had a full understanding of the risks of the investigation. But this left plenty of room for the pharmaceutical industry to explore new avenues of unethical conduct involving the growing avalanche of electronic— and often suspect—data. Drug companies fund most of the US-based research—in 2013 it was 90 percent—and they require that academic researchers grant ownership and final say on publication to the companies. The companies provide additional funding to many of the authors through consultant fees, speakers' bureaus, and advisory boards.[12]

In 2007, researchers at the University of California, San Francisco, examined 192 studies of statins used to lower cholesterol and found that positive results were 20 times more likely if the study had been sponsored by the parent company than if the study had been independently conducted.[12,13] In the case of statins, the same physician "thought leaders" who run academic cardiology departments and serve on governmental advisory boards that define the range of normal for cholesterol levels are often listed as primary investigators and advisory board members for companies that produce the cholesterol-lowering drugs. For example, in 2013, when the American Heart Association and the American College of Cardiology published more stringent levels of blood cholesterol, pushing more people into the "danger zone" and thus vastly expanding the number of patients requiring drugs, they failed to highlight that 12 of the 25 expert cardiac physicians on the advisory board who published their recommendations in the journal *Circulation* were on the payrolls of pharmaceutical companies that produce cholesterol-lowering medicines.[14]

Similar patterns of selectively publishing only positive results, and authors with conflicts of interests aggressively recommending drug therapy, also appeared in a 2010 review of over 500 clinical trials. Industry-funded studies were positive 85 percent of the time compared with positive results in only 50 percent of the government-funded studies.[15]

Studies that were never published are equally revealing. Also in 2008, a group of researchers from Oregon Health Sciences University and Harvard decided to explore a collection of studies registered with the FDA seeking approval for new antidepressants between 1987 and 2004—74 studies in all that included 12,500 patients. Thirty-eight had positive results. Thirty-six had negative results. All but one of the positive studies was published in full, yet only three negative studies were published in full and unbiased form. Of the remaining 33 negative studies, the 11 that were published were structured to convey a positive outcome, and the remaining 22 were never submitted for publication.[16]

Bottom line: The American system of research is rife with unethical conduct and financial conflict of interest. All too often, the physician thought leaders who direct academic medical departments are the same individuals who staff government drug review panels, and the researchers who conduct studies receive checks from the very companies whose potential products they are reviewing.

*   *   *

Increasingly, studies funded by US multinational companies do not involve US citizens and are often performed with less stringent oversight. Again, in 2008, there were more than 9,000 clinical research studies with over 2 million human subjects from 115 countries around the world, and here "ethical lapses" can all too quickly descend into outright criminality, as defined by the Nuremberg tribunal.[17]

One such extraterritorial study is believed by some to have served as the basis for John Le Carré's book (and the subsequent film) *The Constant Gardener*.[18] In a clinical trial conducted by Pfizer in Nigeria in April 1996, the ethical lapses ranged from deceptive and fraudulent recruitment to experimentation on children who were in no position to grant their consent.

Nigeria is a country of 356,000 square miles, separated into 36 states, one of which is Kano.[19] Except for brief episodes, the central African nation had been under military dictatorship since declaring its independence from the United Kingdom in 1960. Civil war erupted in 1967, and over the next three years, warfare, combined with disease, hunger, and starvation, claimed up to 3 million lives.[20]

In the early 1970s, the oil industry brought Nigeria into membership in OPEC, but the wealth never trickled very far beyond an inner circle of military leaders. The country had 170 million or so inhabitants, with Christian dominance in the south and central portions, and Muslim dominance in the north and southwest. On its way to becoming the largest economy in Africa, Nigeria was defined by corruption, deprivation, and human suffering.[21]

One cause of suffering was meningococcus bacteria carried through the air in the dry, dusty season and known to cause acute swelling of the brain. Outbreaks have been recorded every 3 to 10 years dating back to the late 1880s. People who survived exposure benefited from naturally acquired immunity, but that protection kept the immune system activated and alert to this infection for only three years.[22] After that, absent vaccination, individuals were once again vulnerable to reinfection.

Vaccines for the three variants of meningitis were developed and were rushed into service at the first sign of a problem. But chaos and corruption are not ideal partners for a mass public health undertaking. In the early 1990s, 13 million Nigerians were vaccinated, with the help of relief organizations such as the World Health Organization (WHO), UNICEF, Médecins Sans Frontières (MSF; Doctors without Borders), and the International Red Cross. Up to 85 percent of those affected by the disease were below the age of 20 and most were treated with chloramphenicol, which had been available since 1949. It was effective, but its use had been greatly restricted because of its tendency to suppress the bone marrow production of blood cells, a consequence that could be especially severe and deadly in 1 out of every 24,000 cases.[23]

In 1995, the overall antibiotic market was $11 billion strong. In Pfizer's central research facility in Groton, Connecticut, infectious disease expert Scott Hopkins had been working on a range of clinical trials that, in less than two years, would support the approval and release of an über-antibiotic called Trovan. Approved already for 11 different indications, it would briefly threaten the dominance of Bayer's blockbuster antibiotic Cipro (ciprofloxacin).[24]

Trovan was strong, but some doctors were concerned that it was too powerful. It took a scorched-earth approach to killing microbes—the ultimate broad-spectrum antibiotic—and Pfizer's strategy was to recommend it for as broad a swath of conditions as possible, including some that affected children and some that were rare (at least in developed countries), such as meningitis. Whether driven by missionary zeal or entrepreneurial passion, Dr. Hopkins saw opportunity in the out-of-control epidemic in Nigeria. Trovan could save lives, Pfizer reasoned, and at the same time, data supporting Trovan's use in children could be gathered quickly and included in the portfolio soon to be presented to the FDA. Moreover, in just a few short weeks, the company could complete a clinical study that would take years in the US, if it would ever be approved at all.[24]

Pfizer gave the green light and used its contacts, including company managers in Nigeria, to clear the path for a study involving children who were often gravely ill, undernourished, and highly vulnerable. Most of their parents were illiterate, which made their consent for their child's participation dubious. Rules for engagement, including standard protections for human research subjects and procedures for governmental approval of the experiment, were not codified, and graft and corruption greased every palm on the way to approval. In short, one could hardly have chosen a set of conditions more ripe for ethical catastrophe.

Scott Hopkins and five other Pfizer researchers arrived in Kano, Nigeria, on April 2, 1996, aboard a chartered DC-9 packed with medical equipment. They were armed with a research plan, and their destination was the Infectious Disease Hospital, a series of one-story cinder-block buildings with metal roofs. They claimed to have authorization for this "philanthropic mission," and for the study, but the quality and legitimacy of the clinical-study authorization would be contested in court for the next decade. What is clear and beyond dispute is that the group was made to feel uncomfortable by volunteers from Médecins Sans Frontières, who were already at the hospital vaccinating citizens and treating the ill with the standard chloramphenicol, which was approved by the WHO.[25]

Hopkins and the others found a public health response that was breaking down. As the hospital director later said, "In March, when things were at their worst, each patient had four or five visitors looking after them. It was so crowded that you couldn't walk through the wards."[24] According to one WHO official, "Things were made worse by the fact that the disease broke out in a great number of places all at once, spreading resources thin. There has not been enough vaccine to go around, and medical personnel have really been badly taxed." The deputy director of MSF summed it up with this: "The meningitis epidemic of 1996 is by far the worst that Sub-Saharan Africa has ever seen. The death toll just keeps going up, and it is pretty certain that the official figures underestimate the size of the problem."[26]

One Pfizer physician, Juan Walterspiel, formerly an infectious disease physician at Yale, believed the company would live to regret its decision to wade into this minefield. He sent a letter to Pfizer CEO Bill Steere, asserting that the study was in violation of ethical rules for the conduct of medical experiments in humans. Some of the children were in critical condition, and their undernourishment meant that oral absorption would be highly unpredictable. "At least one died after a single oral dose," he wrote. "Such a patient . . . should never have received an experimental antibiotic orally."[24]

Walterspiel was fired the day after his letter arrived. Some months later, he was compensated with a favorable ruling in a wrongful-termination suit, but how much he received was shrouded in the nondisclosure provisions of the settlement.[24]

Later, as part of a lawsuit filed against Pfizer by the Nigerian government, depositions disclosed that the validity of the documents Hopkins carried authorizing the study were challenged by local officials at the hospital. A local ethics committee's approval, provided months later to the FDA as part of a package for approval of Trovan for pediatric use, would prove to be a backdated and fraudulent document for which the company would be forced to offer a public apology. Strained relations between Pfizer clinicians and MSF physicians were in part responsible for the Pfizer team's decision to move their center of operation soon after their arrival into a separate building next door, where they could do their job without ongoing criticism.[24,25,27]

The study itself lasted only two weeks and involved 200 children aged 3 months to 18 years. All had clinical meningitis, confirmed by blood tests and spinal taps. The 200 were selected from thousands of children arriving during that time with their parents or guardians. Some parents and guardians, at least, were unclear that the children were being entered into a clinical study sponsored by the pharmaceutical industry. Others clearly thought the effort was part of the MSF-run medical relief program. Pfizer later testified that illiterate parents gave permission through local, multilingual nurses who explained the study in detail, clarified the patients' rights, and crossed all t's and dotted all ethical i's. But quite a few parents didn't remember it that way. Several parents of dead children claimed that they were never shown or read a consent form, were not informed of the risks of the study, and were not informed that an MSF treatment center was right next door.[24]

As for the study design, the 200 randomly selected children were split into two groups. One hundred received a full daily weight-adjusted dose of Trovan, orally if possible, or by injection if necessary. The other

100 received a third-generation cephalosporin antibiotic, Rocephin, produced by Hoffman–La Roche. The full-dose injection of Rocephin was delivered the first day, but only a one-third dose was used on subsequent days. Pfizer lawyers later contended that this was an on-site decision made by one of the Pfizer team who had helped develop the drug at Hoffman–La Roche. Allegedly, this team member knew that the painful, prolonged injection was more than effective against meningitis at one-third the amount.[24] In the years that followed, clinical studies would actually prove this to be true, confirming that the amount of Rocephin that was used was more than adequate to kill the meningitis bacteria.[28] But at the time, there was no proof of this. And a panel of Nigerian medical experts wasted no time in broadcasting that the use of a comparator at suboptimal dosing was an "old trick" designed to make your new offering look good by comparison.[24,29,30]

Other variables were challenged and answered by litigants years later, but the raw facts were that the experiment left 5 of the 100 Trovan-treated children dead, while 6 of the 100 Rocephin-treated children died. Likely both regimens saved lives, but other children never fully recovered. Whether this was as a result of their drug treatment or the disease itself is up for debate. What is incontestable is that dozens of the study participants suffered paralysis, deafness, blindness, and a range of other disabilities.[24,28]

For the first 10 years of the suit, Pfizer did nothing, and all three copies of the official Nigerian report of the case somehow disappeared. Clearly the government was outmatched by a multinational company with near-unlimited financial and legal resources. Then, in May 2006, a copy of the original Nigerian report suddenly appeared on the doorsteps of the *Washington Post*, which reported that the local government in its original investigation had determined that "Pfizer violated Nigerian and international law in the experiment."[30]

In July 2007, two months before I resigned from Pfizer, the company posted the "Summary Trovan, Kano State Civil Case—Statement of Defense" on its website.[28] It stated in part, "Pfizer contends that there was no regulation or law in Nigeria requiring ethical committee approval before conducting a clinical trial or investigative study. Therefore, there was no need to obtain what the law did not require. In addition, there was no formal ethics committee sitting at either Kano's IDH [Infectious Disease Hospital] or at the nearby Bayero Teaching Hospital. There were, however, numerous other forms of approval by local physicians and government officials authorizing the study to go forward including, but not limited to, the head of the IDH and Dr. Idris Mohammed. At no time was patient care compromised in any way."

After more than a decade of exhausting litigation, in 2009 Nigeria agreed to a settlement. Compensation came in the form of a no-fault settlement in which Pfizer offered up $75 million. Of this, $10 million was delivered to Nigeria's Kano State as reimbursement for the legal expenses the government had incurred in support of its injured citizens. Another $30 million went to health care activities considered worthy of funding by the local government. And $35 million was provided to those participants in the study who were injured or to relatives of the dead. That put an end to the legal battle in which Nigeria's government lawyer, Babatunde Irukera, had originally requested $9 billion in damages and that 31 criminal counts be brought against Bill Steere and nine other company employees.[29]

In a final bizarre twist forecasting tactics used in the 2016 election, the WikiLeaks release of US State Department cables in 2010 documented a conversation between Pfizer's Nigerian country manager, Enrico Liggeri, and US officials at the Nigerian embassy, admitting that the company had hired private investigators to dig up dirt about the federal attorney general, Michael Aondoakaa, and had released some of that material to the local press to pressure the official to settle the case.[31] If Aondoakaa did not act, Liggeri promised, he had "much more damaging information" to support more negative coverage that would follow. As part of the settlement, all parties were bound by a confidentiality clause. Pfizer admitted no wrong, and the medical records of study participants, formerly held by the Kano State Ministry of Health or the Infectious Disease Hospital, appear to have been destroyed.[32]

Pfizer's unfortunate clinical trial in Nigeria was actually bucking a growing pharmaceutical industry trend in the late 1990s to outsource this type of research. In response to tighter legal controls on studies involving human subjects, and at a time when financial pressures had already prompted drug companies to downsize, Big Pharma began to off-load liability to contract research organizations (CROs), the newest thread in the Medical Industrial Complex.[33,34]

The earliest CROs appeared in 1980, in North Carolina, where a few entrepreneurial scientists offered statistical and preclinical drug-testing services to pharmaceutical clients. During the 1990s, the pharmaceutical industry was focusing on the sales and marketing of blockbuster drugs, and the costs of research and development were exploding. Companies began to off-load increasing numbers of research studies to such outside firms. From 1995 to 2005, major pharmaceutical CRO spending as a proportion of total research and development services grew from 4 percent to 50 percent.[35]

Drug companies that had long outsourced large portions of their marketing, PR, and government relations found that they could select a CRO with specific specialty skills or a geographic presence in an under-developed country where, in part because there was little legal oversight, a trial could be run at half the cost of doing the same study in the US. The US had no system in place for regulation or certification of CROs until 2009, when the FDA made clear that these organizations would be subject to the same regulatory constraints as the companies that engaged them. But even without an "arm's length" liability firewall, studies conducted in emerging nations, notably China, where "volunteers" earn one-tenth what they might in the West, are growing at twice the rate of those in the US or Europe.[33,34,36]

Historically, "volunteers" for research in the US, lured by the promise of free treatment and payment for enrollment if they fell into the study's experimental group, have been seven times more likely to be uninsured than nonvolunteers. When the Affordable Care Act expanded American health coverage, this pool of study participants shrank, and even more drug trials moved overseas.

Trials do occur in the US today, but they are generally early phase 1 studies, limited to a few individuals and designed to establish fundamental safety and effective dosing schedules. The individuals who submit to these tests, primarily college students, the unemployed, or the disadvantaged, are now termed "paid volunteers," receiving from $200 to $400 a day to place their bodies at risk. In 1996, when Lilly was exposed for recruiting homeless alcoholics from a shelter, its director tried to deflect accusations of exploitation by saying, "These individuals want to help society."[36] But in 2005, GlaxoSmithKline CEO Jean-Paul Garnier seemed more to the point in admitting that the use of lower-income subjects was key to the company's profitability. He noted that the cost of a single participant in the US was $30,000, compared with just $3,000 in Romania.[35] Logically, then, US-based companies, which in the past performed only 15 percent of their clinical trials overseas, now do the majority of their studies beyond US borders.[36] Enrollment in US multinational-funded studies is growing by 20 percent per year in India and by nearly 50 percent per year in China, while US participants in such studies continue to decline by a rate of 6 percent a year.[35]

The growth curve has been especially steep in the past decade. In 2008, CROs ran more than 9,000 clinical trials worldwide in 115 countries and enrolled some 2 million participants, most of them overseas.[35] By 2016, the top 10 global CROs had revenues of $21.4 billion. By 2020, over half of all clinical trials run under the auspices of major pharmaceutical companies will be outsourced to CRO companies whose total revenues will exceed $40 billion.[36]

The rise of these organizations in the new millennium coincided with financial pressures related to failing drug pipelines and the expiration of patents on 1990s blockbusters—pressures that had already prompted drug companies to downsize. Emerging in the same era as military contractors like Blackwater that service the military-industrial complex, CROs offer the Medical Industrial Complex both cost benefits and the ability to gather data quickly in countries with less regulatory oversight.[37,38,39]

Rich in information technology expertise, CRO contractors now manage the full range of "preclinical services" such as drug safety and toxicity tests in laboratory animals, DNA analysis, and specialized laboratory analytics, as well as more than half of pharmaceutical phase I, II, and IV trials. Over the past decade, the field of players has been consolidating, staying one step ahead of competitors through mergers, acquisitions, and formal collaborations. The top five firms—Quintiles, PPD International, Parexel, ICON, and PRA Health Sciences—were responsible for 41 percent of all CRO revenues in 2016. The top 20 firms that year earned 61 percent of total CRO revenues.[40,41]

Medical device companies, foundations, and even the US government outsource various functions to CROs, while drug companies create strategic partnerships, sharing equity in new products in return for CROs' running the clinical trials and getting FDA approval. Some CROs now provide a sales force for a drug or a device, meaning that these organizations are fast becoming the pharmaceutical companies and device makers of the future. But while the structures may shift, the incentives for putting profits over people remain the same.[41]

Under conditions that favor low cost, speed, and delivering packages of data ready for immediate FDA submission and review, oversight of the studies and the rights of human subjects participating can easily be neglected. Not surprisingly in these environments, critics have scrutinized data integrity, trial execution, and ethical standards for human subjects. And with trends like these, it is easy to see how a Nigerian study on critically ill children might quite easily proceed. But setting aside the ethical questions surrounding the use of low-income citizens of other countries, testing overseas may also deliver skewed results. While body chemistry may vary little with geography, cultural variances can be significant. For example, a study of a new selective serotonin reuptake inhibitor for depression using Chinese subjects might measure success through a 10-question US survey instrument that does not take into account cultural differences that could affect patient responses.[35]

In US-based studies, outright fraud—the fabrication of results—is uncommon. Nonetheless, adjusting design and the reporting of results to put a best foot forward in the name of competition, or to achieve rich financial or academic rewards like publications and career advancement, is more than common; it's pervasive.

The most common ploy is to do studies on "ideal" patients—young, healthy, active, and on no medications—while the product, on approval, will be used by older patients with chronic disease who are on multiple medications.[36]

Drugs historically have been judged by means of a placebo control group of subjects who receive a treatment that resembles the real medicine being tested but in fact lacks any active ingredients. Judging drug effectiveness against a sugar pill, when you think about it, is a low bar for performance, as it shows, not that a product is better than the best treatment currently available, but just that it's better than nothing. In the past decade, this approach has been challenged by independent comparative-effectiveness research, where a new drug's performance is measured against an existing therapy, and some of the drugs tested have performed poorly indeed.[42]

In 2013, a thorough exploration of pharmaceutical-industry research practices, *Bad Pharma: How Drug Companies Mislead Doctors and Harm Patients*, by physician and investigative journalist Ben Goldacre, reviewed dozens of studies in which results were corrupted. Trials were cut short if good results appeared early, prolonged to dilute the effect of early adverse reactions, or designed to test multiple outcomes with reports emphasizing the few positives while ignoring or downplaying the negatives. Trials also ignored dropouts, which led to undercounting of drug failures and complication rates among those who had chosen to discontinue participation in the study. Some of the trials Goldacre reviewed weren't trials at all—they were simply modern versions of the old 1950s strategy meant to familiarize practicing physician "researchers" with a new treatment option and socialize them to it. Physicians were provided with samples of investigational drugs and asked to try these on their patients and report back their impressions of the drugs' effectiveness.[42]

To combat fraud by increasing transparency, in 1997 Congress passed the FDA Modernization Act, requiring that studies for lifesaving drugs be registered on a new website, ClinicalTrials.gov, when the studies were initiated. The FDA broadened its criteria for which studies needed to be registered. After four years of experience, it was clear that companies were not rushing to the land of transparency. So, in 2004, the International

Committee of Medical Journal Editors, which included editors from *JAMA* and the *New England Journal of Medicine*, elected to use their own power to force early disclosure of all studies. Their lever was a declaration that they would no longer publish research papers based on studies that had not first been formally registered on ClinicalTrials.gov.[43]

When the $700 billion pharmaceutical industry threatened to cut off millions of dollars of advertising revenue, these editors folded like paper tigers. They knew all too well that drug money, paying not just for ads but for bulk reprints of individual favorable articles, which their reps distributed to doctors, kept these journals alive. Debate and critique played out in critical articles in the journals themselves. For example, a *JAMA* article in 2009 criticized editors for purposefully vague directives such as "We *encourage* the registration of all interventional trials." Authors also shared their analysis of the results of 323 clinical drug trials in the 10 top medical journals in 2008 and found that 176, or 55 percent, were inadequately registered.[44]

In 2007, Congress ramped up oversight with an FDA Amendment Act requiring that all pharmaceutical trials, at any stage in the development process, be registered. It further required that all results, positive or negative, be posted on the site within one year of completion. Five years later, only one in five studies had met itsobligations.[45] A review of 8,907 studies that underwent mandatory registration on the government site over a three-year period (2009–2012) found that less than half had reported any results of those trials at all on the site.[46] Five years later, a 2018 investigation revealed that barely three-quarters of the ongoing clinical trial studies had been registered to the site, and journals have not fully embraced the role of policemen for the government's trial transparency efforts.[38]

In some cases, academic researchers need only lend their names and credibility. For example, a 2011 study that analyzed 630 publications in *JAMA*, *Lancet*, the *New England Journal of Medicine*, *Annals of Internal Medicine*, *Nature Medicine*, and *PLOS Medicine* determined that, based on the voluntary admissions from the 70 percent of authors contacted who agreed to participate in the confidential survey, industry-hired consultants (ghostwriters) were involved in manuscript preparation in 12 percent of the research articles, 6 percent of the review articles, and 5 percent of the editorials—and that is without considering the 30 percent of authors who chose not to participate in the survey.[47] The numbers on first glance may appear to be small, but they are more than enough to undermine the credibility of these premier medical journals and undermine public trust in the medical evidence presented in these publications.

Problems with collusion in scientific studies are part of a continuum that spans a century of profiteering and cover-up, from Williams Radam's 1890 "Microbe Killer" elixir to Big Tobacco's co-opting Hans Selye's stress program and the creation of "type A" personalities to Arthur Sackler's invention of the medical condition "ataraxia" to primary care physicians in West Virginia identified as "soft target" high prescribers of opioids and to Richardson-Merrell's unapproved distribution of thousands of thalidomide tablets to doctors under the guise of a research study. In all these cases, the common threads are pursuit of profit and the willingness of physicians to be co-opted in exchange for professional and financial gain.

For physicians seeking academic accolades, power, profit, and prestige, the clinical investigation machinery is often the shortest route to entry into the medical aristocracy. Playing along with the deep-pocketed drug, biotech, and medical device industries not only provides investigational grant funding; it nearly ensures publication (especially if the trial results are positive), along with opportunities to present your findings at prestigious meetings and serve on well-paid industry advisory committees and even governmental scientific bodies—including expert FDA panels. The game also allows young physicians to flex their leadership muscles by heading up new "specialty" organizations within the AMA Federation, whose creation traces back to industry funding and industry advocacy.

It's a daisy chain of self-interest that keeps the Medical Industrial Complex rolling along.

Chapter 12

Viagra: "Everything That Rises Must Converge"

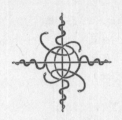

C orruption of research may be the most morally offensive aspect of the Medical Industrial Complex, but it's the MIC's raw power that is truly jaw-dropping. In global business, in domestic politics, and in the shaping of public opinion about what a disease is and how best to treat it, the MIC and its data consuming and interlocking hospital, insurance, and pharmaceutical branches have long been able to make seemingly anyone "an offer he or she can't refuse."

Perhaps the most dramatic example of concentrated MIC power in action in the 20th century, a shiny object familiar to almost all Americans, is a story I know well because I was a part of it. It began innocently enough in the 1980s, with Ian Osterloh, a mild-mannered Pfizer scientist based in Sandwich, England, who was investigating a nucleotide he hoped would reverse the narrowing of coronary arteries and thus lead to a drug for the treatment of high blood pressure and the chest pain called angina.[1]

Osterloh's research had focused on blocking the effects of an enzyme called phosphodiesterase type 5 (PDE5), which occurs naturally in humans and is present both in smooth muscle cells and in blood platelets.[1] Early studies had shown that inhibiting this enzyme led to the dilation of blood vessels and decreased clot formation.[2] After three years, Osterloh and his colleagues had isolated a compound that reliably did the job of shutting down PDE 5. Scientists rather than marketers, they called their discovery UK-92480.

In 1992, the research team launched their first phase I study of UK-92480 to see how it functioned clinically. Pfizer paid volunteers to stay for a 10-day stretch in a hospital clinical research wing and receive—depending on which card they drew—either 25 milligrams, 50 milligrams, or 75 milligrams three times a day.[3] Osterloh and his team monitored the subjects closely, and the scientists were underwhelmed by the compound's cardiovascular performance.[3] In addition, there were side effects—mostly muscle pain and backaches. It looked as if a dose that could effectively dilate coronary vessels and treat chest pain would be so high that the aches and pains would outweigh any benefit.

Quick to cut its losses, Pfizer determined to drop further cardiac studies. But in reviewing the patient follow-up forms, Osterloh noticed something both striking and completely unexpected. Three of the nine men who had taken the 50-milligram tablet and five of the eight who had taken the 75-milligram tablet reported massive, long-lasting erections.

More than 5,000 miles away, a UCLA research team led by pharmacologist Louis Ignarro had been intentionally studying the same territory that Pfizer had stumbled upon by accident—they were working to explicate all the biochemical steps that lead to an erection. Their research, first published in 1990,[4] and further amplified in a *New England Journal of Medicine* article in 1992,[5] showed that the process was much more complex than moonlight and roses. Sexual stimulation causes nerves to release nitrous oxide, which activates an enzyme that increases the messenger nucleotide cyclic guanosine monophosphate (cGMP), which dilates penile arteries, which then causes the penis to stiffen.

For this work in uncovering the critical role of nitrous oxide in relaxing vascular smooth muscle, Louis Ignarro would be awarded the Nobel Prize in 1998.[6] More immediately, it helped Pfizer scientists realize that they might be on to something as they designed further studies for their unexpectedly intriguing new compound. But perhaps even more important, this "real science" gave Pfizer a defense against future claims that it was creating a "lifestyle drug"—a mere aphrodisiac—that could be trivialized and abused. Subsequent studies revealed that for UK92480 to work, nerve endings first had to release nitrous oxide, which meant that the subjects had to be sexually excited *already*. The drug's role, which came into play only after stimulation had formed the messenger cGMP, was merely to prevent its degradation and to keep it in the area longer. Furthermore, the drug did not enhance erections in patients who did not need pharmacological help in achieving one.

In 1993, Pfizer did another study involving 16 men in Bristol, England. The group was split in two, half receiving a dose of 25 milligrams of UK92480 three times a day, and the other half receiving identical-appearing placebos.[7] For one week the men were instructed to keep diaries at home and record the number and quality of their erections. At the end of the week, they were brought back to the study site and encouraged to spend two hours exploring specific pornographic magazines and videos—termed the "blue materials"—as they wished. Meanwhile, the men were hooked up to an apparatus called the RigiScan.[8] Developed in 1985, this device measured the changing thickness of the penis, allowing doctors to measure erections during periods of sexual excitement and stimulation. In addition, men normally have one or more erections during deep sleep. The device worn at night could document the presence or absence of these erections as a baseline before and after treatment.

The results were very good news for Pfizer, with over three-quarters of research participants responding to sexual excitement and stimulation with erections.[7] By the time a second study was completed in May 1994, the researchers had proved that the drug was effective in a single daily dose.[8] By late 1995, daily dose levels had been set at 25, 50, and 100 milligrams, and a green light was given for large phase III trials that took on pretty much any men except those on nitroglycerin, those who'd had a cardiovascular event in the previous six months, and those with a spinal cord injury, who would be studied separately.[9]

In tandem with this study, marketers had already made a business case for continued investment. The Massachusetts Male Aging Study in 1994 confirmed that the incidence of complete impotence tripled from

5 percent to 15 percent between the ages of 40 and 70.[10] Most of the men affected had not sought a doctor's help, because the treatments at the time involved painful injections or surgery and were only marginally effective. The introduction of a simple pill to address the problem would clearly dominate the marketplace.

Over the next two years, working with some 4,500 subjects in 13 countries, Pfizer researchers were able to prove 82 percent effectiveness in initiating erections overall—and this included men with cardiovascular disease, diabetes, spinal cord injury, hypertension, postsurgical dysfunction, depression, and multiple sclerosis. The subjects' average time to erection after they took the pill was 25 minutes, a delay deemed acceptable by the company for all but the most impatient. The pill had minimal side effects and was well tolerated in men drinking alcohol or taking medicines, including antihypertensives, antidepressants, aspirin, lipid-lowering medications, diabetes drugs, and antacids.[11]

One challenge researchers did not have to face was in recruitment of subjects.[12] Quite the contrary—in addition to the quantitative results, the Pfizer researchers could report qualitative endorsements: patients saying, "Please send more tablets."[7]

By 1995, I had left private practice to serve as senior vice president of academic affairs at Pennsylvania Hospital. One day a recruiter called me up saying that he represented a major Fortune 100 health-related company and was looking for a physician-spokesperson to engage with the medical community, health organizations, and the media.

Later in the conversation, when he revealed the name of the client and the nature of the product, I realized why he had thought to call me. I was a urologist, a "real doctor" with hands-on clinical experience. I also had considerable media experience. But more than that, in a 1980 textbook I wrote for Cambridge University Press, I had made an extended appeal for physicians to drop the lay term "impotence" in favor of a more scientific label, "erectile dysfunction."[13]

My first exposure to the kind of resources being wielded in support of this new potential blockbuster drug was when the recruiter sent a helicopter down to Philadelphia to pick me up and had a limousine waiting for me at the 34th Street Heliport in New York. Instead of going directly to Pfizer headquarters, though, I was taken up to 75 Rockefeller Plaza to a meeting with 44-year-old Linda Robinson, chair of the Expert Advisory Committee for Pfizer's new product—no longer UK-92480, but Viagra.[14] (How exactly the company arrived at the name remains in dispute, but one popular explanation is that it was chosen to evoke an association with Niagara Falls.)

Linda's remit was to identify every controversial issue that might arise in the public forum with Viagra's approval and develop an in-depth strategy to manage each and every one of these issues. Her committee was packed with not just scientists but also sex therapists, ethicists, theologians, and representatives of four of the largest public relations firms in New York, including her own company: Robinson Lerer & Montgomery.[15]

If helicopters and limousines were the outward trappings of power, Linda Robinson was its very embodiment. Already well known for her role in the leveraged buyout of RJR Nabisco, the story at the center of the book and film *Barbarians at the Gate*,[16] she had been featured in a 10-page cover story in *Vanity Fair*.[17] This piece described her as a world-class crisis management professional and the most powerful public relations broker in the country. Her husband, James D. Robinson III, was the chairman of American Express, and she was on first-name terms with most of the major players in media and politics in New York. Her father, Freeman Gosden, had been a radio personality (Amos of *Amos 'n' Andy*) and a longtime Hollywood fixture close to many political figures, including Ronald Reagan.[18] When Reagan entered the 1980 presidential race, Linda became assistant to the campaign's press secretary. After Reagan's victory, she became press secretary to the secretary of transportation just as America's air traffic controllers went on strike, and the showdown between them and President Reagan became one of the lead stories of the year.[17]

At Pfizer, Linda's work was overseen by another power player, Lou Clemente, the lawyer who had worked throughout the 1970s and 1980s with former Pfizer CEO Ed Pratt to achieve intellectual property protections for American corporations as part of the 1994 General Agreement on Tariffs and Trade.

As part of that decades-long intellectual property campaign, Lou had assembled an incomparable public affairs war room that brought together resources in government relations, investor relations, media relations, public affairs, and shareholder relations.[19] He also coordinated the activities of Pfizer executives who had allies in key positions in influential organizations such as the American Enterprise Institute, the Brookings Institution, the Heritage Foundation, and the Hoover Institution. Together they were able to enroll these "thought leaders" in support for a trade-based approach to intellectual property that had become harder and harder for governments to resist.[20]

Traditionally, at Pfizer, as well as at other major pharmaceutical companies, messaging had taken a back seat to product promotion. Each drug was supported by its own marketing team, which in turn supported its product release in the US and around the world as the drug gained country-by-country approvals. Overall pharmaceutical operational leadership at Pfizer was divided into sections including the US, Latin America, Europe, and Asia/Africa/Middle East/Japan. However, after the patent wars of the 1980s, in the face of the burgeoning consumer movement as well as the threat of health reform focused on cost containment and managed care, outgoing Pfizer CEO Ed Pratt had helped engineer the move of Lou Clemente from his corporate counsel position to a new department, Corporate Affairs, reporting directly to the new CEO, Bill Steere.

In creating this Corporate Affairs juggernaut and assigning Clemente to develop a comprehensive public affairs campaign, Steere was completing an important and highly controversial power shift emblematic of the pervasive reach of the Medical Industrial Complex as it neared the end of the 20th century. Pfizer's US Pharmaceuticals division usually planned and executed the messaging and the marketing rollout of any new product released in the US. But for what was soon to be Pfizer's most famous product, Lou—reporting directly to the CEO—would oversee public affairs, federal government relations, state government relations, shareholder relations, corporate governance, investor relations, internal communications, information technology, media relations, and medical relations, coordinating all messaging to all Pfizer's external constituencies.

Steere's motivation in shifting resources and the locus of control of messaging for this new drug reflected his desire to carefully protect the future of two brand names: Viagra and Pfizer. Viagra itself was a complex product being launched at a time of increasing criticism of the overmarketing and overpricing of drugs. Since the FDA approval of Rogaine to treat baldness in 1988, insurers and academic critics had lobbied against the use of precious resources to support the purchase of drugs for what were viewed as frivolous lifestyle problems. Viagra could easily get caught up in that debate, which could vastly undercut the drug's potential profitability. There was also the potential for accusations of promoting sexual promiscuity and abuse. One additional concern was the nagging knowledge that compared with being in a resting state the exertion required for sexual intercourse carried twice the risk of sudden death.

But if anything, Steere was more concerned about the Pfizer brand. As the approval of Viagra approached, Pfizer was on a trajectory to become the largest pharmaceutical company in the world. It ranked number eight when Steere had taken it over, and now the company fielded six blockbuster billion-dollar-a-year drugs. He had built the future of the company around an extensive expansion of his sales force and the highest investment in research and development in the industry. Steere's Pfizer was high science all the way, and the company had already received hundreds of media requests ahead of this new product's release. A poorly managed launch of Viagra could turn Pfizer into the "sex company." Steere's strategy was to publicly engage and lead the debate on the drug, and in engaging New York's top crisis-management professional, Linda Robinson, and directing Corporate Affairs himself through Lou Clemente, he signaled that anything less than perfect communications management would be unacceptable.

Clemente's team included experienced professionals in state and federal government relations, public policy and communications, media relations, investor relations, shareholder relations, and now medical relations. They already had contacts at the NIH, the FDA, conservative think tanks, and a wide range of elite academic medical centers, whose researchers were paid advisers to Pfizer. What I added were relationships with the leadership of the American Medical Association, the American Hospital Association, the American College of Surgeons, and the Association of American Medical Colleges. To achieve Pfizer's goals, we would be pulling on every thread within the Medical Industrial Complex simultaneously and then some.

In resigning my post at Pennsylvania Hospital, I left behind an increasingly contentious medical environment that was deteriorating day by day. I was also embracing a new challenge in an industry and a role for which I was not fully prepared. Lou Clemente gave me an office on the 11th floor and a list of some 50 internal people I should meet and cultivate. Before coming to Pfizer, I had never had a job in which mingling was the only thing I was asked to do for the first six months. Then again, I had never before had a job that involved the global sway and the money that were at Pfizer's command.

I was asked to offer opinions from my perspective as a clinician. How would urologists react if men with this embarrassing, age-old problem abandoned specialist consultation and saw instead a primary care physician who could simply prescribe a pill? What was the consensus of urologists on whether the condition was more physiologic or psychological? How likely was it that a standard evaluation of erectile dysfunction would reveal underlying chronic conditions such as diabetes or hypertension or heart disease? How often did men lie about how often they had sex? If they lost the ability at 65 or 70, did they really care enough to seek treatment?

Clemente knew that to be effective as the "professional" voice of Viagra, I would need a noncommercial platform, as well as a fancy title, not just to engage the public and physicians but also to attest to my independence and integrity. To develop the right strategy for showcasing this integrity and independence, he turned me over to a young and aggressive public relations team, Bob Chandler and Gianfranco Chicco.[21]

Our initial conversation led to questions about the patient-physician relationship, which led to Chandler and Chicco's bringing in the Yankelovich Group, national pollsters in health care, to find the answers. They discovered that, while differences existed between the views of doctors and patients, more than 90 percent of both parties in the examining room agreed that the patient-physician relationship consisted of three things: compassion, understanding, and partnership.[22] In a few more weeks, Chandler and Chicco came up with a name and logo for my platform: the Pfizer Medical Humanities Initiative. "Medical" suggested professional authority; "Humanities" implied something caring, inclusive, noncommercial; "Initiative" spoke to action over words. The logo was a circle with two pairs of interlinked doctors and patients, and three words in the margins—"compassion," "understanding," and "partnership."

It was a high-minded-sounding program arrived at through the same tried and true polling apparatus used to test-market new shades of lipstick.

Working with the staff from Chandler and Chicco, I finalized a national survey instrument designed to answer the question "Was the patient-physician relationship evolving, and if so, in what direction?" The stated goal was to empower me, as the new director of the Pfizer Medical Humanities Initiative, with the most advanced, proprietary social science knowledge on a relationship that was central to the interests of the leadership of organized medicine nationwide. Practically speaking, however, being director of the Pfizer Medical Humanities Initiative, a lofty-sounding endeavor designed to enhance my prestige as a "thought leader," would also make me more effective in helping sell Viagra. The initial distribution of our research findings about doctors and patients would create "buzz" as we announced the new program and my association with Pfizer.

I burned through most of my first-year budget of $650,000 in the first six months in order to learn that, in 1997, this core relationship in American society was indeed evolving, moving from paternalism to partnership; from "doctor says" to shared decision-making; and from individual to team-based approaches to care.[23] As predicted, these were insights valued by organizations like the AMA, which were struggling to absorb the implications of consumerism and anxious to position themselves as part of the future rather than the past.

Meanwhile, the commercial product that was the point of all this lofty-sounding activity continued to move through the system. The official new drug application was filed with the FDA on September 29, 1997, and three weeks later, Viagra became a beneficiary of the compromise agreement that had been reached during the AIDS crisis. It was granted priority review status based on the fact that it represented a "major advance" and served an "unmet need." Six months later, on March 27, 1998, it received FDA approval.[24]

Big Pharma as a whole was already on a tear with wholesale drug revenues up by 60 percent since 1994. The population was aging, and attempts to curtail health care costs had met stiff resistance from the AMA and hospitals. The discovery drought that had marked the 1970s and much of the 1980s had been relieved by faster FDA drug approval and the release of government patents. Me-too drugs were all the rage, with five nearly identical products on the market just for lowering cholesterol by the early 1990s.

Pfizer was hitting operating profit margins in 1997 above 32 percent on $12 billion in sales, 90 percent of which came from drugs. When Bill Steere became CEO in February 1991, drug sales represented only 50 percent of the company's revenues, but then he declared all non-pharmaceutical holdings a "distraction" and sold them off. Steere doubled his sales force to an industry high of 5,400 in the US alone, stocking it with gung-ho ex-military people, including 1,000 veterans of Operation Desert Storm. These reps were energized by hefty bonuses and multiple quotas and ruthlessly weeded out if they didn't make the grade.[25]

Direct-to-consumer advertising, severely curtailed since the Kefauver-Harris Amendment of 1962, had been greatly liberalized by 1997 as part of President Bill Clinton's pro-growth agenda. TV advertising, previously outlawed, was ramped up in support of a glut of blockbuster me-too drugs. But Steere took the new reliance on image making one step further, actually putting marketers in charge of research and development teams, thus giving them authority over scientists who might not know the difference between "a good scientific idea and a good new drug idea." Product concepts were put to the test early, with elaborate revenue modeling and scenario building that helped predict the cost of one side effect or another.[25]

With all this muscle behind it, Viagra looked to be a cultural watershed, a media extravaganza, and a big, big seller. On the other hand, it carried the risk of becoming a punch line delivered with a smirk—the worst example of a lifestyle drug, a trivial, profit-driven enterprise that was beneath the dignity of a proper maker of medicines. Unless handled perfectly, everyone involved knew, Pfizer's embrace of this one product could undermine a half century of image building regarding the pharmaceutical industry's commitment to true innovation, and thus could undermine both physician and consumer support. Most of all, this one drug could relocate the 150-year-old pharmaceutical research company squarely in "the sex business."[26]

One week before FDA approval was to be announced, ABC Television's newsmagazine *20/20* aired an exclusive feature on the drug reported by its medical correspondent at the time, Dr. Timothy Johnson.[27]

I knew Tim from medical media circles, and the morning after Bill Steere saw Johnson on TV, he called me into his office and handed me a sealed envelope of very classy, custom stationery and said, "I want you to deliver this to Tim." Taken aback, I said, "You want me to take this to him in Boston?" He said, "Yes. I liked his piece last night, and I want to thank him. Take it up to him this morning."

I was still adjusting to the imperial grandeur of a corporation that could throw money at such gestures, but in little more than an hour, the Delta shuttle delivered me to a waiting Town Car that carried me directly to the WCVB-TV studios just west of Boston, where Johnson was based.[28]

As I entered Tim's office, he, too, needed a moment to adjust. Smiling, he rose, extended his hand, and said, "Mike, what are you doing here?"

"Well, Tim, Bill Steere really liked your piece last night, and he asked me to bring this to you."

I handed him the envelope.

He sat down with a befuddled smile, then said, "He had you come all the way up here to give me this?"

To which I replied, "Yup, he wanted me to personally deliver it to you."

So he sat back in his chair, opened it slowly, read the enclosed small note in silence, smiled again, and with a slight shake of his head, carefully replaced the note in its envelope.

"Thanks, Mike. Tell Bill I appreciate it."

A short time later, I was back in the air, returning to the media and financial capital of the world, and to the hot, burning center of the Medical Industrial Complex in action.

Viagra was approved by the FDA on March 27, 1998. A few days later, I had my debut as a Viagra spokesman on FOX News. Some of Linda Robinson's people had been embedded in our 11th-floor "Viagra war room" and, working with the Viagra Advisory Committee, had identified and researched nearly every issue that could possibly arise. As a result, I had been thoroughly briefed on the line FOX would take that day—Viagra for women. My simple response: Viagra had not been studied for women, and should not be used for women.

Meanwhile, women's advocates, as well as organizations ranging from the Planned Parenthood Foundation to the American College of Obstetrics and Gynecology, duly noted that, as insurers buckled under Pfizer's demands for coverage of Viagra, these same insurers were still not covering the cost of contraceptives. American women at the time were also paying 31 percent more in out-of-pocket expenses for their health care than men.[29] If Pfizer could argue that Viagra was cost-effective because it coincidentally spurred earlier treatment for various chronic diseases like heart disease, diabetes, and hypertension, certainly women's health advocates could make the case that with at least one of every three pregnancies a year being unintended, this far more costly phenomenon could be avoided by covering contraceptives. Pfizer responded by updating its own employee coverage of contraceptives and offering a full-throated endorsement of insurance coverage of women's birth control. By August 1998, bills were making their way through Congress to require coverage of birth control pills for 2.4 million federal employees.[30]

During the first six weeks of the Viagra launch, Pfizer addressed more than 3,000 media requests, including *Newsweek*,[31] the *New York Times*,[32] *CBS Evening News*,[33] *USA Today*,[33] the *Wall Street Journal*,[34] and

US News & World Report.[35] Prior to this burst of activity, Pfizer's unaided name recognition with the general public was 8 percent. Industry leader Merck, with its famous *Merck Manual*, sat at 18 percent. After the initial launch period, Pfizer's name recognition had skyrocketed to 34 percent.[36] Viagra's unaided name recognition exceeded 90 percent, and this was before any direct-to-consumer advertising.[37]

During that six-week launch some 50,000 doctors wrote more than 1.5 million prescriptions, far exceeding the numbers for any new drug launch in history. Less reported was the fact that the Pfizer manufacturing machine had managed to stock all US pharmacy shelves with the product within 10 days of its March 27, 1998, approval, and that materials and packaging were globally uniform.[38] Like Coke, Viagra was now a worldwide brand.

The risk with such rapid expansion was of course product safety, but the biggest concern was that some older men, engaged in sex with the help of Viagra, would die. The company had sounded the trumpet early and often—"absolutely contra-indicated in men taking nitroglycerin for heart disease"—hoping to immunize itself against liability. Nitroglycerin's ability to dilate vessels was amplified by Viagra, and taken together, the two drugs could initiate life-threatening drops in blood pressure. The company had even gone to the trouble of communicating to hospital staffs that before administering sublingual nitroglycerin, they should ask men who came to the emergency department with chest pain if they had recently taken Viagra. But none of that addressed the risk for men who didn't know they had coronary artery blockage.[39]

As the numbers of Americans on Viagra rapidly rose, some men did die while having sex, and the FDA took the unprecedentedly transparent action of listing coronary deaths of men on Viagra in real time. By late 1998, 6 million Viagra prescriptions for 4.5 million men had been written, and the FDA website had listed 128 associated cardiac fatalities.[39] The culprit, as it turned out, was not primarily the drug itself but rather its capacity to make sex possible for these men. A person with a hidden coronary artery disease has double the chance of a heart attack from the exertion of sex as compared with being at rest.

As the sales numbers on Viagra initially soared and the data rolled in, Pfizer had a very good sense of who was taking the drug. Ninety percent were over the age of 40 (which helped address the charge that the drug was an aphrodisiac to be widely abused by young men trying to enhance normal function). The most common accompanying diagnoses of men taking the drug for erectile dysfunction were hypertension, cardiovascular disease, diabetes, and cancer of the prostate.[40]

Meanwhile, down in the trenches, Pfizer's governmental relations team was engaged in hand-to-hand combat to achieve insurance reimbursement in all 50 states and around the world.

California-based Kaiser Permanente was one of the major insurance players that persisted in viewing Viagra as a "lifestyle drug" and in refusing to cover the cost. By taking the position that the drug was essentially trivial, Kaiser found itself at odds not just with Pfizer but with the Catholic Church and its popular pope, John Paul II. Linda Robinson and her Advisory Committee had approached the papacy months earlier to get a reading prior to drug approval. As a Pfizer spokesman commented matter-of-factly, "We thought it was the responsible thing to do. They felt that impotence can hurt relationships and couples. Viagra can help in improving marital relations."[41]

On August 20, 1998, I was dispatched to Los Angeles to testify before Dale Bonner, commissioner of the California Department of Corporations.[42] The state regulatory body had oversight responsibility for laws governing HMO coverage of benefits. Kaiser, along with PacifiCare Health Systems, Health Net, Aetna, and US Healthcare had requested of the Department of Corporations that they be permitted "to offer the drug as a supplemental benefit for which employers would pay an additional premium." The department's position was that "if a doctor prescribes Viagra as being medically necessary, plans have an obligation to provide it" with full coverage.

Commissioner Bonner called the public hearing to air the dispute after several California citizens, some of whom were disabled, charged that Kaiser had indiscriminately refused to cover Viagra based on its cost to the plan. Pfizer's government-relations staff packed the media-filled hearing room with proponents of the drug, so it was more Bambi versus Godzilla than a fair fight. Industry-friendly state legislators had already worked over the commissioner. For reasons only Kaiser might explain, it had decided to send a visibly uncomfortable female pediatrician to argue the case against us. Even more unfortunately for Kaiser, speaking just before me on behalf of Pfizer was a mother of a paralyzed young man who testified that her son's only hope for parenthood was Viagra.

I had come with a long, written commentary that I had submitted to the panel, but as I began to read it, the commissioner cut me off, then proceeded to ask me questions about the drug for the better part of an hour. He was especially interested in the information I provided to support the claim that this was not a "recreational drug."

My answer drew on my own clinical experience and knowledge of the drug:

"When I was a urologist in private practice, my patients . . . weren't looking for an enhanced sexual performance; they were hoping to restore the ability to have an intimate relationship with a loved one . . . It is clear that Viagra is providing very real benefits to men and their partners."[43]

But then I went on to enhance the case for Viagra by recasting erectile dysfunction as a "marker disease," meaning a disorder that reflects another hidden underlying disease that needs to be investigated. Utilizing data from the famous 1994 Massachusetts Male Aging Study, an academic urologist had published a paper that listed the incidence of various urologic conditions, as well as their more common accompanying chronic diseases.[44] From those figures, I was able to see that, in very loose statistical terms, for every 1 million men who saw a doctor for help with erectile dysfunction, gave a medical history, then took a basic physical exam and had blood work done, approximately 30,000 would be found to have diabetes, 50,000 would harbor heart disease, and 140,000 would have hypertension. Laying out the numbers, I was able to confidently make the case that if Viagra was able to get men off the couch and to come see a doctor a couple of years before they otherwise would, their chronic diseases would be diagnosed, treated, and managed earlier—which would save insurers like Kaiser a great deal of money over the long run.

Finally, I noted that the alternative therapies, like vacuum pumps and penile injections and silastic rod implants, were invasive, painful, less effective, and two to three times more costly.[45]

The commissioner's decision came down in late December 1998, and it was a huge win for Pfizer.[46] He ruled that Viagra was not recreational but medically necessary, that insurers did not have the right to arbitrarily limit coverage of medical treatments based solely on cost, and that Kaiser must cover the cost. The insurer was also required to provide coverage and to make restitution to its members who had been denied coverage over the prior six months. Kaiser also agreed to pay a fine of $250,000 to the state for the cost of the commissioner's summer gathering.

The results were widely reported and sent a message to other insurers still considering tactics to avoid covering the drug. Within another year, nearly all insurers would fall into line, although with limitations on the number of pills, and often with high co-payments for motivated Viagra users, a compromise Pfizer was more than willing to make.[47]

As Pfizer waited for the response from California, it commissioned a Harris Poll on October 26, 1998, that showed broad public support for Viagra reimbursement in all categories of patients, including those with spinal cord injury, diabetes, multiple sclerosis, hypertension, and cancer of the prostate.[48] Pfizer appeared well on its way to having its seventh billion-dollar-a-year blockbuster seller—with, as of yet, no advertising.

What state and federal agencies and insurers had underestimated was the number and the power of the strings being pulled not just in Washington, but in state capitals across the nation, by my colleagues on the 11th floor in Pfizer's state and federal government relations departments.

The team split the country into six regions: Mid-Atlantic/New England, Northeast, Central, Southern, Southwest, and Western. Statehouses were divided up among 20 full-time state government relations managers, nearly all with prior local legislative experience.[49] These Pfizer employees were, in turn, supported by numerous local lawyers, lobbyists, and advocacy group organizers, capable of delivering a community-based response like the one that had been on full view in the Viagra hearings in California.

Moreover, Pfizer had been aided at every step along the way by weak analysis by opponents of Viagra reimbursement. This was most obvious in exaggerated early claims that coverage would break the backs of insurers. For example, Kaiser initially predicted that the annual cost of coverage would be at least $100 million.[50] The National Governors' Association pegged the yearly Medicaid coverage cost at $100 million.[51] And the Veterans Administration said that coverage for veterans would hit $280 million a year.[52] Pfizer financial experts dug into the numbers and demonstrated that they were off by some 20-fold.

Before long, even Medicaid patients became eligible in 39 of 50 states. One that did not extend coverage was Arkansas, whose then governor Mike Huckabee, a fundamentalist minister before entering politics, was said to have remarked that he was "not sure that welfare recipients should be treated to a more active sex life at the expense of hard-working taxpayers."[53]

Despite the tremendous success of its initial muscle-flexing rollout, Pfizer's US Pharmaceutical group's concerns were rising with the first-year anniversary of the launch still three months away. Revenues, while still strong, were flattening, with over 50 percent of sales going to existing customers. The trend line suggested a significant slippage in new sales. Originally projected to hit $1 billion in sales with ease, Viagra now looked as if might peak that first year at $800 million.[54] Of even more concern was an estimate that only about half the men with severe erectile dysfunction had so far sought care, and this number wouldn't budge.[55] The marketing department did a survey and came to the conclusion that most men with the problem were just too embarrassed to mention it.

Linda Robinson and the Pfizer in-house marketers were discussing strategies to embolden men with the problem when someone recalled an appearance on CNN by former senator Bob Dole. On the evening of May 6, 1998, on *Larry King Live*, the senator had mentioned out of the blue that he had participated in a Pfizer trial and considered Viagra "a great drug." Dole was now fully recovered from his unsuccessful presidential run, and had become a popular celebrity guest with a wry sense of humor, a bit of age under his belt, and a scar from the surgical removal of his cancerous prostate. A few days after his appearance, his wife, preparing for a run for the presidency, appeared in New York with Rudy Giuliani and was asked about her husband and Viagra. She supported both.[56]

With Viagra now underperforming, Pfizer defined the challenge as getting men who had not yet seen a doctor off the couch, and it believed an ounce of encouragement from Bob Dole might do the trick.

It wasted no time, and by December 1998, the contract was signed, with Dole agreeing to appear in commercials on behalf of Viagra throughout 1999, and to dedicate up to two days each month to follow-up events that year promoting men's health.[56] For those events, he would be ferried about in the company's Gulfstream IV jet or helicopter, and be accompanied by a Pfizer executive—namely me. In return for these services, he was to be compensated with a handsome fee rumored to be in the million-dollar range. Also part of his package was a year's supply of Viagra, which I delivered to him in a brown paper bag to protect his anonymity—the only prescription for the drug I ever wrote.

The ad began to appear early in 1999, and it received an overwhelmingly positive response inside the company and in the media. Dole was described as "forthright, honest, and even dignified." After noting all the ways the subject might make viewers uncomfortable, he told the audience, basically, to grow up.[57] With what looked like one of the corridors of power as a backdrop, Dole appeared vibrant and youthful, dressed in red, white, and blue. He never mentioned Viagra. He merely said:

"Courage. Something shared by countless Americans. Those who risk their lives. Those who battle serious illness. When I was diagnosed with prostate cancer, I was primarily concerned with ridding myself of the cancer. But secondly, I was concerned about post-operative side effects like erectile dysfunction, ED, often called impotence. You know, it's a little embarrassing to talk about ED but it's so important to millions of men and their partners that I decided to talk about it publicly."[58]

Accompanying the television spot was a full-page print ad that seemed to appear everywhere overnight and featured a screen grab of Bob Dole in the spot with stylized white type reading, "It may take a little Courage to ask your doctor about Erectile Dysfunction. But everything worthwhile usually does." The text below Dole's photo talked about ED and directed the reader to a toll-free number for more information. A small Pfizer logo appeared in the lower-right-hand corner. But again there was no specific mention of Viagra, reflecting Pfizer's extreme concern about being accused of marketing a sex drug, rather than spreading awareness about a serious medical condition.[59]

The ads won praise, but multiple surveys continued to document unmotivated males. In June 1999, a CNN survey found that some 4 out of 10 men said they would be reluctant to seek help if they had erectile dysfunction.[60] An AARP survey around the same time found that the incidence of severe erectile dysfunction in men under age 60 was only 2.5 percent, while the rate in men age 60 to 74 was 16 percent. Just under 6 percent of all men surveyed were being treated for ED, with about half on Viagra.[61] All these results were lower than previously thought.

Undaunted, Pfizer reached into its MIC bag of tricks to develop a series of professional and consumer education strategies. By now, 60 percent of prescriptions for Viagra were being written by primary care physicians, so Pfizer reached out to its allies at 15 of the top medical schools in the US with funding—a direct intrusion of commerce into medical education—to encourage the expansion of their curriculum in "sexual health/sexual dysfunction." More than half took the funding.[62] In expanding the education of medical students and residents, the intention was to routinely include questioning about sexual function in patient encounters. The hope was that growth in the numbers diagnosed would result in higher numbers of those treated with Viagra. In addition, Pfizer continued to roll out "brochures, slide kits, anatomic diagrams and models," not to mention the paid speakers, expert advisers, and a wide range of continuing education seminars that were in reality little more than tax-deductible vacations at palm-shaded resorts.

With growth curves still flat, marketers detected that the physician-patient conversation about sexual function was sufficiently awkward that the topic rarely if ever surfaced in the annual physical exam. Having had success in introducing an office-based, patient self-administered simple "survey test" for depression in order to increase the number of antidepressant prescriptions for the Pfizer drug Zoloft, the company, with the help of urologists and sex therapists, now developed a similar instrument for ED.[63] It was derived from a longer, more elaborate survey that had been used in the clinical trials. But this one had only five questions, with grades of 0 to 5 for each question. The lower the score, the more likely you had ED.[64]

The five questions:

1. How do you rate your confidence that you could get and keep an erection?
2. When you had erections with sexual stimulation, how often were your erections hard enough for penetration (entering your partner)?
3. During sexual intercourse, how often were you able to maintain your erection after you had penetrated (entered) your partner?
4. During sexual intercourse, how difficult was it to maintain your erection to completion of intercourse?
5. When you attempted sexual intercourse, how often was it satisfactory for you?

The company also funded research grants to academicians to study ED as an indicator of underlying disease, with this intended takeaway: "Viagra-Inspired ED Checkups Save Lives."[65] Researchers were able to establish underlying disease in patients presenting with ED, but long-term studies to prove that uncovering these conditions extended the life span were lacking. Urologists supported by Pfizer grants announced at the 1999 annual meeting of the American Urological Association that men presenting with ED were more likely than normal men to have cancer of the prostate detected.[66] The Minneapolis Heart Institute Foundation did its part, finding that 40 percent of men with ED had underlying atherosclerosis.[67]

By the end of 1999, 99 countries around the world had given the drug the green light.[68] But even as the numbers of US men treated with Viagra rose to 7 million, with 10 million being treated worldwide, Pfizer still viewed the drug as a serious underperformer.[69] The company was initially pleased with Bob Dole's "Courage" ad, but here was one of the most famous products of all time, one whose messaging was being directed out of the CEO's office, and it was currently only the seventh-best seller in Pfizer's vaunted stable of products and struggling to break $1 billion after its first year on the market.[70] Pfizer marketers now had the ammunition to seize back control and felt the product strategy needed a total redo.

To make matters worse, in January 1999, Elizabeth Dole, Bob's wife, stepped down from her role as president of the American Red Cross to dip her toe into other presidential waters, crisscrossing America with frequent stops in Iowa.[71] Early polls gave her reasonable odds of winning the Republican nomination, but by summer 1999 her numbers were sliding. Her advisers blamed Bob Dole's "Courage" ad for costing Mrs. Dole votes, and they wanted Pfizer to pull it.

Even though Pfizer's contract with Bob Dole allowed the company to run the ad for a full year, Pfizer bowed to direct pressure from the former Senate majority leader, pulling the ad off the air five months early. But Elizabeth Dole continued to lose ground to George W. Bush, and in October 1999, with the "Courage" ad already sidelined, she bowed out of the race.[72]

Bob Dole continued to devote two days a month to public appearances at consumer health and veterans' conventions on behalf of the company, and we made the most of those. On one day alone, relying on a company jet, I left New York at 7 a.m., picked up Dole at Reagan National Airport in Washington, hit five different cities across the country, and was back home by 7 p.m.

But Pfizer was not happy that Dole had reneged on his contract, and was not above dumping the war hero and former presidential candidate. Pfizer marketers had all but given up on getting more older men motivated to see their doctors and were now after a younger demographic, which is why they decided to sponsor a NASCAR Winston Cup Series team and cover the car with the Viagra logo.[73] As a tie-in, the marketers embraced a new strategy they called "Tune Up for Life." They emblazoned this line on a tractor trailer parked at NASCAR racetracks, inside which they provided free screening for high blood pressure, diabetes, and cholesterol, along with their five-question ED screening. In 2001, they did an estimated 25,000 screenings, but results of these efforts were never published.[74]

Viagra left a bad taste in the mouths of Pfizer marketers—the missteps with Bob Dole breaking his contract, the embracing of tactics like NASCAR and associated screening sideshows, the battles for control with Lou Clemente's Corporate Affairs department, and especially the fact that its most famous product seemed to have underperformed in the marketplace. Nonetheless, CEO Bill Steere had achieved his objectives. He was now the most visible and admired personality within an increasingly organized and profitable Medical Industrial Complex, a sector that was attracting Wall Street investors hand over fist.

Viagra might be number six in sales for the company, but in a few more months the company itself would be valued number one worldwide in industry revenues. The Pfizer brand celebrated science, not sex, and the organization's decision to establish the integrated Corporate Affairs juggernaut would shortly deliver financial benefits beyond Steere's wildest dreams.

Viagra was a "shiny object" offering a distraction from a wide range of intractable problems. Even though it was an accidental discovery, it was viewed by nearly all as a concrete and crowning example of the power and utility of private enterprise in American health care. Arising as it did at the peak of the pharmaceutical "blockbuster" era, it entertained and enriched in equal measures, reinforcing the myth that scientific progress is synonymous with human progress.

During the decade of Viagra, health care costs continued to rise at double the rate of inflation. Attempts at health reform under President Clinton failed. Forty-four million or 16 percent of the US population were uninsured. The Human Genome Project was launched. Nearly 140,000 were diagnosed with HIV/AIDS in a single year, with a 60 percent mortality rate. Nearly 500 hospitals closed nationwide, 40 percent of those being rural hospitals.[75] And United Healthcare received $2.3 billion for the sale of its original pharmacy benefit management company, Diversified

Pharmaceutical Services, after mining patient databases to create "Report Cards" to steer customers' health choices.[76]

As the new millennium dawned, prices of health benefits were continuing to rise out of control, and large employers who were increasingly managing the burden of self-employed health benefit plans were launching cost-control strategies like restrictive hospital and physician panels, higher deductibles, and more patient co-pays. Health insurers followed suit, and at the same time they competed with each other through expansions and mergers while conducting hand-to-hand combat negotiating annual pricing agreements with their doctors and hospitals. Public access to services, especially in rural areas, was in steep decline. Not only were rural hospitals closing in droves, but 16 percent of independently owned rural pharmacies disappeared between 2003 and 2018.[77]

In public, dustups and finger-pointing between the AMA, PhRMA, health insurers, and hospital leaders were occurring with some frequency. But behind the scenes, leaders of the various camps were in firm agreement on one common objective—maintaining the status quo. To accomplish that, they would have to work cooperatively and below the radar screen to establish hidden vehicles for future profit sharing.

What was significant about Viagra was that it instigated the structured reorganization of Pfizer's corporate public affairs toward heavy investment in federal and state government relations. This evolution was mirrored not only by its pharmaceutical competitors, but also by the giant health insurers, medical associations, and hospital systems nationwide. As the various companies and their trade associations and patient support groups migrated toward Washington and one another, the next ten years would offer them an unparalleled opportunity to work together on a common future.

Chapter 13

New Rules

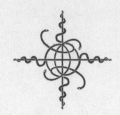

On the surface, the 1990s, "decade of the blockbuster," looked like the best of times for the Medical Industrial Complex, and especially for the pharmaceutical sector, with Pfizer on its way to becoming lead dog. Along with its celebrity drug Viagra, it had also amassed six other billion-dollar market leaders: the antihypertensives Procardia, Cardura, and Norvasc; the antidepressant Zoloft; and two anti-infectives, the antifungal Diflucan and the antibiotic Zithromax. When these were combined with its hyperaggressive sales force and direct-to-consumer advertising, it was earning revenues that all its competitors envied.

But as the turn of the century approached, Pfizer and its competitors entered what would become an extended research-and-development slump that made continued double-digit profitability questionable. While Pfizer confidently issued quarterly reports reassuring investors that its rich and overflowing pipeline of emerging discoveries would soon pay off big, senior management meetings were overflowing with concern based on trend analyses that pointed to patent cliffs approaching for each and every blockbuster. The major chronic diseases were already under treatment, and the blockbuster fields were now overcrowded with me-too drugs that were cannibalizing one another. Cures for cancer, Alzheimer's disease, multiple sclerosis, and other diseases were nowhere on the immediate horizon. In addition, the genomic revolution was gaining steam, with new and aggressive biotech companies focused on promising the biologic cures of the future.

Financial analysts had seen the problem coming. In the late 1990s they pointed to three critical weaknesses in the pharmaceutical industry: the decade-long investment necessary to achieve approval of a new discovery, patent protection that bred overconfidence and eventually disappeared, and an overreliance on concentrated sales of a few blockbuster drugs. Combined, these factors created boom-and-bust cycles. The 1980s couldn't buy a discovery, but focus and determined investment eventually paid off in the spectacular decade of the 1990s. However, the first decade of the new millennium was far less certain.

Not everyone would agree with Lou Lasagna when he pegged the cost of bringing a new drug to market at something close to $1 billion, but few disagreed that drug development was an exceedingly high-risk, high-reward business. The process from first identifying a new chemical entity to gaining FDA approval could easily consume 10 years, requiring complex laboratory experiments to define safety, dosage, and basic properties, before progressively larger and more expensive clinical trials were conducted to prove effectiveness. And anywhere along the way, the potential new drug compound could fail, and 4,999 of every 5,000 did.[1]

No wonder, then, that the drug companies were scrambling to find shortcuts to profit through alternative means.

At Pfizer, the war room that Lou Clemente and Linda Robinson had built was repurposed in November 1999, not to launch another blockbuster, but to pull off a hostile takeover aimed at acquiring Lipitor, a cholesterol drug that would yield profits exceeding Viagra's 10 times over.[2] As the book *Barbarians at the Gate* had carefully documented a decade earlier, Linda was a seasoned veteran and a central figure in the hostile takeover of RJR Nabisco in 1988.

The current target was Warner-Lambert, founded by a Philadelphia pharmacist named William Warner at roughly the same time that the Pfizer cousins were setting up shop in New York. Its first big moneymaker had been a sugar shell that could hide the bitter taste of certain medicines. Over the next century, the company gained a footing in confectioneries like Trident, Chicklets, and Certs and in consumer health products like Rolaids, Lubriderm, and Listerine; and then moved into prescription drugs.

In 1970, Warner-Lambert acquired Parke-Davis, a once power-ful name in pharmaceuticals that had held the number one position in total revenues during the 1950s but then began to slide. By 1990, the merged company's early-generation cholesterol pill had gone off pat-ent and manufacturing irregularities had caused it to recall eight drugs, resulting in the loss of $130 million in sales. That left Warner-Lambert at number 22 in the pharmaceutical industry. With health care reform-ers making demands and profits slipping, the company severely cut back its sales force and shuttered most research divisions, electing to focus on cardiovascular disease, and specifically on a new statin compound called atorvastatin.[3] This new statin blocked the enzyme that creates cholesterol and indirectly promoted the reuptake of cholesterol deposits in the body.

In the 1990s, coronary artery disease was America's number one killer, with nearly a million heart attacks in the country each year—half of them fatal.[4] The Framingham Heart Study in 1980 had identified smok-ing, high blood pressure, and high blood cholesterol as major risk factors in heart disease. In 1985, the National Heart, Lung and Blood Institute at the NIH launched the National Cholesterol Education Program and identified cholesterol as a major cause of the plaque buildup that blocked the small arteries to heart muscle. Two years later, the group issued recom-mended blood levels for cholesterol, declaring levels below 200 milligrams per deciliter safe, 200 to 239 milligrams per deciliter borderline high, and more than 240 milligrams per deciliter high risk. In 1987, having worked on the issue for 45 years, Merck researchers discovered the first statin, Mevacor. Bristol-Myers Squibb followed in 1991 with Pravachol, which was followed by a second Merck entrant, Zocor, in 1992. Finally, Novartis surfaced a fourth derivative, Lescol, in 1994.[5]

To many within the investor community, being number five in the crowded statin field seemed like a bad bet.[3] But a phase I study in 1992 revealed that Warner-Lambert's new compound reduced the bad LDL cholesterol levels by 50 percent. A phase II study in 1995 showed a drop in total cholesterol of as much as 60 percent.[6] These results were dramatic enough to qualify the drug for FDA's new fast-track service, and a phase III study, focused on the rare familial hypercholesterolemia, earned it a "priority status review."[7] Head-to-head trials showed this new drug to be far superior to Merck's Zocor, and in December 1996, the company received FDA approval a year ahead of schedule. Atorvastatin, brand name Lipitor, was ready for market.[8]

Even though this was clearly the most effective statin available, Lipitor was widely criticized as a me-too in a crowded field. Warner-Lambert's powerful competitors had significant professional allies in cardiology who were both well-established and committed loyalists. Unwilling to fold, Warner-Lambert's president made the calculation that by taking on a partner, it could beef up its inadequate sales force and stay in the game. It considered five companies and in 1996 chose the marketing juggernaut Pfizer, which paid $205 million for the rights to sell Lipitor, while agreeing to split the costs for advertising, promotion, sampling, and sales, as well as sharing the cost of more than 100 ongoing phase IV clinical trials involving some 100,000 patients.[9] In return, Pfizer received 48 percent of net sales. Lipitor was aggressively priced to undercut Zocor and Mevacor by 27 percent and 34 percent, respectively.[10]

A national cholesterol-education program paved the way for the new entrant. In true MIC fashion, the campaign was funded by Pfizer and Warner-Lambert but administered through the nonprofit American Heart Association. Beginning in January 1997, samples fell like rain, with an astounding 7 million distributed in the first year, delivered to 91,000 prescribers by 2,500 commission-primed sales reps. In that first year, the sales force cataloged a total of 831,000 "medical community contacts," which translated into just under 30 percent of all "detail time" logged in doctors' offices.[10] The American Heart Association remained a reliable ally in the years ahead, with its advisory committees supporting a more restrictive definition of "normal" cholesterol levels and acceptable blood pressure readings in America's aging seniors, thus greatly expanding the number of patients who would be prescribed statins and antihypertensive drugs.

By October 1997, Lipitor was the market leader in its class, with a 30 percent share. Its $1 billion in first-year sales was 10 times greater than the $100 million Warner-Lambert had projected, and the drug was being sold in 50 countries.[10] Competitors poured money into the newly approved direct-to-consumer television advertising, but that seemed primarily to have the effect of increasing patient flow to doctors who then prescribed Lipitor. Midway through 1999, worldwide annual sales revenues for Lipitor were projected to approach $4 billion, and analysts were now saying that the drug, in its final patent year, 2010, would be likely to bring in $10 billion.[10]

As part of the co-marketing agreement with Warner-Lambert, Pfizer was prohibited from attempting to acquire the smaller company without its permission.[11] But Pfizer had heard rumors of a development that could undermine its co-marketing arrangement. Warner-Lambert was said to be considering a merger of equals with American Home Products.[12,13] Founded in 1926, AHP purchased the drug manufacturer Wyeth five years later. Over the next half century, it grew by acquiring numerous companies including Ayerst Laboratories and Ayerst's estrogen product Premarin in 1943, and A.H. Robins with consumer products ChapStick, Dimetapp, and Robitussin in 1989.[14]

Pfizer CEO Bill Steere approached Warner-Lambert chairman Lodewijk J.R. de Vink about acquiring his company, but the Dutchman had no interest in being courted.

Then, on November 3, 1999, the *Wall Street Journal* broke the news that a merger between Warner-Lambert and American Home Products were imminent, a marriage that, if consummated, would create one of the largest pharmaceutical companies in the world.[15] This reflected the enormous escalation of Warner-Lambert's valuation to $72 billion tied to its celebrated drug. That evening, despite several calls from Pfizer board members urging it not to act, the Warner-Lambert board voted to approve the American Home Products merger.[16]

Knowing when and where the signing and joint press conference were to take place, the Pfizer team organized a strategically timed communications offensive that had Linda Robinson's fingerprints all over it. As Warner-Lambert's Lodewijk and American Home Products CEO John Stafford delivered their carefully orchestrated performances, they received word, onstage, that Pfizer had just announced an unsolicited $82.4 billion stock offer for Warner-Lambert.[14,16,17]

Perhaps the most skilled of all MIC wheelers and dealers, Pfizer had spent years mastering a real-time, message-driven strategy to ensure that all vital constituencies would be engaged in unison. But here the targets were not state insurance boards or the Vatican but rather the owners of large blocks of stock, including big Wall Street players like Goldman Sachs and large pension managers like CalPERS. These investors were able to signal support for the deal through their stock purchases of the two companies, with rises in Pfizer's price per share and declines in Warner-Lambert's sweetening the Pfizer deal. Meanwhile, the public affairs chief and the head of media relations and investor relations kept the general and financial press, as well as individual shareholders, on Pfizer's side with positive articles appearing in the *Wall Street Journal* and *New York Times*.[17,18]

Finally, an integrated campaign driven by Pfizer's federal and state government relations departments, faced with two US senators requesting that the Federal Trade Commission examine the antitrust aspects of the proposed merger, reinforced in political circles the advantage of a Pfizer takeover—shareholder earnings, US domination of pharmaceuticals worldwide, explosive innovation, and jobs. As had been the case in the battle to gain Kaiser Permanente's agreement to support Viagra, this was not a fair fight.[18]

According to J.P. Morgan & Co., the company seeking to acquire another in the prior year had prevailed three-quarters of the time.[13] Three months later, Lodewijk de Vink was out and Pfizer was in.[18]

Warner-Lambert stockholders were richly rewarded with a deal worth $90.2 billion. John Stafford's American Home Products was $1.8 billion richer, thanks to a negotiated settlement agreement that had been built into its marriage plan with Warner-Lambert before Pfizer had disrupted it at the altar. Seven years later, Stafford and AHP, now renamed Wyeth, would be rewarded again with a $64 billion buyout deal from the very same Pfizer. But for now, Bill Steere was the head of both Pfizer and Warner-Lambert, owning Lipitor outright with more than 10 years of patent life left.[18]

Steere now oversaw 87,000 employees. His sales force was 7,500 strong, and his 12,000-plus researchers, housed in their state-of-the-art laboratories, were busy trying to come up with the next blockbuster.[18] The largesse of Pfizer and its pharmaceutical competitors was now flowing freely. High profitability helped fund academic clinical research institutes, medical education grants, journal advertising, and large-scale reprint purchases, as well as funding thought-leader physicians as speakers and advisers. Goodwill also flowed to hospitals nationwide in the form of corporate philanthropic grants and highly publicized overseas efforts to address everything from HIV to malaria to guinea worm and trachoma. The flush of cash also took the edge off negotiations between insurers and the drugmakers, which had additional wiggle room to compromise to meet the needs of their MIC partners and their employer clients.

The only cloud on their horizon was that investors were looking for a continuation of the spectacular rate of return that had far exceeded 20 percent over the last few years. To accomplish that feat for a company with Pfizer's valuation was unlikely. Steere was saying that the new company would cut $1.3 billion in overhead and deliver 25 percent growth per year over the next three years.[18] But with the Warner-Lambert merger, the huge market capitalization base of the "new Pfizer" meant that more dollars in earnings would be necessary to match institutional investors' high expectations.

On the day of the deal, February 8, 2000, the Pfizer stock price closed, with investors' great optimism, at $37 a share. Choosing his moment well, on August 11, 2000, with the stock price hovering at $43, Bill Steere announced his retirement. At the end of the year, Steere stepped down, and Hank McKinnell, then president, assumed the top post. Steere's parting words were unintentionally ironic: "It's the perfect time to leave. I've done my part. We're No. 1. Now Hank has to figure out how to keep us there."[19] Almost immediately the share price began a relentless march downward. A decade later it would dip into the mid-teens before finding its bottom.[20]

Lou Clemente looked to assume the same trusted adviser role for McKinnell that he had enjoyed with Steere, but the new CEO never embraced the idea of an independent, muscular, Corporate Affairs department reporting directly to the CEO. Six months after Steere retired, Clemente announced that he, too, would be stepping down within a year.

To address the fears of his board and his executive team, McKinnell leaned on his strategic planners for analytics that would quantify the risks they faced in the coming years. What he and others saw was not at all reassuring. Every blockbuster that had carried Pfizer to the top was now heading toward patent expiration, and the increasingly aggressive generic manufacturers were licking their chops in anticipation.

Traditionally, when major pharmaceutical drugs went off patent, the company would abandon production, and generic companies would pick up production at a small fraction of the cost—often 20 to 30 percent of the original price. Pfizer had three choices. It could continue to roll the dice and hope that its researchers would finally generate a major commercial discovery, or it could continue to produce and market its own branded generic. In this scenario, Lipitor wouldn't disappear as a trusted brand, but it would now be heavily advertised and outcompete the generic brand that was a bit cheaper but not as familiar to patients. The third choice was to do both of these things, a course Pfizer and its major competitors increasingly embraced.

As 2002 arrived, Pfizer had produced only two new drugs since the 1998 approval of Viagra and the hastily removed broad-spectrum antibiotic Trovan, which lawsuits had proved caused liver damage and death in some patients. These were the antischizophrenic Geodon, which contributed a mere $150 million in 2001; and a minor antifungal drug, Vfend. Seeing the need for an immediate transfusion, McKinnell chose a two-prong plan: pursuing new products through acquisition and new policies.[21]

On the product side, McKinnell went in hot pursuit of Pharmacia, Pfizer's marketing partner for arthritis all-star Celebrex, part of a brand-new class of pain relievers called cycloxygenase-2, or COX-2, inhibitors. Merck already had the COX-2 market leader, a drug named Vioxx. COX-2 enzymes normally increase the amount of prostaglandin, a chemical that promotes inflammatory responses in the body. When COX-2 production is inhibited, inflammation and pain decrease. The drugs had a low addiction profile and were projected to reach as many as 50 million arthritis sufferers over the next seven years.[22]

Pharmacia CEO Fred Hassan had resisted McKinnell's advances for more than a year, but on July 16, 2002, the two companies announced a $53 billion all-stock transaction. The prize was not only Celebrex, already a billion-dollar blockbuster, but the son of Celebrex, Bextra, which was waiting in the wings.[23]

But then the wheels began to come off the entire COX-2 bandwagon. Merck's Vioxx was pulled off the market after it was revealed that the company had concealed a secondary effect of the drug that was responsible for close to 30,000 heart attacks.[24,25] Declaring nobly that it was reaffirming the company's mission of "putting patients first," Merck set aside some $5 billion to settle the claims of US patients alone.[26]

The FDA subsequently declared the entire class of drugs, including Pfizer's Celebrex and Bextra, fundamentally dangerous.[27] This meant that the drug's packaging now carried the dreaded "black box warning" alerting consumers and health care providers to safety concerns including life-threatening risks. Two months later, the FDA asked Pfizer to pull Bextra off the market, which it did.[28] But after learning that the Celebrex safety profile was somewhat better than either Vioxx's or Bextra's, the company fought to save the one drug left standing in the class.[29] Pfizer pulled its direct-to-consumer advertising for the product so as to not further upset clinicians and patients, and sales slipped accordingly.[30] But the company quietly reinforced sales-rep visits on behalf of the product, and after looking at their other options, none of which were risk-free, a sizable proportion of doctors remained supportive. A few years later, after both print and television ads were revived, sales of Celebrex were once again over $2 billion, but this was far below original projections.[31]

For several years, McKinnell and other pharmaceutical CEOs had recognized that new product discoveries were not "just around the corner," as optimistic scientists had predicted. They had already begun to pull back on their R&D support, which in the days of Viagra had been approaching 20 percent of revenue, and by 2006 would be slightly below 15 percent.[32] At the same time, industry spending on direct-to-consumer advertising, meant to squeeze every last dime out of existing products, was on the rise. Between 2000 and 2005, industry-wide direct-to-consumer advertising

spending increased by 330 percent, with total US pharmaceutical promotional spending exceeding $30 billion in 2005.[33]

In addition to the COX-2 product challenges, the purchase of Pharmacia had brought a very significant liability tail. Pfizer would pay close
to $1 billion to settle initial suits related to the two drugs, and would be
forced to pay $2.3 billion to the government to settle charges of cherry-
picking data and misleading the public about Bextra and other products.[34]
The company also paid $1.4 billion for the rights to a flawed inhalation
device for insulin that, when it failed, led to a total write-off of $2.8 bil-
lion.[35] During the same period, Pfizer bet on an antismoking drug that
allegedly caused psychiatric crises,[36] as well as a cholesterol drug that
would soon be found to cause a 60 percent increase in cardiac deaths
among those using it in clinical trials.[37]

With product-oriented profit strategies failing, McKinnell and other
pharmaceutical CEOs embraced policy changes as their potential salva-
tion. They were not alone. The new millennium was a wake-up call for
members of the Medical Industrial Complex. In the 1980s and 1990s,
Reagan's wave of deregulation and broad industry support, and Clinton's
economic policies during his second term, combined with an increasingly
aging population, had sent health care prices soaring.

Employers and insurers had instituted a range of cost-control measures under the mantra of "managed care," which by the end of the 1990s
had accomplished little beyond sending the AMA and its members into
open revolt, claiming intrusion on their sacred professional autonomy.
Hospitals, at the same time feeling the economic pressures, were creating
vertically integrated networks and alliances in an effort to eliminate regional
competition. This required heavy investment in buildings, technology,
and information systems. The large academic institutions were pursuing
industry investment and partnerships in on-campus research facilities to
support hoped-for NIH grants. Meanwhile, NIH director Francis Collins
was promising Congress and the American public a "new age of genomics,"
with a wave of new cures on the immediate horizon. Industry and academic
medicine were happy to accept his money but were far less optimistic.

Under these pressures, members of the MIC began to look inventively at new solutions to maintaining control of their profitability, and what they discovered was one another. Whereas in the past, each of the major pillars of the Medical Industrial Complex was content to go its own way, engaging now and then in intramural pricing skirmishes in pursuit of an ever-growing percentage of the nation's resources, all of them now realized that they were approaching a possible ceiling at 20 percent of GDP.

At the same time, a widely publicized government report claiming as many as 190,000 avoidable safety-related hospital deaths per year, and a World Health Organization comparative national health report showing the US at the bottom in a range of quality measures, raised the uncomfortable question, "What exactly is America getting for its health care dollar?"

As the 2000 presidential election approached, the pillars of the MIC found common ground in the expansion of their federal and state government relations operations, which increasingly embraced well-coordinated political activism.[38] They found plenty of room for agreement in support of unencumbered free enterprise, high returns on investment, intentional complexity and opacity when it came to patient billing, and proprietary control of patient data for all MIC members.

Key to the success of all these objectives was the election of George W. Bush, who had courted major leaders from medicine, pharmaceuticals, hospitals, and insurers and expressed interest in privatizing the management of Medicare and Medicaid, as well as covering pharmaceutical costs for seniors over 65.

Bush's election in 2000 provided the MIC proof of concept that quietly colluding and cooperating with one another in Washington, DC, while publicly appearing to compete with one another around the country in support of patients' interests, was a winning strategy. Along the way, their loose coalition was drawing new converts. For example, the AARP leadership had begun preliminary discussions with UnitedHealthcare on how they might share the spoils of members' purchases of future Medicare Part D drug plans, as well as privatized Medicare Advantage plans, and industry-supported patient advocacy groups had been quick to mobilize when called to action during the 2000 election.

After Bush's victory, the number of MIC lobbyists grew exponentially. Pfizer government relations funded 82 lobbyists in 2000 to support Republican control of Congress and the White House.[38] A year later the pharmaceutical industry as a whole spent $78 million on lobbying activities and employed 623 different lobbyists.

In the run-up to the 2002 midterms, Pfizer's New York headquarters had the look of a Republican campaign office, with candidates, pollsters, and consultants wandering the halls, strategizing, comparing notes, and making presentations. At Pfizer, both state and federal government relations were being run by the Republican former speaker of the New Jersey state assembly, Chuck Hartwick, who had also served as vice chairman of the Republican National Convention Platform Committee. After Lou Clemente's departure, Hartwick had been put in charge of Corporate Affairs, but his shop was less the intricate, interdepartmental, strategic, and holistic public affairs machine of the past and more government relations on steroids. The fact that Chuck, a longtime employee of a major pharmaceutical company, had simultaneously headed the main legislative body of the state with the largest concentration of pharmaceutical company multinationals in the world, along with the fact that he had held an official leadership role for the Republican Party, raised no eyebrows. Business as usual within the Medical Industrial Complex was also business as usual at the New Jersey statehouse.[39]

The GOP spent just under a billion dollars on the midterm elections, ran 1.5 million television ads, and gained eight seats in the House. More important, in achieving a net gain of two seats in the Senate, Republicans now enjoyed a majority of 51 to 49 and controlled both houses of Congress.[40,41]

Democratic leadership wasted little time in laying some of the blame at the feet of the pharmaceutical industry. The day after the election, House minority leader Dick Gephardt told the *New York Times*, "What you've got to look at is the incredible amount of special interest money that was on their side. There were races where we were outspent 4 to 1, 5 to 1, the pharmaceutical companies probably spent $60 million across the country."[40]

The MIC list of legislative objectives now was focused on Medicare prescription drug coverage and the privatization of government health plans. Funding drug insurance coverage was a high priority since it would expand sales for the pharmaceutical industry, reimburse hospitals for drug costs, and provide new sales opportunities for insurers as legions of seniors purchased Medicare Part D plans and partially privatized Medicare Advantage plans.[42,43]

There was also a growing recognition that health care resources were not unlimited and that, if cost control were to be part of their combined future, the MIC was best positioned to manage and profit from the process. As for the Bush team, they were already focusing on a second term, which required staying below the radar and neutralizing the claim that Bush secretly wanted to privatize Medicare.[44]

The MIC had made the calculation that it simply needed more paying customers for its existing products. Insurers would profit from sale of the policies, doctors and hospitals would have fewer "no pay" customers, and drug companies would sell more drugs. Ironically, this ploy, the expansion of federal insurance coverage, was a complete reversal of the Medical Industrial Complex position for over a half century. Historically, the MIC had viewed encroachments by government into direct health services, and especially those requiring the support of American taxpayers, as a slippery slope toward rationing and price controls.

But winning the election turned out to be easier than expanding prescription coverage under Medicare.

Ten years earlier, when President Bill Clinton first proposed the idea, expanded prescription coverage had been defeated by a coalition of the health insurance and pharmaceutical industries, which were then still so profitable that they didn't see the value of sharing further control of their activities with government. But now all were convinced that the government's interests and their own were aligning. Also, there was real money to be made in managing, or appearing to manage, cost and data, and they were already partway there.

In 1993, Merck had invested in a data management firm that was able to track the pricing, distribution, and sale of drugs, while supporting the fulfillment of patient prescriptions on a retail level. By automating the system and directing patient purchasers toward preferred lower-cost products like generics or Merck's own brand-name drugs, it hoped to turn a profit on the operation.

This new MIC player was called a pharmacy benefit manager. Merck's PBM was called Medco, and within a few years it had become more profitable than Merck by inserting itself into the middle of the pharmaceutical supply chain.[45] CVS and UnitedHealthcare also parented their own PBMs. While unified government relations initiatives provided a common planning site and meeting ground for socializing MIC members, PBMs increasingly filled a structural need to support a new era focused on patient data mining and opaque profit sharing within the increasingly organized MIC syndicate.

The Bush administration pushed legislation called the Medicare Modernization Bill, intended to put the popular entitlement program on firmer financial footing while expanding prescription coverage. Most of Washington now agreed that reform was necessary to bring the cost of managing seniors with illnesses under control, but the bill's proponents were hammered from both sides with arguments that private-sector incentives had gone either too far or not far enough.[46] By June 2003, budget resolutions in the House and Senate committed $400 billion for Medicare reform.[47]

The battle centered on the Medicare Advantage or Medicare Part C plans that had been created in 1997.[44,48] These federally subsidized Medicare plans offered seniors who voluntarily chose them, rather than choosing traditional fee-for-service Medicare, additional benefits like health maintenance and wellness offerings and, in varying amounts, prescription coverage. Private insurers had been recruited by the Clinton administration to manage these plans, and shared in any profits derived from management efficiencies. But absent price controls, as costs of hospitalization and drugs rose steeply in the late 1990s, insurers pulled back on extra benefits, especially pharmaceuticals, and the numbers choosing Medicare Part C declined.[44,49]

Bush's original plan was to provide his new prescription benefit only to seniors within Medicare who chose his partially privatized Medicare Part C—Medicare Advantage. But when the administration was presented with an outcry of unfairness from both Republicans and Democrats, he backed down and decided that a freestanding drug benefit, dubbed Medicare Part D, should be available as a voluntary choice for those who decided to stay with traditional Medicare as well.

To protect the interests of his key pharmaceutical and insurance industry supporters, Bush agreed that the plans would be administered through private insurers which, in turn, would negotiate against one another and with the newly empowered intermediary pharmacy benefit management companies like Merck's Medco and CVS Caremark over pricing. Insurers would be allowed to use various formularies that generally grouped drugs into two or three categories or tiers, with the best prices for consumers restricted to cost-effective drugs in column one, and higher-price options dropping into column two or three and costing consumers considerably more. Protecting the industry's need for choice and coverage of me-too drugs, the legislation also required that each category of drug have at least two options available. With this scheme, Bush committed to no direct government negotiation on Medicare drug purchases. In addition, he declared importation of Canadian low-cost drugs illegal, based on the dubious assertion that the safety of the drugs and the absence of counterfeit products could not be ensured, even though they were supplied by U.S. multinational companies.[50]

Canadians paid roughly half of what Americans paid because of the role of referee played by the Canadian national health care system. Each year, it collected pricing information from six European nations (France, Germany, Italy, Sweden, United Kingdom, and Switzerland) and the United States for all drugs on its approved drug list, and then used a formula to establish what the average price would be in Canada for each drug in the coming year. The entire procedure was conducted in the open, and middlemen profiteers were kept to a minimum.[51]

To further sweeten the deal for pharmaceutical companies, Bush agreed to a rule that would force 6.5 million "dual eligible" individuals (those then covered by both Medicaid and Medicare as a result of disability or extreme poverty) into Medicare drug coverage.[52] This group was currently receiving its drugs through state Medicaid programs. Pharmaceutical companies were required under federal law to set their prices for Medicaid programs at the lowest market price available to any and all plans nationwide. This rule, termed the Maximum Allowable Cost (MAC) provision, greatly curtailed pharmaceutical companies' profitability in supplying this poor and vulnerable segment of the population. In transferring dual eligibles to the Medicare Part D plans, where drug costs had no government controls, Bush assured the pharmaceutical companies of an additional markup of 25 percent on drug revenues from these patients.[49]

Conservatives worried about the cost, which they felt the administration had understated, and which they placed at $410 billion over 10 years.[52] Consumers worried about the complicated design that left them to pay a portion—dubbed "the doughnut hole," sitting as it did between initial purchases that were covered and higher thresholds that, once reached, also triggered coverage.[53] Overall, the government was committed to covering three-quarters of the bill, and consumers, through deductibles and co-payments, would have to manage the rest.[54]

Traditionalists within the MIC, like the American Medical Association, were early supporters. AMA members generally believed in expanding coverage for their patients, but their primary concern was the long-standing anxiety that any changes would be a foot in the door for socialized medicine. Once Bush established that there would be no direct government negotiation with drug companies, others lined up as well, including the American Association of Health Plans, the American Hospital Association, and the Business Roundtable. The health insurance industry saw the legislation as a source of new revenue, and as a solution to the deteriorating Managed Medicare (Medicare Part C) situation. By establishing another source of federal dollars to cover their pharmaceutical cost, industry sponsors of Managed Medicare (Medicare Part C) plans could once again offer a range of extra benefits that would entice seniors into these lucrative options and away from less profitable traditional Medicare. If the MIC coalition held, Medicare Part D and its new drug benefits could reinforce Managed Medicare and ensure a bright future.[44,46,47]

One serious concern remaining was the AARP, which had managed to scuttle Reagan's catastrophic care bill years before. That experience taught everyone that politicians messed with older Americans' beloved entitlements at their own risk. Seniors felt they had earned the privilege of health care coverage in their golden years; on the other hand, rich seniors had little interest in paying a premium to support poor seniors.

In addition, the media was not giving a pass to this complex sweetheart deal in which the MIC was paid in full and patients were saddled with partial coverage and ever more billing complexity. E. J. Dionne, in a *Washington Post* story titled "Medicare Monstrosity," wrote, "How do you know this bill is such a great deal for the drug companies and HMOs? On word of an agreement last week, share prices soared."[55]

There also was evidence of a more widespread dissatisfaction far beyond the Beltway. A 2003 poll taken shortly before the bill was passed found that 47 percent of seniors opposed the change, while only 26 percent approved. Their opposition derived from the fact that the president's original proposal offered drug coverage only to seniors who opted for the privately managed Medicare C plans. Seniors feared this was the first step toward dismantling Medicare as they knew it. But Billy Tauzin (R-LA), chairman of the House Energy and Commerce Committee, announced, "You couldn't move my mother out of [fee-for-service] Medicare with a bulldozer. She trusts in it, believes in it. It's served her well." Then he suggested that his colleagues "almost certainly will want a strong and adequate prescription drug benefit within fee-for-service Medicare," and the president reinforced once again that the program would include all Medicare recipients.[54]

Bush's advisers had cautioned that the Iraq invasion that spring would distract Congress from focusing on the bill, and yet the Senate Finance Committee produced a "bipartisan agreement" in June. Seven days later, the two-page outline had taken on flesh, thanks to some heavy lifting by

MIC lobbyists, and from there it emerged as a rather complete 90-page tome, which passed out of committee on June 13.[54,56]

AARP remained the big unknown, but now led by Bill Novelli, the cofounder of the huge health care PR firm and Pfizer favorite Porter-Novelli,[54,57] clearly it was not the same organization that had turned Reagan's catastrophic health plan on its head. Having sealed a profit-sharing deal with the fastest-growing national health insurer, UnitedHealthcare, to provide its members with supplemental health insurance, AARP was now more than ever heavily invested in the commercial side of the Medical Industrial Complex and positioned to be a major beneficiary of Medicare Advantage Part C and Part D plans that carried the new pharmaceutical subsidies.[58]

Novelli's reach inside government had been expansive, extending all the way from an assist to the Nixon reelection campaign against George McGovern to a cordial relationship with 1990s Republican superstar and Clinton's nemesis Newt Gingrich. Even so, it surprised the Democratic leadership to discover on the morning of November 17, 2003, that AARP had committed $7 million to a public campaign in support of the Bush bill.[58] "The endorsement provides a seal of approval from an organization with 35 million members," one analyst noted. "Republicans also hope it provides political cover against charges by some Democrats that the bill would undermine the federal insurance program for the elderly and disabled."[59]

Novelli and the AARP leadership justified their move as the best opportunity they had to advance pharmaceutical coverage for their members. Even so, 60,000 members were suspicious of the profit-sharing arrangement between AARP and UnitedHealthcare and sufficiently worried about potential threats to their Medicare that as a result they either resigned or declined the annual renewal of their membership by the end of Bush's second term.[59]

Five days after the AARP announcement, at 3 a.m. on a Saturday, after a full day of arm-twisting and dealing, the House bill was allowed to come up for a vote. After 15 minutes, Bush's supporters were 15 votes behind, and the bill was held open. After further concessions to individual holdouts, it was still two votes short at 216–218. With everything at stake,

HHS secretary Tommy Thompson was sent to lobby on the House floor, an action seldom taken. President Bush himself, just back from a visit with the queen of England, was awakened at 4 a.m. to lobby the few remaining undecideds. The "longest roll call vote in history," lasting just under three hours, came in at 220–215 in favor. Three days later, after some political maneuvering, the bill passed in the Senate.[60]

On December 8, 2003, with great fanfare, President Bush signed the Medicare Modernization Act in a heavily staged event. Declaring the legislation "a victory for America's seniors," he went on to say, "I'm pleased that all of you are here to witness the greatest advance in health care coverage for America's seniors since the founding of Medicare." With no evidence of irony, and no acknowledgment that within living memory the Republican Party had called Medicare a threat to the American way of life, he added, "And today, by reforming and modernizing this vital program, we are honoring the commitments of Medicare to all our seniors."[60]

With the help of Big Pharma and Big Business generally, Bush comfortably won reelection over John Kerry. The AARP and its partner, UnitedHealthcare, secured a hefty chunk of the expanding Managed Medicare (Medicare Part C) and Medicare Part D business, and the pharmaceutical industry indulged for the moment in a self-congratulatory, if short-lived, celebration.

But the most lasting impact of the deliberations that led up to the Medicare Modernization Act was the conversion of the MIC from a loose network of major sectors with casual connections to health delivery, and a penchant for joining forces only when its own status quo was threatened, into a complex, still loosely strung syndicate committed to self-control and distributing the profits secretly among its members in the form of opaque negotiated rebates, invisible to the consumer, at the point of sale. In the center of the food chain were the MIC's newest creations, the pharmacy benefit managers, or PBMs, designed as vehicles to organize the movement of data, drugs, and money throughout the MIC supply chain.

When PBMs began, insurers and employers believed that this new entity might contribute to cost control by efficiently processing prescriptions, maintaining approved drug formularies, and holding down prices. But they soon realized that ownership of a PBM by a drugmaker, an insurer, or a giant retail pharmacy allowed the owner to coordinate pricing decisions, see competitors' pricing information, and favor some drugs over others in return for kickback payments, even if the consumer unknowingly was forced to pay more.

There are now about thirty different PBMs. But three major companies control 78 percent of the PBM market and service 180 million Americans.[61] These opportunistic middlemen emerged from three different MIC industry sectors: a physician managed care group, a pharmacy corporation, and a pharmaceutical manufacturing company.

The first one, Diversified Prescription Delivery, was developed in 1988 by UnitedHealthcare, the insurance company that grew out of a physician-run managed care medical group called Charter Med, incorporated in 1974. United Healthcare was the first to recognize that new information technology would revolutionize the health care industry. Whereas the WHO owned the ICD-9 diagnosis billing code databases, and the AMA owned the CPT procedure billing code databases, United-Healthcare had far more expansive ambitions—to control and mine actual patient databases. From this perch, it was the first to develop pharmacy drug formularies, hospital admission pre-certification requirements, physician office software that predated electronic medical records, and tight controls on utilization beyond those of other HMOs at the time.[61]

The realization that data now was king spread rapidly. A second PBM, PharmaCare, appeared as an offering from CVS in 1994, and in 2007 was renamed CVS-Caremark.[62] The third dominant PBM, mail-order giant Express Scripts, has a complex parentage. It was formed from the purchase of a SmithKline Beecham's PBM in 1999 and the addition of Merck-Medco in 2012.[63] Five years later, in 2017, Express Scripts reported revenue of over $100 billion compared with Pfizer's $52 billion of revenue that year.[64]

The PBMs' sphere of influence and market power derive from the fact that approximately 4.5 billion prescriptions are filled in the US each year. Americans' appetite for legal drugs is close to insatiable. Just under

50 percent of US residents have filled a prescription in the last month, and 10 percent of our population currently take five or more prescription medications. Approximately $50 billion is expended each year in the manufacturing of these drugs, which move primarily through three giant wholesale distributors in the US—AmerisourceBergen, Cardinal Health, and McKesson—on the way to the retail pharmacy. Their combined revenue in 2015 was $378 billion for distributing the drugs to 60,000 pharmacy outlets, 63 percent of which are part of large retail chains. By 2017, their combined revenue reached $481 billion.[65]

PBMs are now the Grand Central Terminal of the legal trade of drugs and the primary processors of patient and insurance enrollee data. They negotiate the deals for each and every drug with pharmaceutical companies, the placement of those drugs on insurers' and employers' tiered insurer formulary drug lists, and the integration and management of utilization and cost strategies with pharmacies, insurers, and hospitals nationwide. Their cutouts and givebacks to the drug and the insurance industries, and negotiations with hospital systems, involve sharing the profits and are nontransparent. Nearly everyone is in on the deal—except the patient.

What makes it all the more shocking is the fact that this bloated financial system of drug and data distribution frequently fails to provide drugs when and where they are needed. In 2006, the FDA listed 55 drugs as being in short supply. By 2011 that number had grown to 350, and in 2018 it hovered around 110. While in the past five years there has been a focused effort to improve the system, when Hurricane Maria all but destroyed production facilities in Puerto Rico, a manageable shortage of sodium chloride intravenous fluids became a medical emergency.

Breaks in the supply chain are common enough that they support an army of gray-market price gougers—off-line distributors functioning as commodity traders outside the normal supply chain, which try to predict coming shortages, rush in to buy up a supply, and then resell it at exorbitant prices to desperate hospitals and pharmacies. Add to this a surprising number of gray-market U.S. counterfeiters. For example, in 2003, Pfizer was forced to recall millions of Lipitor tablets that had been counterfeited and packaged to be indistinguishable from the real product. But the product didn't come from China or India. It came through a variety of U.S. gray-market distributors including Med-Pro in Nebraska, Albers Medical in Missouri, and Alliance Pharmaceutical in Illinois.[65,66,67]

An American Hospital Association survey in 2011 revealed that 82 percent of its hospital members had delayed therapies because of drug shortages. In May, 2018, 9 out of 10 emergency room doctors reported a shortage of a critical drug in their department over the previous month.[67,68,69] That same month, Ruth Landau, an obstetric anesthesiologist at New York-Presbyterian Hospital, received a request from the hospital pharmacist to ration the use of bupivacaine, the main drug used for epidural anesthesia during childbirth. At the time, her frustration was evident in her comment to *Fortune* magazine. She said, "Suddenly, we're being told this one drug—the one we've been using for decades, that we know best how to give, how fast it kicks in, we can do it with our eyes shut—suddenly, we're being told we won't have that drug."[70]

While PBMs quietly orchestrate the movement of immense amounts of drugs, money, and data in the MIC network, with a supply chain that includes wholesalers supplying pharmacies across the nation, they play a minimal role in oversight. This became abundantly clear in 2016 when the major drug wholesalers AmerisourceBergen, Cardinal Health, and McKesson were charged by the Department of Justice and the DEA with receiving $17 billion for supplying 423 million tablets of OxyContin to 55 counties in West Virginia between 2007 and 2012. Nine million pills were shipped to one pharmacy alone over a two-year period. Six of the 55 counties had the highest opioid overdose rates in the United States, and over 2,000 of their citizens died from the drugs.[71]

As the human carnage of the opioid epidemic continues to pile up, the MIC syndicate is now focused on formalizing its territorial control through cross-sector integration and mergers and acquisitions. Cigna CEO David Cordani said as much to investors when Cigna offered $67 billion to purchase Express Scripts in 2018. "When we think about Express Scripts," he explained, "it has PBM capabilities, but it has 27,000 individuals and a significant number of consumer touch points around health and well being. It expands our service portfolio beyond that of a PBM. Having the capabilities to serve an individual whether they are healthy, healthy at risk, chronic or acute is important."[72] Meanwhile, CVS, the parent of PBM Caremark, went the other way. That same year, the retailer made a $69 billion offer to purchase health insurer Aetna.[73]

President Bush may have inadvertently spawned the early development of a more formally integrated MIC, but his successor, Barack Obama, solidified the control of these inside players over the health care status quo. Whereas the bargaining chip with the former president was the expansion of drug coverage for seniors, the payoff for his successor was the expansion of health insurance coverage to America's most vulnerable citizens. The MIC would exact a heavy price for its support, and then sit silently by as Republican leaders supported by a Russian intelligence–led social media criminal enterprise worked diligently to collapse the very patient protections and coverage that had anchored the legislation.[74]

Chapter 14

Time to Deal

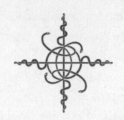

B y 2006, when the MIC had fully aligned with the administration of George W. Bush and Medicare Part D, Pfizer had 110,000 employees and a $7 billion annual research budget. It was also generating $8 billion a year in profits on $51 billion in sales, derived primarily from a combination of aging 1990 blockbusters and drugs like Lipitor and Celebrex that had been picked up through the acquisition of former competitors. Expanded government coverage of pharmaceuticals might provide a hedge against a few setbacks, but there was nothing in the works to replace Lipitor, which alone generated more than $12 billion a year in sales. The large numbers of employees and the bloated valuation of the company were not a reflection of true financial health, or of any immediate breakthrough discoveries on the horizon, but the simple result of Pfizer's having ingested Warner-Lambert and Pharmacia. The drug business was fundamentally different, with generics having grown from 36 percent in 1994 to represent 63 percent of all pharmaceutical sales in 2007.[1]

The basic business model, which relied on a steady stream of new discoveries whose profits could be reinforced by direct-to-consumer advertising and compliant physician prescribing, had imploded. With no new blockbuster discoveries, and nothing new to sell, cost cutting seemed to be the only tool at a CEO's disposal, and Pfizer wielded it by eliminating the employees and manufacturing and research sites of acquired companies. Pfizer employees themselves were not immune, especially the sales force, which had nothing new to sell or promote. Meanwhile, the political atmosphere inside Pfizer was turning it into a shark tank.

The feeling at Pfizer that the party might be over was shared throughout the Medical Industrial Complex. In 2007, health care inflation overall was 5.2 percent while the consumer price index measure for all inflation rose by only 2.8 percent. Economists blamed the cost of hospitals, drugs, and medical devices for the majority of the rise. Hospitals were overwhelmed trying to address safety and quality concerns. Doctors and patients were struggling to adjust to new electronic medical record systems and receive the payments they were due from insurers—a situation leading nearly half of all physicians to become employees of rapidly expanding health care systems. And employers, seeing rising employee health premiums, leaned heavily on insurers.

As prospects turned south, and Pfizer struggled to identify a path for its future, so did the leadership of all the various MIC segments. Pfizer's travails, repeated and amplified by the financial press, provided a cautionary tale absorbed by health executives of all stripes concerned about their own standing in their organizations.

Since the heady days of 1998, Pfizer had expended $180 billion in acquisitions and $55 billion in research to develop only nine marketed new medicines and only a single billion-dollar blockbuster. Two of its old standards—Norvasc for hypertension and Zoloft for depression—had already lost patents, and Lipitor for high cholesterol would follow in 2011. With those and other losses, Pfizer sales were projected to decline by 40 percent by 2012, leaving the company with a projected $18 billion decline in sales in five years.[2]

By 2006, research operations seemed to have ground to a halt. Pfizer's lawyers were now discovering all the hidden liability that came with its megamergers, including suits filed by patients and by internal whistle-blowers exposing illegal marketing practices tied to new products it now owned. The previous four years had witnessed a long, continuous, and contentious battle to limit the liability inherited from acquired firms. Leading that battle had been a confrontational trial lawyer and former executive of GE and McDonald's, Jeff Kindler, hired as the general counsel by Hank McKinnell in January 2002.[1,3]

On July 29, 2006, the Pfizer board, with the encouragement of former CEO Bill Steere, released McKinnell and elevated Jeff Kindler to be the new CEO. At the time, roughly 25 percent of Pfizer's revenue was attributable to sales of Lipitor. Kindler placed most of his hope for a replacement for that aging star on a substance called torcetrapib, which had been found to raise HDL, the "good cholesterol." His research team had been so confident that raising HDL would lower the risk of death in high-risk cardiac patients, and that torcetrapid would compensate for the loss of Lipitor, that they had designed a study to test the new drug against Lipitor itself. They enrolled 15,000 patients and embarked on the two-year project.[4] If the results turned out to be as good as the company hoped, Pfizer's long discovery drought would be over, and finally there would be an answer to the financial analysts' persistent question, "What are you going to do after Lipitor goes off patent?"

As one top executive told me, "As torcetrapib goes, so goes Pfizer." In late November 2006, Kindler staked his claim, saying publicly that the drug "will be one of the most important compounds of our generation."[3] But a week later, on December 4, 2006, the sky fell in. Early analysis of results from the clinical trial demonstrated that the drug raised "good cholesterol" as predicted, but it inexplicably killed off patients at an alarming rate: Study subjects taking the drug had a 60 percent increase in cardiac deaths over the control group. For a company that had spent the past five years fighting off an ever-increasing mountain of lawsuits, pulling the plug was a no-brainer.[2,4,5]

Kindler slashed 10,000 jobs, including 20 percent of Pfizer's sales force.[6,7] These were challenging times for drug reps in general. In 2005, an organization led by internist Bob Goodman, called No Free Lunch, had applied to have an exhibit booth at the annual convention of the American Academy of Family Physicians (AAFP). Goodman's organization was encouraging physicians to limit sales visits and refuse any gifts from pharmaceutical reps. The AAFP, in deference to its pharmaceutical supporters, refused to allow the exhibit. No Free Lunch went public with the snub, and one week later the AAFP reversed its position and rented exhibit space to the organization.[8] During the next 10 years, the numbers of general and specialist physicians willing to see drug reps would drop from 80 percent of doctors to 50 percent.[9]

Given this trend, and given the fact that Pfizer had very little new to sell, firing sales reps was a fairly obvious step. The more questionable move for a company looking to the future was eliminating six R&D sites as well as research projects in 10 disease areas. Pfizer investment in R&D had now declined from nearly 20 percent of its top-line revenues to just 11 percent by 2007, even as the actual cost of research continued to grow. And Pfizer was facing 14 patent expirations by 2014 that carried a projected loss of revenue of $35 billion over those seven years.[10]

Kindler had watched how McKinnell's political gamesmanship—assuming the helm at Pharmaceutical Research and Manufacturers of America (PhRMA) and championing all things Republican in two George Bush administrations—had helped secure Medicare Part D. The next election seemed likely to go to the Democrats, and Kindler was a Democratic Party activist and a substantial contributor to Democratic causes. In spring 2008, he gave the maximum allowable to Hillary Clinton in the Democratic primary, then deftly shifted support to Barack Obama when it became clear he would be the candidate.[11,12] His trips to Washington were frequent enough that active rumors spread throughout the company that he had more interest in joining a new Democratic administration than in running Pfizer.

Also that spring, Kindler made a friendly call to Bernard Poussot, the CEO of Wyeth, the company that had been spun off by American Home Products during the battle for Warner-Lambert. This led to talk of a merger, but then the financial industry collapsed in 2007–2008, and along with it the global economy.[10]

But like most elements of the MIC, Pfizer had a way of making even hard times work for itself. With competitors unable to secure financing from any of the large banks (all of which were struggling merely to survive in the wake of the 2008 banking collapse), Pfizer was able to drive down the price of Wyeth. The only wrinkle was that much of Pfizer's vast stockpile of cash sat overseas in places like Ireland, where it was taxed at 5 percent. If the company brought that cash back inside the US to finance this deal, it could be taxed at 34 percent.[10]

Armies of lawyers and accountants found a way around some of the tax issues by paying for Wyeth overseas properties with Pfizer overseas money. But that left $22.5 billion in loans to be secured from a jittery group of bankers that included Goldman Sachs, JPMorgan Chase, Citigroup, Bank of America, and Barclays. Ultimately, the acquisition went through and was announced on January 25, 2009, with a price tag of $68 billion, the first big deal since the economic collapse. That price was considered by analysts to be a good deal since the combined companies were expected to generate $20 billion in cash annually.[10]

There was considerable duplication between Pfizer and Wyeth, which meant that Pfizer could sell pieces and use the cash to pay off debt. And of course, there were redundant R&D sites and employees that could be cut. Another 20,000 people got the ax, half at Pfizer, along with 4 more of its remaining 46 manufacturing sites.[13,14]

Even so, Kindler predicted "flat earnings for the next three years" and cut Pfizer's quarterly dividends in half. Providing some hope, the combined entity would have several billion-dollar-a-year blockbusters, as well as Wyeth's experience in high-tech biologic and vaccine businesses, which were seen by most to be the future of the industry.

As Barack Obama prepared to assume the presidency, Kindler was on deck as chairman-elect of PhRMA. At that time, the organization's day-to-day operations were directed by Billy Tauzin—the same Washington player who as a congressman from Louisiana had sponsored the 2003 legislation that would become Medicare Part D. An adroit politician who had started out as a Democrat and switched to the Republican side, in part to gain a congressional leadership post, he made another strategic leap in leaving Congress to become the CEO of PhRMA at $2 million a year. In that role, Tauzin was the director, while Kindler, the incoming chairman of the CEO board, was "the boss." But when it came to their political objectives, they were entirely simpatico. The message: Play every angle to get every possible advantage.[15,16]

During the 2008 campaign, Obama had doubled down on his voting record in favor of health care reform, in favor of reimportation of inexpensive drugs from first-world nations, and in favor of federal negotiation of drug pricing within Medicare Part D. Each of these was anathema to the pharmaceutical industry, but Kindler and Tauzin managed to find one area of common ground. That was the new president's desire to expand insurance by employing a model that Republican governor Mitt Romney had established in Massachusetts, which, in turn, was modeled on a proposal that Bob Dole and other Republicans had advanced in the early 1990s as an alternative to the proposed Clinton health care initiative.[17]

The plan required mandatory participation in health insurance plans, organized on both federal and state levels, with financial penalties for those with means who did not participate. Whatever its concern for its fellow Americans' access to health insurance, PhRMA calculated that such a federal program could mean an additional 35 million customers and as much as $117 billion in additional revenue for the pharmaceutical industry over the next decade. In total, the industry's worth, as projected, would grow by one-third, from $359 billion to $476 billion.[16]

Six weeks after President Obama's inauguration, on March 5, 2009, Kindler and Tauzin came to the White House for the first of five meetings to iron out a deal.[16] The president was willing to wager all his political capital early in an effort to achieve what no other president had ever achieved—the passage of substantive health reform. As a student of history, he believed that this was impossible if the pharmaceutical industry opposed it. At the same time, his two guests representing the industry knew that picking up 35 million new customers would be meaningless unless they could secure pledges from the Obama administration that the government would not press for price negotiations as part of Medicare Part D, would not allow drug reimportation from Canada, and would provide patent protection for new high-tech biologic drugs.[18,19]

Industry analysts were caught off guard when, on May 11, eight weeks after the original meeting, President Obama announced that a deal had been struck.[20] The very next day, PhRMA launched what would be a $150 million television advertisement campaign in support of the new health care bill.[16] Another five weeks passed before details of the complex negotiations and their movement away from price controls would be revealed by Senate sponsor Max Baucus (D-MT).

In return for industry support, the White House agreed not to pursue federal price negotiations, and the administration's Department of Health and Human Services declared that the product safety of reimported medicines could not be ensured, and therefore would not be allowed. Finally, the administration agreed to allow 12 years of patent protection to a new class of biologic drugs, those very expensive biotech creations that were being increasingly customized for small targeted groups of desperate patients. As one result of these actions, Celgene, a biotech company which produced biologic drugs for select cancer patients, would see its stock rise by 74 percent in the next three years.[19]

What the industry pledged in return was not insignificant. First, it agreed to an additional $20 billion, beyond concessions already made, in price cuts to the government on Medicaid drugs over the next decade. During the same period, it blessed $30 billion in new excise taxes on its patented products. Finally, it ponied up an additional $30 billion to cover part of the Bush administration's Medicare Part D "doughnut hole" that had been confusing and exasperating for senior citizens. In total, this amounted to an $80 billion giveback, more than was palatable, especially considering that PhRMA in-house projections were for additional profits before givebacks over the same period to approach $200 billion.[15,16]

But this was not all that had been conceded. Big Pharma had turned its back on its historic patrons in the Republican Party, and as Republican John Boehner, then Speaker of the House, had promised Tauzin, "There's gonna be hell to pay."[16]

The Republicans had been following the money trail leading up to the recent presidential election, and they were not at all happy with what they saw. For the first time since 1990, by a 57 percent to 42 percent margin, pharmaceutical industry donations had tilted Democratic.[16] In 2009, PhRMA employed 165 lobbyists in Washington, with 83 percent of these being former employees of the legislative and executive branches.[20,21] Nearly all were focused on passing the Obama health care bill, and their very presence up and down congressional hallways was an ongoing irritant and a reminder of the switch in allegiance.

As part of the agreement, the industry also acquiesced to public disclosure, on a new open-access website, of all financial payments it provided physicians; but here the AMA cried foul, well aware that a portion of physician members believed their financial support from industry should remain confidential.[22] Obama, without knowing it, was testing the bonds that MIC, envisioning an increasingly organized common future, had been strengthening over the previous eight years. Public protests aside, the MIC would survive the stress test intact, and MIC members would move en masse to support the Obama reforms.

Even so, the Obama administration had to contend with conservatives who strongly opposed three new organizational entities proposed as part of the legislation. The first two were the Patient-Centered Outcomes Research Institute (PCORI) and the Independent Payment Advisory Board (IPAB).[19] PCORI was charged with independently assessing the effectiveness of various treatments such as individual pharmaceutical drugs, including those competitors in the same me-too class. Its findings would then be provided to the IPAB, whose mission was to control Medicare cost. The third entity, the Accountable Care Organization, was a subsidized new legal entity authorized to provide insurance policies following benefit rules embedded in the legislation. In all three cases, conservative critics saw tremendous potential sources for future backdoor price controls. But given that they were not truly ceding control, the pharmaceutical, insurance, and hospital industries initially felt confident that they were in control. Most of the individuals proposed to serve on these boards were well-known collaborators or members of the MIC.[19]

Even with PhRMA's active support, the Patient Protection and Affordable Care Act almost failed. On September 10, 2009, President Obama addressed a joint session of Congress, during which he quoted Ted Kennedy, who had died of a brain cancer three weeks earlier. "What we face," the president said, "is above all a moral issue; that at stake are not just the details of policy, but fundamental principles of social justice and the character of our country."[23] The bill passed in the Democrat-controlled Senate on December 23, 2009, and was immediately endorsed by the AMA and AARP.[24] But the struggle would go on in the House of Representatives until late March 2010 as members from both sides of the aisle carefully weighed the presence or absence of local support for fundamental change in the health care system.

That battle did not prevent Billy Tauzin and Jeff Kindler from celebrating an early victory at the 2010 annual meeting of PhRMA on March 18, 2010, with Tauzin underscoring the obvious: "This PhRMA team is a Super Bowl championship team of advocacy."[25]

On March 21, the House passed the Senate bill 219–212. Thirty-four Democrats, who considered the political price of opposition at home too great a price to pay, and all 178 Republicans had voted against it.

The Republican Party would turn this government program, which had originated in a Republican think tank and had first come to fruition under a Republican governor, into the Great Satan, a scheme that it said was every bit as threatening to the American way of life as it had once claimed Medicare to be. On the evening of the law's passage, Senate minority leader Mitch McConnell (R-KY) went to the podium and drew angry murmurs from Democrats when he declared it "one of the most consequential votes any of us will take. If the people who wrote this bill were proud, they wouldn't be forcing this vote in the dead of night."[26]

The first victim, though, was Billy Tauzin himself. A number of CEO members of the PhRMA board felt that they had been strong-armed by Tauzin and Kindler. Their anger was fueled behind the scenes by Thomas Donohue, president of the US Chamber of Commerce, who had been a vocal opponent of what he saw as Tauzin's folding to the demands of the Obama administration and allowing government intrusion into local private insurance markets. Under pressure from dissenting PhRMA CEO board members energized by Donohue, Tauzin was forced to abandon his post a month before the bill passed.[27] Eight months later, less than a year after the Wyeth deal, on Sunday, December 5, 2010, Jeff Kindler announced his early retirement. Pfizer's stock price had declined by an additional 36 percent during his four-year tenure, ensuring a loss of confidence on the part of the board member who had been instrumental in putting him in the corner office, Bill Steere.[3,28] Kindler's demise demonstrated that shareholders were not willing to celebrate policy success in the face of declining profitability. Rigor, relevance, and focus—these were still the leadership values Steere and his cohort sought.

Profitability was also paramount for the pharmaceutical industry as a whole. Though some leaders remained upset by the shift of party allegiance and signaled the same in releasing Tauzin, few could argue against the legislation in financial terms. The bottom line was that the bill as negotiated would give the industry access to significant revenues derived from those newly insured while preventing government interference in the profit sharing and self-management of its still loosely defined syndicate.

Obama's three-legged design of the Massachusetts law included (1) insurance for all, with prohibitions on exclusions for any reason including prior conditions; (2) mandated coverage, with financial penalties managed by the IRS for those employers who failed to provide insurance and those otherwise uninsured individuals who failed to purchase insurance on new federal and state insurance exchanges; and (3) financial subsidies for those who could not afford insurance, up to incomes of 400 percent of the poverty level.

The pharmaceutical industry's projected additional profit over 10 years before givebacks was pegged at $200 billion. After receiving rock-solid assurances that Medicare Part D drug prices would remain unchallenged, and that drug importation from other countries would continue to be prohibited, the industry ultimately settled on added concessions that pushed calculated givebacks over the next 10 years up to $120 billion from $80 billion.[16,29]

The insurance industry agreed to contribute $102 billion in initial lower-premium adjustments, an amount dwarfed by future premium subsidies for new enrollees of up to $500 billion, as well as annual rate hikes over the next five years including those of Humana, Cigna, UnitedHealthcare, and Aetna that ranged from 8 to 10 percent.[30] The insurers also negotiated protection of Medicare Advantage plans and wiggle room in the medical loss ratio, which defined what percent of a premium could go to administrative costs (read profits), as well as how large the premium price variance could be between healthy "young invincibles" and older, sicker patients with complex chronic diseases. Insurers wanted a five-to-one spread. The administration insisted on a two-to-one spread. They settled for three-to-one.[31]

Finally, the hospital industry with its academic medical centers predicted profits between $200 billion and $250 billion over 10 years. It settled on a giveback of $155 billion in the form of reduced annual increases in Medicare payment rates and penalties for failures—such as high 30-day readmission rates for discharged Medicare patients—to meet quality measures. It also received assurances that federal research dollars would continue to flow to the NIH, an important source of grants to academic centers, and that the government would continue to generously underwrite the costs of residents and fellows engaged in graduate medical education programs. Finally, reimbursement formulas for the care of uninsured poor, sick patients would remain intact.[32]

The size and similarities of these 10-year profitability figures underscored the fact that the Medical Industrial Complex is supported by three powerful pillars—the drug companies, the insurance companies, and hospitals—which share and exchange and compete for resources. And at the center of all this commerce is the physician—the one who writes the prescription, who orders the tests, who admits and operates on and treats the patients, and who processes and accepts the insurance payments. Studies repeatedly confirm physicians' central role in generating the greatest part of all health care costs in America.[33]

Republicans would expend boundless energy over the next decade trying to repeal and replace the Affordable Care Act, at times "in the dead of night," but they have as of yet not been able to convince Americans that stripping the vulnerable of protections and repealing the coverage of over 20 million previously uninsured Americans would improve America's health care system.[34] A 2017 *Economist*/YouGov poll found that approximately 60 percent of those surveyed favored federally funded health insurance for all, as well as a public health insurance option, including the availability of Medicare for all. The majority of Americans increasingly recognize that the status quo, while serving the needs of an ever-expanding MIC, no longer serves them.[35] Yet the MIC's tangled web of mutually reinforcing relationships still exists. It will be difficult to untangle, but it is by no means impossible.

Chapter 15

The MIC—
"Tapeworm of American
Economic Competitiveness"

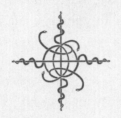

L ate in 2017, a small biotechnology firm based in Philadelphia, Spark
Therapeutics, received approval from the FDA for voretigene nepar-
vovec, a therapy to correct a defect in the human gene *RPE65*. This genetic
site directs the production of a protein that serves to activate light recep-
tors in the retina. A defective *RPE65*, inherited by one in 81,000 persons,
results in progressive deterioration of sight and eventual blindness.[1]

The novel therapy consists of attaching corrected versions of the
RPE65 gene to a benign adenovirus carrier, then injecting the genetically altered material beneath a patient's retina. A trial of 29 patients ages
4 to 44 with varying degrees of impaired vision led to improvements in
light sensitivity and improved vision. The only catch: it's expected to cost
$850,000 for the single injection therapy.[2]

No other nation can match America's record for scientific "star
turns." Our academic labs and pharmaceutical research facilities continue
to make startling advances, but much of the focus is on miracle cures like
Spark's gene therapy, which, more often than not, benefit a very small
population and are prohibitively expensive.[3] In 2017, for the third straight

year, lawmakers voted to increase the budget of the National Institutes of Health by $2 billion, rejecting cuts proposed by President Trump.[4] It's been said that our lawmakers, many of whom are well on in years and perhaps seeing intimations of their own declining health, are infatuated by "the charisma of the cure."[5]

But simply stated, pouring huge sums of public money into the search for elusive cures while recklessly overmarketing pharmaceuticals is not the same as running an effective and efficient health care system. In a recent *New York Times* public debate, Craig Garthwaite, a conservative health economist from the Kellogg School of Management at Northwestern University, said, "The US system is a bit of a mess." At the same event, Harvard School of Public Health associate professor Austin Frakt added, "It's very hard to justify the very high level of US spending based on innovation alone."[6] I would submit that both these comments seriously understate the case.

As Americans bear the brunt of high cost and low performance, every other developed nation far exceeds our rate of progress in dealing with such basics as infant mortality, immunizations, infectious disease rates, malnutrition, and sanitation. In 2017, the *Washington Post* highlighted the work of University of Washington researcher Christopher Murray, who had just completed a study of what is called amenable mortality—"deaths that theoretically could have been avoided by timely and effective medical care." He examined the incidence of 32 causes of death in 195 different countries from 1990 to 2015, publishing the results in the *Lancet*. Many of the most highly developed nations had the lowest death rates—countries like Canada, Australia, and Norway. In preventing these unnecessary deaths, the US ranked 80th, where our performance neighbors included Estonia and Montenegro.[7]

Digging into the data, Murray discovered that the US did well in the battle against infectious diseases preventable by vaccines, but had disastrous results in nine of the conditions measured, including lower respiratory infections, neonatal disorders, diabetes, and hypertensive heart disease. As Murray put it, "America's ranking is an embarrassment," not simply because of the performance, but also because of a declining trend line over the 25 years. In contrast, other nations, from Peru to South Korea to Niger and Jordan, registered steep rises in performance over the 25-year period. Murray also mentioned that the US spends more than any other nation in the group analyzed—an average of $9,000 annually for each person.[7]

These reports help explain a dawning awareness—still at the margins but growing—that our "business-centric" system of health care is fundamentally flawed, particularly our unique system of leaving something as fundamental as health insurance to the private sector.

As a physician who entered medicine not primarily to make a buck but to perform a meaningful service, I find a central-planning model that is logical and transparent, one that emphasizes universality and solidarity, and that integrates with other social services that affect health and wellness—the kind that exists in every other industrialized nation except the US—to be much more in keeping with the values that drew me to the profession in the first place.

The facts leave no doubt that our health care system wildly overspends taxpayer resources and underperforms at every turn except in speculative research. It is also clear from the preceding chapters how our nation arrived at this sorry state, and that incremental reform, with its predictable political blowback, has proved ineffective. Everyone seems to agree that our health care system is in crisis, and that it burdens the national economy. And yet the threads of the Medical Industrial Complex that keep us enmeshed in extravagantly expensive failure simply become stronger and more intricately intertwined.

Warren Buffett, a man who knows something about sustainable growth, said recently: "The health care problem is the number-one problem of America and of American business. . . . Medical costs are the tapeworm of American economic competitiveness . . . The cost of supporting the American health care system—hospitals, HMOs, doctors' visits, prescription drugs, medical devices, insurance companies, Medicare, Medicaid—is rising at an alarming rate."[8,9]

Buffett is acutely aware of demographics, especially the fact that America's 76 million baby boomers are adding to the population at a rate of 10,000 babies per day. He also appreciates that nearly 17 percent of Americans have past-due health care bills on their credit reports, a total debt burden nationwide of $81 billion.[10,11]

Oddly enough, though, even after compiling this long account of our stupendously wasteful and self-serving system, I remain—like him— optimistic when I consider the assets we have available, should we ever truly commit to achieving "the best health care system in the world."

These formidable assets include the nearly $4 trillion already committed, even if misallocated, to the nation's health; a remarkable array of educational institutions devoted to the creation of a highly skilled health-professional workforce; an incredibly dedicated network of public health schools and practitioners; a well-distributed but underutilized group of pharmacists anxious to contribute at their full potential; and a rapidly expanding primary-care army of nurse practitioners and physician assistants. The United States also possesses a testing ground of 50 different states offering the ability to customize various approaches to care within conditions set by the national government. A majority of the population now supports health care as a right, and a move toward a single-payer authority/multi-plan model, in national polls. The nation has a first-class and highly profitable scientific research and development community that could well stand on its own without diverting resources from health planning or patient care, and an enormous number of health system middlemen currently involved in non-real work who could be redirected toward strengthening services that would contribute positively to the social determinants of health—including improvements in nutrition, education, housing, transportation, and safety.

In a polarized society like ours, though, trying to drive change solely by a communitarian ideal that prioritizes social cohesion is probably not a winning proposition. So in closing, I'd like to briefly examine American health care from a dollars-and-cents perspective that everyone, including small-business owners as well as fair-minded lawmakers, both liberal and conservative, might appreciate.

If our citizens are increasing their understanding of the choices for health insurance, they also are increasingly aware of the true impact of spiraling health care costs and the secondary effects—including stagnant wages, income inequality, a lack of job mobility, high rates of medical bankruptcy, the closure of rural hospitals, an inability to invest in infrastructure repairs, and our growing national debt, which, on a percentage basis, is now the fifth highest in the world after Japan's, Greece's, Italy's, and Portugal's.[12]

In 2017, Republicans went out of their way to praise the virtues of changes in federal tax laws that most economists concede will further aggravate the nagging problem of income inequality in America.[13] On February 3, 2018, Speaker of the House Paul Ryan denied there was a problem, and chose to celebrate a secretary at a public school who he said had told him that "she was pleasantly surprised her pay went up $1.50 a week . . . she said [that] will more than cover her Costco membership for the year."[14] What more and more Americans are realizing is that access to affordable, high-quality, universal health care would be of far greater value to her and her family than a subsidized entry card to a big box retailer.

Were we to manage to be as efficient as the average developed nation and reduce our health costs as a proportion of GDP from nearly 20 percent to 14 percent, which would still place us above the national health care expenditure of Germany, Switzerland, France, Australia, Canada, Britain, and Singapore, we would immediately free up more than $1 trillion for a range of infrastructure improvements, jobs, and services that would contribute to advancing all Americans' health and well-being.[15]

I think as a companion to Warren Buffett's "tapeworm" assessment, the following cautionary tale is worth considering. From the 1940s to the 1980s, the Soviet Union maintained its status as a world power only by pouring a huge proportion of national financial resources into its military-industrial complex. The best estimates were that the Soviet Union in 1980 spent 27 percent of its gross domestic product on its military, up from 22 percent the year before.[16] As Nikolai Leonov, a KGB general, later recounted regarding the Soviet economy, "There was a visible decline of the rate of growth, then its complete stagnation. . . . It was a frightening and truly terrifying sign of crisis."[17] By the time Ronald Reagan came to the White House, the Soviet system was under severe strain, and when Reagan sped up the arms race, the entire Soviet structure gave way, and the Soviet Union collapsed.

Our spending curve in support of the Medical Industrial Complex is closely tracking the Soviets' 1980s expenditures on its military-industrial complex. Our society is already showing the strain, and the health care needs of our rapidly aging population could well be the jolt that causes the entire structure to collapse.

Another disturbing parallel with the Soviet Union should be a warning to us: From 1965 to 1985, as the Soviets diverted resources away from human needs and toward the military, the mortality rate for Russian men rose by 30 percent. This was mainly due to increases in cardiovascular and respiratory diseases, lung cancer, suicides, and homicides.[18] Today, as we divert resources away from the real needs of our people toward a wasteful, inefficient, and woefully illogical profit-based Medical Industrial Complex, our own mortality statistics are on a similar track, fueled in part by an opioid epidemic and Adderall for all created and reinforced by corrosive marketing, along with MIC collusion in rigged science, rank profiteering, and sloppy prescribing.

Our life-expectancy figures have consistently declined each year since 2016. The CDC's National Center for Health Statistics reported in 2018 that the new average life expectancy for Americans is 78.7 years, 1.6 years behind the average in developed nations (including Canada, Germany, Mexico, France, Japan, and the UK), which is 80.3. As Dartmouth economists Ellen Meara and Jonathan Skinner remarked about the downward reversal of US life expectancy, "It is difficult to find modern settings with survival losses of this magnitude."[19]

Making this sharp decline even more dramatic—in a nation where people of color have traditionally lagged behind in health outcomes—in this case, those at the center of the downward spiral of life expectancy are poorly educated white males. From 2000 to 2013, the death rate for this cohort had increased 22 percent to 415 per 100,000, compared with 200 per 100,000 in Sweden, 240 per 100,000 in Canada, and 300 per 100,000 in Germany.[20]

But digging further, Caleb Alexander and his team at the Johns Hopkins Bloomberg School of Public Health uncovered yet another pattern very similar to that of the Soviet Union just before its collapse: opioid overprescribing with subsequent addiction, amplified by alcohol poisoning and suicide.[21] The two most common traits that preceded opioid overdose deaths in our country were pain and mental distress. The final tolls have shown that more than 100,000 lives have been lost in the past decade. As we have seen, this epidemic is not an anomaly but rather a by-product of a deeply flawed national health care system that focuses on spectacular cures while largely ignoring "the social determinants of health."[21,22]

The Hopkins study in 2017 made operatives in the Medical Industrial Complex, including the AMA and PhRMA, squirm by asking why an overwhelming majority of the prescription drug abuse in this opioid epidemic originated from legitimate physician prescriptions; why 1 in 10 Tennessee teenagers since 1999 had been prescribed opioids; why prescription opioids were frequently diverted to others illegally; why 70 percent of those abusing prescription opioids accessed their most recent supply through a friend or family member; and why it hadn't been possible to track this "abuse trail" from health prescriber to prescription to patient to acquaintance in the early days when it began. Why had huge drug wholesalers like McKesson, a critical partner in the PBM data-rich syndicate, knowingly provided mountains of OxyContin without a single red flag to tiny storefront pharmacies in hardscrabble, low-density communities in Kentucky and West Virginia?[23,24]

But even for those not in dire straits in economically depressed regions of the country, our current, profit-oriented system reinforces citizens' sense of vulnerability and the feeling that they lack control over their immediate destiny. Many Americans avoid seeing a doctor because the costs are beyond their ability to pay. In July 2018, a story went viral about a woman whose leg was crushed in a Boston subway accident who pleaded with bystanders not to call an ambulance, saying, "I can't afford it."[25]

Lack of early intervention leads to deteriorating health that leads to even higher costs later on, which lead to health care emergencies as the leading cause of bankruptcy in the US.[26] These are not the makings of a vibrant workforce and a thriving economy. This is also not an environment that inspires entrepreneurial risk-taking or meaningful career development, let alone family formation or stability.

The 2018 statistics portray a nation on the wrong track, with a national birthrate dropping to a historic low, down for a third consecutive year. A lower birthrate means a declining tax base, an inadequate workforce, and fewer healthy young people to pay into insurance risk pools.[27] And again, one of the major reasons for this low birthrate is the failure of our society to address some of the social determinants of health by providing the kind of prenatal care and child care support that makes parenthood seem not only feasible but also something to be optimistic about.

According to a recent study by the Institute of Medicine and the National Research Council, the US also ranks in the bottom quartile among 30 industrialized nations in terms of workdays lost to disability.[28] Moreover, while our economic competitors are improving their health outcomes, ours are declining. A report by the Joint Center for Political and Economic Studies estimated the cost of our health care deficiencies due to reduced productivity, lost wages, and lack of worker mobility for the years between 2003 and 2006 as being $1.24 trillion.[29] A 2012 Institute of Medicine study was somewhat more conservative, pegging losses at $750 billion, with 25 percent of the losses due to excessive administrative costs and 28 percent due to unnecessary services driven by the redundancies and absurdities of the MIC.[30]

In the US, the total insurance sector (including life insurance, property and casualty insurance, and health insurance) is a branch of the financial industry, one-third of which is tied to the health insurance industry, with some 500,000 direct and indirect employees.[31] The quest for profitability and love of secrecy in this sector translate into financial stress for older Americans, 11 percent of whom, in a 2014 study, reported difficulty in paying their medical bills. For comparison, only 4 percent of seniors were similarly affected in Canada, 2 percent in France, 3 percent in Germany, 2 percent in Switzerland, and 1 percent in Sweden.[26] This system embodies the worst kind of featherbedding and protectionism, and our maintenance of it flies in the face of the modern trend toward eliminating the middleman.

Not only does our insurance system employ far too many people performing tasks that are not constructive; it has also triggered the creation of a second clerical workforce housed in hospitals and doctors' offices simply to manage the intentional complexities of billing and payment. This "arms race" between insurers and providers gives us 16 nonphysician health care workers for every physician, with half of these being nonclinical clerks and administrators, not medical technicians or nurses.[32]

In a similar fashion, senior management administrative costs in US hospitals now consume 16 percent of the average hospital budget, compared with just 7 percent in Canada and 9 percent in France and Germany.[33] And all this while our entrepreneurial health care system ignores the most basic needs of vast numbers of people.

In the most recent Bloomberg rankings of health care, in 2016 the US came in 50th out of 55 countries in efficiency and cost management, and it's a simple truth that the higher the overhead in delivering a service, the smaller the pool of resources available for the actual service.[34] This is why most nations control the centralized back-office functions and financial administration through single-payer oversight authority.

Efficient use of central services does not have to mean top-down, command-and-control, or one-size-fits-all thinking. Canada uses flexibility and choice by allowing provinces significant leeway in delivering services as long as the basics of its benefit package are honored. Offerings vary from province to province, as defined by budgets and priorities set by provincial governments from year to year. Hospitals are funded by the provinces, and doctors (who on average make more than American doctors!) are largely reimbursed via a fee-for-service model.[35,36] As is the case with the recent Medicaid expansion under the Patient Protection and Affordable Care Act, ample leeway is offered to allow each region a reasonable amount of experimentation and choice. If we simply had the political will, we could use our 50 states as laboratories in similar fashion.

Efficient use of central services also does not mean letting individual consumers off the hook. The Canadian, British, Swiss, German, French, and Australian national health plans all cover on average only 70 percent of the total cost of care, leaving citizens the option to purchase additional services on their own. Canada's plan does not cover pharmaceuticals, optical needs, or dentistry, but these services are covered by private supplemental insurance that citizens can purchase. The same is true in France. In both countries, approximately 90 percent of citizens reach into their own pockets and purchase supplemental insurance. In Switzerland, all citizens must buy health insurance, but there is a wide range of choice among public nonprofit and private for-profit plans that are permitted to vary benefits, premiums, and coverage. In Australia, some citizens choose to pay extra for private hospitals, thereby gaining access to additional services not available at publicly funded institutions.[6]

The Republicans' recent attempts to dismantle the Affordable Care Act by focusing the public's attention on the specific provisions of the legislation have inadvertently clarified what citizens value in responsible health care plans. After nearly a decade of listening to those who proclaimed it a sacred duty to repeal the legislation, then seeing the slapdash plans proposed to replace it, the majority of Americans realize that while the Patient Protection and Affordable Care Act has its flaws (including voluntary participation of states in the expansion of Medicaid and the fact that drug prices are allowed to soar in the absence of government negotiations), it has demonstrated its value. The legislation has expanded access, prevented discrimination against those with prior illnesses, permitted coverage to travel with the individual if one changes employment, and delivered the security of knowing that needed care will not be delayed, nor will an unpredicted illness or injury lead to a medical bankruptcy. The debate has also made clear that rising costs and declining quality cannot go on forever.

On a more philosophical level, the debate has reinforced the proposition that access to health care should not be a privilege available only to those with enough cash to pay for overpriced private insurance. Increasingly, Americans realize that a segment of our population cannot afford insurance, and that costs for their care must be subsidized by the rest of us. (And that the desperate visit of an uninsured citizen at an emergency room, where he or she won't be turned away, costs much more than a planned visit to a primary care physician.) More and more Americans also realize that a healthy insurance system requires full participation, meaning a contribution to the "risk pool," which in turn requires some form of enforcement. As these learnings sink in, our combined willingness to overpay to be underserved while providing opportunities for entrepreneurs to bolster their profitability on the backs of everyday Americans may be wearing thin.

This new openness to changes in health delivery has been reinforced by glimpses of far more successful systems elsewhere, including their subtle intricacies. Many Americans, maybe the majority, now realize that no national government anywhere has a centralized, one-size-fits-all system, and no country pays for all health care services used by its citizens. What well-developed nations have in common is universal coverage, but each uses a variety of methods to pay for it, including government taxes, private expenditures, and often both. No two countries do this in exactly the same way, but the key point is that every developed nation except our own has made an up-front commitment to universality, cost containment, thoughtful health planning, and equitable access to care.

The expansion of Medicaid as part of the Patient Protection and Affordable Care Act has also placed governors in the 36 states that chose to participate in a position to integrate health care with other social services that are critical to ensuring a healthy and productive population. Some innovative interventions are remarkably low-tech. For example, 541 vacant lots were identified in Philadelphia and approximately 200 chosen for trash removal and the planting of grass and trees. In neighborhoods where average income was below the poverty line, these simple improvements were accompanied by a 70 percent drop in depression rates.[37]

Findings like these come as no surprise to the governors who chose to accept Medicaid expansion and now have considerable discretion in how to apply these resources. Eleven of the participating governors are Republican and took political heat for cooperating with President Obama. But none is expressing regret. In fact, three additional Republican governors are currently considering dropping their opposition. Governors like John Kasich of Ohio are fast becoming students of health reform, and for the first time they are comparing reform notes with one another. In Kasich's state, Ohio, 700,000 citizens living at or below 138 percent of the poverty level, the established level below which health insurance costs are subsidized, have gained insurance since January 2014. The uninsured rate in Ohio has declined from 15 percent to 6.5 percent. For Kasich, participation was an easy leadership decision. Following 2017 congressional testimony, he said, "If they don't get coverage, they end up in the emergency room, they end up sicker, more expensive. I mean, we pay one way or the other. And so this has been a good thing for Ohio." As for "repeal and replace" efforts by his party, they earn from Ohio's governor a curt, "Can't do that."[38]

In studying the complex challenges, Kasich and his fellow participating governors are gaining a better understanding of the many social determinants of health. England, for example, has far better health outcomes than the US, but a significant factor is that only 10 percent of its citizens fall below the poverty line, whereas 17 percent of our citizens must deal with the economic deprivations—lack of mobility, poor nutrition, compromised environments—that destroy health and well-being.[39] The lesson here is that focusing on poverty as well as the provision of high-quality health care can be a winning combination in any state regardless of its politics.

Governors and their staffs who study the various national health systems quickly realize that none is perfect. For example, the UK system in December 2017 was the subject of widespread reports of excessive wait times for emergency services and specialty consultation blamed in part on three years of underfunding. Still, its commitment to national-level health planning, and its willingness to acknowledge that these services are essential to the strength of the nation, makes surfacing and addressing the challenges of continuously improving these complex human systems more likely. The services do not paper over their weaknesses with claims of "UK exceptionalism."[39]

In the past, the social determinants of health in the US have suffered for lack of funding and support in large part because our wasteful health care system consumes the lion's share of public resources. A recent study of 13 developed nations revealed that the US was the only nation to spend more on health care than all other social services combined.[40,41] Similarly, if Americans want to review the nation's best thought on the social determinants of health, they will not find it carefully integrated on the front end of our national health plan as it is in Health Canada's mission statement or Sweden's statement on equal access and shared responsibility.[42,43] Rather, it is buried on an obscure website sponsored by the Office of Disease Prevention and Health Promotion, which represents the "and Prevention" in the name of the Centers for Disease Control and Prevention.

How and why American medicine arrived at this point is now clear. Instead of embracing a thoughtful approach to strategic health planning following WWII, our nation encouraged a free enterprise and entrepreneurial attack on disease, even as our military built out national health systems for Germany and Japan. Along the way, major health sectors—including the medical profession, hospitals, insurers, and pharmaceuticals—infiltrated government bodies, weakening regulatory control as they pursued self-interest and profitability ahead of the interests of American patients, families, and communities. They were aided and abetted by crooks like Arthur Sackler and Hans Selye, and by well-meaning enablers like Mary Lasker.

Cross-sector leaders like Lou Lasagna, Antonio Gotto, and myself helped the various MIC sectors populate and socialize one another's territories, at times competing, and at other times colluding in the pursuit of career advancement, deregulation, and federal funding. The new information age helped spawn complex insurance and delivery systems focused on mining and monetizing proprietary patient databases. These required expanding nonclinical workforces and encouraged the opaque gaming of the system and diversion of profits. More and more money flowed into an ever-increasing number of derivative organizations, many flirting at the edges of criminality, that figured out how to gain entry into the increasingly complex pharmaceutical, insurance, hospital, patient care, electronic medical record, medical education, and scientific research supply chains.[44]

As we entered the new millennium, players within the various MIC sectors discovered common political ground with the help of their over-lapping lobbyists in Washington and statehouses across the land. PBMs now had their own Washington-based lobbying association, the Pharmacy Care Management Association, which invested about $3 million in political arm twisting in 2018. Add to that the combined investment of the PBM giants—CVS, UnitedHealthcare, and Express Scripts. Together they invested around $13 million in lobbying that year.[45] At the same time, PBMs continued to amass huge patient databases that provided critical intelligence on patient choice and preferences, the sites of care delivery, choice of insurers, numbers and amount of drugs consumed, and pricing history.

Members of the MIC by now realized that data was their future and that active participation and collusion with PBMs were mission-critical. Legal sharing of the spoils was the reward for participating in this remarkably wasteful and inequitable health delivery system. The PBMs, with their hidden kickbacks and rebates, were now an increasingly formalized consortium, on the verge of achieving a permanent stranglehold on the system by acquiring other major sectors of the MIC formerly outside their domain.

The failure of the uniquely American health care system can be summed up in just three words: "uninsured," "outcomes," and "cost." Many of our citizens lack health insurance coverage and therefore delay seeking care when they need it. When our citizens do seek care, the results are highly variable; are based on geography, race, gender, and ability to pay; and in general are inferior to results in most developed nations. Finally, the cost of care exceeds that of all other nations in the world by a wide margin.

So what would it take to move our awareness into action, and for the United States to reverse course and repair our narrowly focused and distinctly irrational system?

There are plenty of instructive models—from Canada to Germany and beyond—that suggest many small, commonsense reforms. Many of these are relatively straightforward regulations that would be no more draconian than the safety standards we currently impose on automobiles and baby furniture.

Basic Steps to Reform the
Medical Industrial Complex

Medical Education:

1. Eliminate all direct and indirect industry sponsorship of all continuing medical education programs, establishing a transparent, taxpayer-supported fund for this purpose.
2. Charge the American Medical Association and the Association of American Medical Colleges to develop a strategic plan for self-funded medical education focusing on virtual training, utilizing faculty without financial ties to industry, and eliminating continuing medical education intermediaries.
3. Require all medical schools to provide an ethics course on the Medical-Industrial Complex that covers our unique history, challenges, and opportunities to improve access to efficient, high-quality health care for our people.
4. Require the American Medical Association to perform and publicly post an annual educational quality review of each of its AMA Federation specialty societies.
5. Require the American Medical Association and the Association of American Medical Colleges to post their 990 forms and those of all affiliate members, including AMA Federation members and AAMC academic teaching hospital members, in an easily accessible location on their websites.

Clinical Research:

1. Establish financial and ethical criteria for defining "industry compromised researchers," and enforce their exclusion from all government medical-product-review advisory boards.
2. Ensure that all trial results are registered on ClinicalTrials.gov before FDA approval, without exception.
3. Suspend and financially penalize companies that falsify, manipulate, or exclude research data.

4. Enhance audits on all overseas clinical research studies by CROs.
5. Actively promote and encourage whistle-blowers, and fund institutional studies for publication that assess and promote ethical research practices.
6. Transparently disclose all contributors to the NIH, CDC, and FDA foundations.
7. Require all academic consultants and advisers to self-declare their primary role as either "researcher" or "clinician/educator."

Publications:

1. Prohibit the publication of submissions that involve writers who hide their authorship, and enforce multiyear suspensions of medical journal authors found to have utilized such ghostwriters.
2. Prohibit the publication of trial results that have not officially been registered on ClinicalTrials.gov.
3. Enforce a lifetime suspension of authors who deliberately manipulate or suppress data.
4. Require an annual public listing by journal publishers of advertisers and purchasers of bulk reprints, with financial details of the transactions included.
5. Require an annual public listing of the total grants provided to journals' parent organizations for any purpose.

Marketing:

1. Suspend all FDA-approved direct-to-consumer advertising. It has no meaningful educational value and plays a critical role in promoting the overuse of pharmaceuticals in America.
2. Establish state and federal health education funds, directed by public health professionals, to promote healthy choices and sound preventive health policies funded by health promotion taxes on industries contributing to poor health.
3. Actively discourage pharmaceutical representatives' visits and the use of promotional drug samples by adding a health tax to

these pharmaceutical marketing outreach activities, similar to the health tax on cigarettes.

4. Eliminate all promotional gifts, including meals.
5. Require that physicians actively select that their identifier number be included in the AMA Physician Masterfile database used to enable drug data mining and prescription profiling, by opt-in rather than opt-out methodology for new and existing physicians.
6. Prohibit the sale and distribution of individual physicians' prescription profiling data to pharmaceutical and medical device companies.
7. Require every patient advocacy group to have a standard "sponsor" link on its navigation bar, and report annually a list of sponsors' total financial and in-kind support, including grants, publication ad buys, funded surveys and research, public awareness campaigns, and organizational or educational meetings.
8. Require the FDA and NIH to publish annually on their public sites an aggregate list of all patient advocacy groups, their sponsors, and total donation amounts.

Even if we could achieve every item on this extensive wish list, most Americans now believe the time has passed for curing America's health care woes solely through such incremental approaches. They have witnessed nearly 10 years of relentless campaigning by politicians who represent a decided minority of Americans seeking to dismantle desperately needed reforms bit by bit.

The majority of Americans now agree that universal health coverage is a central underpinning of a civilized society, essential to creating a stable government, an empathetic culture, and productive healthy citizens.[46,47] Implementing such a program requires careful and thoughtful governmental planning and execution with integration of a wide range of other social services. It must be budgeted with careful prioritization, but it is certainly doable.

The required action now is far more comprehensive and centers on the 800-pound gorilla we must subdue to truly free ourselves from the

MIC syndicate's stranglehold: our perverse, profit-driven, and incredibly wasteful health insurance system. Could the transformation we need be as simple as removing the age restrictions on Medicare and Medicaid, as proposed by some on the left, thereby letting every citizen in on the benefits enjoyed by seniors and the needy during the past half century? Certainly that is one option worth discussing.

But to embrace true reform, we must follow the money and follow the data, and build on progress already made. Clearly the time has come for the US to join the rest of the industrialized world and consolidate health insurance into a standardized single-payer authority/multi-plan delivery system that provides a secure package of basic benefits for all. The first step should be establishing minimum standards and a centralized control system, which would trigger a cascading series of changes leading to more detailed answers to the question "How do we make America healthy?"

Were we to establish universal health care as a right for all citizens and mandate participation based on affordability of all citizens, we would not need to start from scratch to identify the next steps. The Affordable Care Act has already established a basic benefit package that has been accepted by the majority of patients and health professionals in our nation. Majorities also agree with protections from exclusions or price hikes based on prior conditions, the exclusion of skimpy insurance plans that expose clients to unacceptable financial risk, and the ability of citizens to maintain their coverage if they move or change jobs. As for choice of plans, we already have a list of options that meet basic benefit requirements and that could be opened up to larger audiences; these options include Medicare, Medicare Advantage, ACA federal and state insurance exchanges, and Medicaid.

If positioning the government for primary oversight as single payer and restricting private insurers to providing supplemental coverage for services not covered would take us halfway there, what might carry us the rest of the way?

The simple step of allowing reference-pricing of pharmaceuticals on an annual basis—an approach that allows the government to survey prices of drugs on its essential drug list across five to ten comparator nations,

Ten Reasons Why Consolidating Oversight under
a Single Centralized Authority Works So Well:

1. It provides unimpeded universal access to coverage.
2. It lowers administrative costs by at least 50 percent, and overall health care expenses by 15 percent, according to an extensive economic health policy research study published in *BMC Health Services Research* in 2014.[15]
3. It is portable, allowing people to change jobs or geographic locations without worry.
4. It can emphasize prevention by promoting health planning and budgeting priorities.
5. It provides a standard basic benefit package for all, with flexibility for an individual to purchase additional services through private supplemental insurance.
6. It offers a wider choice of doctors and hospitals, with coverage guaranteed, and limits "balanced billing" on essential services that are covered.
7. It prohibits insurers from obstructing access to care with administrative obstacles to payment.
8. By prioritizing care, the system increases wellness, therefore decreasing the cost of sickness.
9. It forces transparent budgeting for outcomes, with a clear definition of goals and priorities, and promotes performance-based payments.
10. It inserts public oversight of patient databases, preventing MIC use of data to maximize profits by steering patient choices and managing opaque MIC profit sharing.

and settle on an average price for each drug in the coming year—would be the next logical step. Using this methodology, already in place in Canada and other European nations, would largely break the MIC's amazingly destructive grip on America's health apparatus. With the role of private insurers diminished by a standardized national approach to delivery of essential health care services, and direct-to-consumer pharmaceutical advertising prohibited as it is in all other nations, there would be little need for PBMs. Pricing would be transparent and kickbacks would be illegal.

What of the other elements of the MIC that currently live off the spoils of this system? If beneficial to society, their functions could be more than adequately supported by the roughly $1 trillion fund created with the savings of health care reform.

This would include a new fund to support lifetime education of not only physicians, but also nurses and all other members of the health professional team. Similarly, a fund to support a new government-run hospital accreditation body would replace the failed Joint Commission on Accreditation of Healthcare Organizations and tackle the nagging problem of safety in our nation's hospitals. A major investment in schools of public health, and support for public health planning on both the state and the national level with a special focus on programs to improve services that support integrating the social determinants of health, would be provided. State-level grants would be used to fund innovations in maternal and child health, early childhood education, new delivery system models, preventive outreach, information system connectivity, housing security, healthy green environments, nutritional upgrades, public transportation, and patient empowerment. Finally, with national oversight and planning of our health care system, patient care databases would no longer be the proprietary marketing tool of the AMA, industry, or PBMs, but would be a secure public resource populated with patient and provider data used primarily for assessing progress in achieving effective preventive treatments and positive health outcomes.

The NIH, FDA, and CDC would continue in their primary oversight and support roles. In addition, a new National Health Planning Department, of equal standing with these departments, would be created and assume annual oversight of strategic health planning, universal coverage, pharmaceutical pricing, and prevention activities. Private health professional advisers or consultants to any of these government bodies would be asked to declare their primary roles as either researchers or clinician educators. Researchers would be managed in the same manner as for-profit industry employees, with rigorous requirements for self-disclosure similar to those required of registered lobbyists. Clinician educators would be prohibited from accepting direct or indirect financial support outside their own institutions if they wished to advise government bodies.

While our current congressional leaders may lag far behind in embracing this action-oriented plan, public opinion has evolved, which means that, despite the challenges, an efficient, accessible, and high-quality national health care system is no longer the "snowball's chance in hell" proposition it once was. Most fundamentally, calling it "socialized medicine," aside from being a gross mischaracterization, is no longer enough to stop the discussion.

Recent disclosures by the *Wall Street Journal* revealed that the 2016 assault on President Obama's health care bill that raged on social media during the presidential campaign was not primarily generated by our own citizens. The vast majority of the 10,000 preelection tweets on the subject originated from one of 600 Russian intelligence-linked accounts determined to sow conflict and confusion that would benefit Republican candidates.[48] This helps explain why, in the wake of the debate over Obamacare and the attempts to "repeal and replace" the legislation, American citizens in decided majorities defended the plan. Clearly they appreciated that a healthy nation requires a healthy population supported with careful health planning and the compassionate delivery of health services to all, especially to our most vulnerable citizens. As nearly all other nations before us have concluded, the right to health care is simply common decency and common sense.

In the Declaration of Independence, our nation's founders proclaimed that equality was self-evident. Nearly 250 years later, what has also become self-evident is that there is no equality without reasonable

access to health care, and that universal insurance coverage is the only
system that truly can provide reasonable access. Rather than resisting
this approach, once seen as "un-American," our citizens are beginning to
see single-payer oversight/multi-plan universal access to affordable and
effective care as the essential next step toward ensuring what should be
every American's birthright—life, liberty, and the pursuit of happiness.

Afterword

I've spent 40 years in medicine, 40 years as an AMA member, a decade in hospital management, and an additional decade as an independent medical journalist, but what solidified my sense of the Medical Industrial Complex was the 10 years I spent inside the largest and most profitable pharmaceutical company in the world. My vantage point extended not only into the Pfizer boardroom but also into the executive suites of the American Medical Association, the American Hospital Association, and the Association of American Medical Colleges, and its premier academic medical institutions; legislative offices in statehouses across America and in Washington, DC; the Christian Coalition, PhRMA, and Lou Lasagna's organization; and TV studios including FOX, CNN, NBC and CBS.

For most of those years, I was convinced that what I was doing—promoting medical humanities—honored my commitments as a physician and served the needs of our patients. I believed in cross-sector leadership and taught others the art.[1] Certainly harnessing the resources of Pfizer and this industry, and applying them to our partner organizations that represented doctors and their patients across this nation, would improve the lot of all our citizens, I reasoned.

But now, with 10 more years of reflection and further research, I realize that along the way I was enabling and solidifying the relationships that are so critical to the hidden functioning of the MIC and was fostering the dismantling of critical checks and balances.

Shortly before I left Pfizer, I ran into Lou Clemente at a special event at the New York Botanical Garden. He was then retired, and I was pleased to see him again. "Mike," he said, "we did so much with you. But we could have done so much more." I remember thinking as I headed home that evening, "There but for the grace of God go I."

Appendix: Time Line of Pfizer's Penalties and Transgressions

While I was employed by Pfizer, I attended a fund-raiser in New York for the International Rescue Committee. At the invitation of Jean Kennedy Smith, I sat next to her brother, Senator Ted Kennedy, who, knowing my background, leaned over and loudly muttered into my ear, "Pfizer is the worst."

Even if this dubious distinction were true, Pfizer would have many rivals in the sweepstakes for disreputable behavior. What the Pfizer record does confirm, when juxtaposed against the evolution of the Medical Industrial Complex, is that penalties and even public disgrace do not necessarily lead to permanent corrective action. In fact, for companies and organizations with the size and power of Pfizer, which directly and indirectly employ hundreds of lawyers and lobbyists, fines, penalties, and public shaming are simply declared a "cost of doing business."

What follows is a partial list of Pfizer's US penalties and transgressions during my lifetime. I offer it as a representative sample of corporate misbehavior in the health care sector—lists such as these exist for every major pharmaceutical and medical device company. The similarly shabby behavior of many hospitals, insurers, drug wholesalers, and physicians is illustrated all too well by the rolling revelations concerning the US opioid epidemic. The Pfizer list should be viewed, therefore, not as the exception but rather as the rule in an MIC system marked by self-interest, complexity, and secrecy.

1950s: Pfizer was heavily criticized for marketing Terramycin directly to hospitals and doctors in a "first of its kind," over-the-top advertising campaign in *JAMA*.[1]

1957: The *Saturday Evening Review* criticized Pfizer for ads including "real doctor" testimonials. The doctors were fictitious.[1]

1958: Pfizer was one of six drug companies charged with price-fixing antibiotics by the Federal Trade Commission. The US Department of Justice also charged the company with making false statements in patent applications.[2]

1961: The Justice Department filed criminal antitrust charges against Pfizer, American Cyanamid, Bristol-Myers, and top executives of the three companies.[3]

1964: The Federal Trade Commission ordered the six companies originally charged with price fixing in 1958 to change their prices. Pfizer was forced to OK production of tetracycline by any company that requested the right.[4]

1968: Pfizer, American Cyanamid, and Bristol-Myers were found guilty in federal court of conspiring to monopolize and guilty of actual monopoly. The companies were each fined $150,000, pending appeal. The judgment was reversed on appeal.[5]

1971: The Environmental Protection Agency formally requested that Pfizer cease hazardous dumping of up to a million gallons of waste each year at its Groton, Connecticut, central research site.[6]

1973: Pfizer, American Cyanamid, Upjohn, Squibb, and Bristol-Myers agreed to a $156 million antitrust settlement for monopolistic price-fixing.[7]

1976: Pfizer, among other companies, admitted to $265,000 in questionable payments to foreign government officials of three countries. The countries were not identified.[8]

1986: Pfizer was criticized in an article in *Progressive Magazine* titled "Death by Prescription" for understating the risk of gastrointestinal bleeding associated with its antiarthritis drug Feldene.[9]

1979–1986: Metal ruptures of Pfizer's Shiley heart valves caused 125 deaths. A 1991 settlement included a $205 million fund to cover thousands of open cases; $10.75 million to the Justice Department for not disclosing problems when originally gaining approval; and $9 million to the Veterans Administration to support ongoing care of veterans with the valve.[10]

1991: Pfizer agreed to a $70,000 settlement with 10 states for misleading advertising for Plax mouth rinse.[11]

1991: Pfizer agreed to a $3.1 million settlement of EPA charges for failing to install pollution-control equipment at plants on the Delaware River in Pennsylvania.[12]

1994: Pfizer agreed to a $1.5 million settlement with the EPA for improper toxic waste disposal in Rhode Island.[13]

1996: The FDA charged that Pfizer ads for its antidepressant Zoloft included false claims and must be withdrawn.[14]

1996: Pfizer and 14 other drug companies paid more than $408 million to settle a class-action lawsuit related to conspiring to fix prices for independent pharmacies.[15]

1998: Pfizer agreed to a $625,000 payment for environmental violations uncovered at its research facilities in Groton.[16]

1999: Pfizer pleaded guilty to criminal antitrust charges and paid a $20 million penalty, admitting that its Food Science Group participated in two international price-fixing conspiracies.[17]

2000: The FDA charged Pfizer and Pharmacia, co-marketers of Celebrex, with producing false and misleading ads and said that the ads must be withdrawn.[18]

2002: After CEO Hank McKinnell was subpoenaed, Pfizer agreed to pay $49 million to settle charges related to defrauding the federal Medicaid program by overcharging for its cholesterol-lowering drug Lipitor.[19]

2002: The FDA ordered Pfizer to stop running ads for Lipitor, charging that they falsely claimed that the drug was safer than competing products.[20]

2002: Pfizer agreed to a $538,000 payment to New Jersey for improper monitoring of wastewater discharged from its plant in Parsippany.[21]

2003: Pfizer agreed to a $700 million settlement for dumping PCBs in Anniston, Alabama. (The original offender was Pharmacia, along with Solutia and Monsanto.)[22]

2003: Pfizer agreed to a $6 million settlement with 19 states for misleading ads for its Zithromax medication for children's ear infections.[23]

2004: Pfizer agreed to a $430 million settlement for paying physicians to prescribe its epilepsy drug Neurontin (inherited from Warner-Lambert) to patients for unapproved indications. (The suit revealed that publication of negative clinical studies was delayed purposefully by the company).[24]

2004: Pfizer agreed to a $60 million settlement of a class-action suit for liver damage associated with its diabetes drug Rezulin.[25]

2004: Pfizer agreed to a $22,500 settlement for failure to properly notify state and federal officials of a 2002 chemical release from its Groton plant, which caused serious injury to several employees.[26]

2005: Pfizer admitted that in 1999, the heart risk associated with use of Celebrex in the elderly had been understated.[27]

2005: The painkiller Bextra was forced off the market by the FDA, which had mandated a "black box warning" about serious cardiovascular and gastrointestinal risks. Later, Pfizer provided $894 million to settle lawsuits for Bextra and Celebrex in 2008.[28]

2005: Pfizer agreed to a $46,250 settlement for charges in connection with Pharmacia and Upjohn federal air-pollution violations at its plant in Kalamazoo, Michigan.[29]

2007: Pfizer agreed to a $34.7 million settlement of federal charges of illegal marketing of its Genotropin human growth hormone (from Pharmacia and Upjohn).[30]

2008: Pfizer agreed to a payment of $975,000 for Clean Air Act violations from 2002 to 2005 at its Groton manufacturing plant.[31]

2009: Pfizer was fined $2.3 billion for illegally marketing the painkiller Bextra. The inspector general of the Department of Health and Human Services forced the company to enter into a corporate integrity agreement.[32]

2009: Thousands of lawsuits were inherited with acquisition of Wyeth, including those involving the contraceptive Norplant and the diet drug fen-phen.[33]

2009: Pfizer agreed to a $75 million settlement to Nigerian courts for its Trovan trials on Nigerian children in 1996. The US case was settled in 2011 for an undisclosed amount. The unlawful-termination suit brought by the whistle-blowing doctor was settled for an undisclosed amount.[34]

2010: Pfizer was charged in federal court with racketeering fraud for its marketing of Neurontin, with the penalty set at $142 million.[35]

2010: Pfizer paid a $1.37 million penalty to a former Pfizer company scientist who contracted a genetically engineered virus and was subsequently fired for raising safety concerns.[36]

2010: Pfizer revealed $20 million in payments to 4,500 doctors and other medical professionals for consulting and speaking on the company's behalf over the prior six-month period.[37]

2011: Pfizer paid a $14.5 million settlement of federal charges for illegally marketing its bladder drug Detrol.[38]

2011: The FDA ordered Pfizer to correct inaccuracies in its "Online Resources" webpage on Lipitor.[39]

2012: Pfizer agreed to a settlement with the US Securities and Exchange Commission to provide $45 million to address charges of bribing physicians and other health care professionals to increase foreign product sales.[40]

2012: Pfizer removed claims related to breast and colon health from its ads for Centrum multivitamins.[41]

2012: Pfizer agreed to a $491 million payment to the Justice Department to settle charges of improper marketing of the kidney transplant drug Rapamune (a Wyeth product).[42]

2014: Pfizer agreed to a $35 million settlement with 40 state attorneys general for improper marketing of Rapamune.[43]

2016: The Obama administration blocked Pfizer from selling itself to Ireland-domiciled Allergan Plc for $160 billion in a reverse merger, or corporate tax inversion, designed solely to escape its US tax obligations.[44]

Acknowledgments

This book began four decades ago in the noontime conference room of Colin (Tim) Thomas, MD, chairman of surgery at the University of North Carolina, where I completed my surgical training in 1978. Tim's pre-op conferences exposed us to his broad knowledge and understanding of medical history and its role in shaping compassionate and empathetic health professionals. Some two decades later, Eli Ginzberg, PhD, the legendary Columbia health economist, generously guided me down the same pathway, and pointed me toward World War II as I struggled to understand how and why the physician had become so entangled in the Medical Industrial Complex.

My father, William P. Magee, MD, who was my professional and personal role model, died of Alzheimer's disease in 1998 during my early tenure at Pfizer. He was a decorated captain in the Medical Corps of Patton's Seventh Army in Europe, one of Dr. William Menninger's "30-day wonders," trained to manage psychiatric casualties in battle zones during the war. Seeking his war records at Eli's urging triggered a decade-long exploration, reinforced by a two-year, Viagra-induced association with one famous World War II casualty, Senator Bob Dole. The five-tier "chain of evacuation," which spanned the distance between battlefield and stateside specialty hospitals, saved the life of Dole and countless others. My father worked in that chain, and Eli Ginzberg helped design it.

These three—the military doctor, the injured soldier, and the wartime administrator—were my silent guides through the early years of unraveling the story of how American health care came to be the global outlier it has become. Since then a long list of critical resources have added context and detail, including Paul Starr's *The Social Transformation of American Medicine*, Eli Ginzberg's *The Medical Triangle*, Marcia Angell's *The Truth about the Drug Companies*, David Blumenthal and James A. Morone's *The Heart of Power*, Thea Cooper and Arthur Ainsberg's *Breakthrough*, Scott Podolsky's *The Antibiotic Era*, Dominique Tobbell's *Pills, Power, and Policy* . . . and later, Barry Meier's *Pain Killer*, Alan Schwarz's *A.D.H.D. Nation*, Steven Brill's *America's Bitter Pill*, Ben Goldacre's *Bad Pharma*, and Elisabeth Rosenthal's *An American Sickness*.

The distance between years of research and final publication of *Code Blue* could not have been bridged without the guidance and constant encouragement of my remarkable agent, Jill Kneerim, a partner at Kneerim & Williams in Boston. The firm's literary agent Lucy Cleland also provided invaluable support.

To aid in the transformation of my original text, I also had the good fortune of working with the brilliant William Patrick, a remarkable developmental editor, who kept me laser focused on the Medical Industrial Complex and on the ties between past and present, always with good cheer.

The choice of Grove Atlantic and its executive editor, George Gibson, proved critical. As Grove Atlantic president and publisher Morgan Entrekin declared, George is "admired here and around the world as a brilliant, gracious, passionate publisher and editor." He has also become a very good friend, and over two years has devoted countless hours to personally and gently guiding and directing the evolution of this book to its final form. Assisting him was the remarkable team at Grove Atlantic including meticulous managing editor Julia Berner-Tobin and talented art director Gretchen Mergenthaler.

My wife, Trish Boggia Magee, was a critical partner, providing thoughtful critique and guidance with each and every draft, and encouraging my first outreach *to New York Times* columnist Perri Klass, who generously read early versions of this text and helped place me in Jill Kneerim's hands. Trish's insistence that this be "an important book" was a guiding star over this complex journey.

There was no shortage of readers during this long developmental process. These included my own four children—Michael, Mitchell, Marc, and Meredith—and their spouses, my ten brothers and sisters, and various colleagues in and out of the health care field. I also benefited from the constant flow of input from my students at the President's College at the University of Hartford and its director, Steve Metcalf. Their encouragement, good humor, and valued insights are embedded in these pages.

Finally, at every step of this process, thoughts of my patients and colleagues over the years were never far away. They are too numerous to name here, but to each I offer my thanks and gratitude.

Notes

Chapter 1—The Constant Gardener

1. *The Constant Gardener*, John Le Carré, 2005. Box Office Mojo. http://www.boxofficemojo.com/movies/?id=constantgardener.htm.

2. Hendersson DR, Hooper CL. Pfizer $2.3 billion-dollar settlement. *Forbes*. September 9, 2009. https://www.forbes.com/2009/09/08/pfizer-bilion-dollar-settlement-fda-opinions-contributors-david-r-henderson-charles-l-hooper.html.

3. Hellmann J. Trump: "Nobody knew that healthcare could be so complicated." The Hill. February 27, 2017. http://thehill.com/policy/healthcare/321318-trump-nobody-knew-that-healthcare-could-be-so-complicated.

4. Carroll AE, Frakt A. The best health care system in the world: which one would you pick? *New York Times*. September 18, 2017. https://www.nytimes.com/interactive/2017/09/18/upshot/best-health-care-system-country-bracket.html.

5. Squires D, Bradley E. U.S. spends more on health care than other high-income nations but has lower life expectancy, worse health. Commonwealth Fund. October 8, 2015. http://www.commonwealthfund.org/publications/press-releases/2015/oct/us-spends-more-on-health-care-than-other-nations.

6. Trends in maternal mortality: 1990 to 2013. World Health Organization and UNICEF. 2014. http://apps.who.int/iris/bitstream/10665/112697/1/WHO_RHR_14.13_eng.pdf?ua=1.

7. Kristof N. The G.O.P. health care hoax. *New York Times*. January 6, 2017. https://www.nytimes.com/2017/01/05/opinion/the-gop-health-care-hoax.html?_r=0 https://data.worldbank.org/indicator/SH.DYN.MORT.

8. Curtin A. US health care ranks last among the 11 developed nations. *Nation of Change*. June 29, 2018. https://www.nationofchange.org/2018/04/13/us-health-care-ranks-last-among-the-11-developed-nations/.

9. McCarthy D, How S, Fryer A-K, Radley D, Schoen C. Why not the best? Results from the National Scorecard on U.S. Health System Performance, 2011. Commonwealth Fund. 10/18/2011. http://www.commonwealthfund.org/publications/fund-reports/2011/oct/why-not-the-best-2011.

10. Du L, Lu W. U.S. health care system ranks as one of the least efficient. Bloomberg. September 28, 2016. https://tmedweb.tulane.edu/portal/files/U_S__Health-Care_System_Ranks_as_One_of_the_Least-Efficient_-_Bloomberg.pdf.

11. Jiwani A, Himmelstein D, Woolhandler S, Kahn JG. Billing and insurance-related administrative costs in United States' health care: synthesis of micro-costing evidence. *BMC Health Services Research*. April 16, 2014. https://bmchealthservres.biomedcentral.com/articles/10.1186/s12913-014-0556-7.

12. Davis K, Stremikis K, Squires D, Schoen C. Mirror, mirror on the wall: how the U.S. health care system compares internationally, 2014 update. Commonwealth Fund. June 16, 2014. https://www.commonwealthfund.org/sites/default/files/documents/___media_files_publications_fund_report_2014_jun_1755_davis_mirror_mirror_2014.pdf.

13. Brill S. *America's Bitter Pill*. New York: Random House; 2015:8.

14. Fung B. How the U.S. health care system wastes $750 billion annually. *Atlantic*. September 7, 2012. https://www.theatlantic.com/health/archive/2012/09/how-the-us-health-care-system-wastes-750-billion-annually/262106/. Institute of Medicine 2012 report: Transformation of health system needed to improve care and reduce cost. http://www.nationalacademies.org/hmd/Reports/2012/Best-Care-at-Lower-Cost-The-Path-to-Continuously-Learning-Health-Care-in-America/Press-Release.aspx.

15. Lewis M. *The Big Short*. New York: W.W. Norton; 2010:254.

16. Nisen M. Pharma gets the worst of both drug-pricing worlds. *Bloomberg News*. February 13, 2018. https://www.bloomberg.com/gadfly/articles/2018-02-13/drug-price-growth-slows-political-pressure-doesn-t.

17. Hospital errors are the third leading cause of death in U.S., and new hospital safety scores show improvements are too slow. Leapfrog Hospital Safety Grade. October 23, 2013. http://www.hospitalsafetygrade.org/newsroom/display/hospitalerrors-thirdleading-causeofdeathinus-improvementstooslow.

18. Kearney MS, Levine PB. Why is the teen birth rate in the United States so high and why does it matter? *J Econ Perspect*. Spring 2012;26(2):141-166. https://www.ncbi.nlm.nih.gov/pubmed/22792555.

19. Mangan D. What Americans don't know about health insurance can—and will—cost them. Yahoo Finance. November 4, 2016. https://finance.yahoo.com/news/americans-dont-know-health-insurance-204032197.html.

20. La Monica PR. John Oliver eviscerates one of Warren Buffett's favorite companies. CNN Money. May 15, 2017. http://money.cnn.com/2017/05/15/investing/davita-dialysis-john-oliver-warren-buffett/index.html.

21. Smallteacher R. DaVita pays $895 million to settle kidney fraud claims. CorpWatch. May 14, 2015. https://corpwatch.org/article/davita-pays-895-million-settle-kidney-treatment-fraud-claims?id=16027.

22. Consumer Affairs. FDA estimates Vioxx caused 27,785 deaths. November 4, 2004. https://www.consumeraffairs.com/news04/vioxx_estimates.html.

23. Smith A. Merck settles Vioxx suits for $4.85B. November 9, 2007. http://money.cnn.com/2007/11/09/news/companies/merck_vioxx/.

24. Brinkerhoff N, Baker V. CEO who oversaw mass Vioxx deaths now teaching at Harvard and on Microsoft board of directors. AllGov. May 16, 2012. http://www.allgov.com/news/top-stories/ceo-who-oversaw-mass-vioxx-deaths-now-teaching-at-harvard-and-on-microsoft-board-of-directors?news=844479.

Chapter 2—Intertwined

1. Davis V. Personal communication with AMA communications coordinator. 2010. http://channelingreality.com/Medical/medical_logo_change.htm.

2. Cancryn A. Azar received millions in compensation from Lilly in last year, disclosures show. Politico. November 20, 2017. https://www.politico.com/story/2017/11/20/azar-eli-lilly-millions-severance-hhs-251107.

3. Elliott J. Alex Azar, Trump's HHS pick, has already been a disaster for people with diabetes. *Nation*. November 21, 2017. https://www.thenation.com/article/alex-azar-trumps-hhs-pick-has-already-been-a-disaster-for-people-with-diabetes/.

4. Grisham S. Medscape physician compensation report, 2017. Medscape. April 5, 2017. https://www.medscape.com/slideshow/compensation-2017-overview-6008547?src=wnl_physrep_170420_mscpmrk_comp2017 &uac=268262SJ&impID=1331481&faf=1.

5. Glied SA, Frank RG. Care for the vulnerable vs. cash for the powerful: Trump's pick for HHS. *N Engl J Med*. 2017;376:103-105. http://www.nejm.org/doi/full/10.1056/NEJMp1615714?af=R&rss=currentIssue.

6. Smith E. Medical association: what's behind its membership surge? Associations Now. February 27, 2015. https://associationsnow.com/2015/02/medical-association-heres-whats-behind-our-member-surge/.

7. American Medical Association. RBRVS overview. https://www.ama-assn.org/rbrvs-overview.

8. American Medical Association. The guidelines for admission of specialty societies to the HOD. https://www.ama-assn.org/guidelines-admission-specialty-societies-hod; AMA specialty organization 5-year review. 2016. https://www.ama-assn.org/5-year-review-hod-specialty-societies.

9. American Academy of Pain Medicine. http://www.painmed.org/ membercenter/about/.

10. Fauber J. Academics profit by making the case for opioid painkillers. *Milwaukee Journal Sentinel*. April 4, 2011. http://abcnews.go.com/Health/academics-profit-making-case-opioid-painkillers/story?id=13284493.

11. Portenoy RK, Foley KM. Chronic use of opioid analgesics in non-malignant pain: report of 38 cases. *Pain*. May 1986;25(2):171-186. https://www.ncbi.nlm.nih.gov/pubmed/2873550.

12. AMA Physician Masterfile. https://www.ama-assn.org/life-career/ama-physician-masterfile.

13. AMA 2014 Form 990. http://www.guidestar.org/FinDocuments /2014/360/727/2014-360727175-0bb01fe9-9O.pdf.

14. Van Zee A. The promotion and marketing of OxyContin: commercial triumph, public

health disaster. *Am J Public Health*. February 2009;99(2):221-227. https://www.ncbi.nlm .nih.gov/pmc/articles/PMC2622774/.

15. Reinberg S. Opioid overdoses nearly triple among kids and teens. WebMD. October 31, 2016. https://www.webmd.com/children/news/20161031/ opioid-overdoses-up-nearly -200-percent-among-kids-teens#1.

16. About the Council on Medical Education. AMA. http://www.ama-assn.org/ama/pub/ about-ama/our-people/ama-councils/council-medical-education.page?.

17. History of medicine. Milestones for health in America—1900s. City University of New York. https://www.cuny.edu/site/cc/health-in-america/1900s.html.

18. Sullivan RB. Sanguine practices: a historical and historiographic reconsideration of heroic therapy in the age of Rush. *Bull Hist Med*. Summer 1994;68(2):211-234. https:// www.ncbi.nlm.nih.gov/pubmed/8049598.

19. Loudon J. A brief history of homeopathy. *JR Soc Med*. December 2006;99(12):607-610. https://www.ncbi.nlm.nih.gov/pmc/articles/PMC1676328/.

20. North RL. Benjamin Rush, MD: assassin or beloved healer? *Proc (Bayl Univ Med Cent)*. January 2000;13(1):45-49. http://www.ncbi.nlm.nih.gov/pmc/articles/PMC1312212/.

21. Woodruff J. Bloodletting and blisters. PBS. December 15, 2014. https://www.pbs. org/newshour/show/bloodletting-blisters-solving-medical- mystery-george-washingtons -death.

22. Ullman D. A condensed history of homeopathy. In: Ullman D, *Discovering Home-opathy: Medicine for the 21st Century*. Berkeley, CA: North Atlantic Books; 2017. https:// homeopathic.com/a-condensed-history-of-homeopathy/.

23. Samuel Hahnemann (1755–1843). Skylark Books. Accessed October 1, 2014. http:// www.skylarkbooks.co.uk/Hahnemann_Biography.htm.

24. Homeopathy timeline: 1900–1924. Biographies and schools. Whole Health Now. http://www.wholehealthnow.com/homeopathy_pro/ homeopathy_1900_1924.html. http://www.homeopathycenter.org/homeopathy-today/homeopathy-today-article-no -title-10.

25. A brief history of osteopathic medicine. American Association of Colleges of Osteo-pathic Medicine. http://www.aacom.org/about/osteomed/Pages/History.aspx.

26. About the Council on Medical Education. AMA. http://www.ama-assn.org/ama/pub/ about-ama/our-people/ama-councils/council-medical-education.page?.

27. Johnson C, Green B. 100 years after the Flexner Report. *J Chiropr Educ*. Fall 2010;24(2): 145-152. http://www.ncbi.nlm.nih.gov/pmc/articles/PMC2967338/.

28. The Flexner Report: medical education in the United States and Canada, bul-letin 4. 1910. Carnegie Foundation for the Advancement of Teaching. http://archive .carnegiefoundation.org/pdfs/elibrary/Carnegie_Flexner_Report.pdf

29. Barzansky B, Gevitz, N. *Beyond Flexner: Medical Education in the Twentieth Century*. New York: Greenwood Press; 1992.

30. Duffy TP. The Flexner Report: 100 years later. *Yale J Biol Med.* September 2011;84(3):269-276. https://www.ncbi.nlm.nih.gov/pmc/articles/PMC3178858/.

31. Gevitz N. From "doctor of osteopathy" to "doctor of osteopathic medicine": a title change in the push for equality. *JAOA.* June 2014;114:486-497. http://jaoa.org/article.aspx?articleid=2094883.

32. Friedman M, Friedman R. *Free to Choose: A Personal Statement.* New York: Houghton Mifflin Harcourt; 1990:238-241.

33. Medicine. Cooperative doctor. *Time.* May 1, 1939. http://content.time.com/time/subscriber/article/0,33009,761173-1,00.html.

34. American Medical Association v. United States, 317 U.S. 519 (1943). https://supreme.justia.com/cases/federal/us/317/519/case.html.

35. Hall TS. Reimagining the learned intermediary rule for the new pharmaceutical marketplace. *Seton Hall Law Review.* 2004;35:193. http://law.shu.edu/Students/academics/journals/law-review/Issues/archives/upload/Hall-2.pdf.

36. Schremmer RD, Knapp JF. Harry Truman and health care reform: the debate started here. *Pediatrics.* March 2011;127:3. http://pediatrics.aappublications.org/content/pediatrics/127/3/399.full.pdf.

37. Merkel H. 69 years ago, a president pitches an idea for national health care. PBS. November 19, 2014. https://www.pbs.org/newshour/health/november-19-1945-harry-truman-calls-national-health-insurance-program.

38. Dickerson J. 50 years before Obamacare, JFK's own health care debacle. CBS News. November 18, 2013. https://www.cbsnews.com/news/50-years-before-obamacare-jfks-own-health-care-debacle/.

39. Howell JD. The paradox of osteopathy. *N Engl J Med.* 1999;341:1465-1468. http://www.nejm.org/doi/full/10.1056/NEJM199911043411910. Accessed October 10, 2014.

40. National Academies of Medicine. Summit on Integrative Medicine and the Health of the Public. 2009. http://www.nationalacademies.org/hmd/Activities/Quality/IntegrativeMed.aspx.

41. Collier R. American Medical Association membership woes continue. *CMAJ.* August 9, 2011;183(11). https://www.ncbi.nlm.nih.gov/pmc/ articles/PMC3153537/.

42. Sears catalog. 1897. https://www.amazon.com/1897-Sears-Roebuck-Co-Catalogue/dp/1602390630.

43. Lipton E, Thomas K. Drug lobbyists' battle cry over prices: blame the others. *New York Times.* May 29, 2017. https://www.nytimes.com/2017/05/29/health/drug-lobbyists-battle-cry-over-prices-blame-the-others.html?_r=0.

44. Burnby J. The early years of the pharmaceutical industry. In: Richmond L, Stevenson J, Turton A, eds. *The Pharmaceutical Industry: A Guide to Historical Records.* Burlington, VT: Ashgate Publishing; 2003:2.

45. Exploring our history: Pfizer history—1919. Pfizer. http://www.pfizer.com/about/history/1900-1950.

46. 1919, Pfizer chemist James Currie. Course Hero. https://www.coursehero.com/file/p3hpb1m/In-1919-Pfizer-chemist-James-Currie-and- his-assistant-Jasper-Kane -successfully/.

47. Development of deep tank fermentation. Pfizer Inc. historic chemical landmark. June 12, 2008. American Chemical Society. https://www.acs.org/content/dam/acsorg/education/whatischemistry/landmarks/penicillin/development-of-deep-tank-fermentation -commemorative-booklet.pdf.

48. Pfizer patent for fermentation process to produce gluconic acid. Free Patents Online. http://www.freepatentsonline.com/1849053.pdf.

49. Pfizer's work on penicillin for World War II becomes a national historic chemical landmark. June 12, 2008. American Chemical Society. http://www.acs.org/content/acs/en/pressroom/newsreleases/2008/june/pfizers-work-on-penicillin-for-world-war-ii -becomes-a-national-historic-chemical-landmark.html.

50. Cooper T, Ainsberg A. *Breakthrough: Elizabeth Hughes, the Discovery of Insulin, and the Making of a Medical Miracle*. New York: St. Martin's Press; 2010.

51. Lilly Library. *Lilly Library: The First Quarter Century 1960-1985*. Bloomington: Indiana University Press; 1985. Referenced in Cooper T, Ainsberg A. *Breakthrough: Elizabeth Hughes, the Discovery of Insulin, and the Making of a Medical Miracle*. New York: St. Martin's Press; 2010.

52. Furman JL, MacGarvie M. When the pill peddlers met the scientists. *Journal of the Economic and Business Historical Society*. 2008;26:133-145. http://smgworld.bu.edu/jefffurman/files/2012/05/FM-Pill-Peddlers-EEBH-2008.pdf. Accessed October 2, 2014.

53. About the International Psychoanalytical Society. http://www.findan analyst.org/ipa.

54. Lynott WA. Bureau of Mines studies of occupational diseases. *Journal of Industrial and Engineering Chemistry*. November 1916:1062. http://onlinebooks.library.upenn.edu/webbin/book/lookupname?key=United%20States.%20Bureau%20of%20Mines.

55. Frenette PS, Atweh GF. Sickle cell disease: old discoveries, new concepts, and future promises. *J Clin Invest*. April 2, 2007;117(4):850-858. http://www.ncbi.nlm.nih.gov/pmc/articles/PMC1838946/pdf/JCI0730920.pdf.

56. Bishop LF. The treatment of arteriosclerosis. *AMA Society Proceedings*. June 14, 1913:1913.

57. Barnes NP. American Therapeutic Society (Louis F. Bishop): the treatment of arteriosclerosis. *JAMA*. 1913;60(24):1913-1916. https://jamanetwork.com/journals/jama/article-abstract/215319.

58. PBS. *The Great War*—World War One: casualties and death tables. Accessed October 2, 2014. http://www.uwosh.edu/faculty_staff/ henson/188/WWI_Casualties%20and%20 Deaths%20%20PBS.html.

59. Achievements in public health, 1900–1999: control of infectious diseases. CDC. http://www.cdc.gov/mmwr/preview/mmwrhtml/mm4829a1.htm.

60. Smith SS. Eli Lilly Jr. made his firm a pharmaceutical power. Investors.com. April 24, 2004. http://news.investors.com/management-leaders-in-success/042414-698276 -eli-lilly-turned-drugmaking-into-science.htm.

61. Lilly JK, Sr. A plan for promoting the affairs of Eli Lilly & company during the years 1920-21-22-23. Lilly Library. Cooper T, Ainsberg A. *Breakthrough: Elizabeth Hughes, the Discovery of Insulin, and the Making of a Medical Miracle.* New York: St. Martin's Press; 2010:123.

62. Lilly JK, Sr. A plan for promoting the affairs of Eli Lilly & company during the years 1920-21-22-23. Lilly Library. Cooper T, Ainsberg A. *Breakthrough: Elizabeth Hughes, the Discovery of Insulin, and the Making of a Medical Miracle.* New York: St. Martin's Press; 2010:120.

63. Madison JH. *Eli Lilly: A Life, 1885-1977.* Indianapolis: Indiana Historical Society Press; 2006. Cooper T, Ainsberg A. *Breakthrough: Elizabeth Hughes, the Discovery of Insulin, and the Making of a Medical Miracle.* New York: St. Martin's Press; 2010:118.

64. *Proceedings of the American Journal of Physiology,* 34th Annual Meeting held December 28–30, 1921, New Haven, CT; February 1, 1922, Baltimore, MD. Cooper T, Ainsberg A. *Breakthrough: Elizabeth Hughes, the Discovery of Insulin, and the Making of a Medical Miracle.* New York: St. Martin's Press; 2010:128.

65. Levinson PD. Eighty years of insulin therapy: 1922–2002. *Medicine and Health, Rhode Island.* April 2003;86:101-106. http://www.ncbi.nlm.nih.gov/pubmed/12751363.

66. Stevenson L. *Sir Frederick Banting.* Toronto: Ryerson Press; 1946. Cooper T, Ainsberg A. *Breakthrough: Elizabeth Hughes, the Discovery of Insulin, and the Making of a Medical Miracle.* New York: St. Martin's Press; 2010:133,134.

67. Cooper T, Ainsberg A. *Breakthrough: Elizabeth Hughes, the Discovery of Insulin, and the Making of a Medical Miracle.* New York: St. Martin's Press; 2010:170,171.

68. *Encyclopaedia Britannica.* Charles Evans Hughes biography. https://www.britannica.com/biography/Charles-Evans-Hughes.

69. Cooper T, Ainsberg A. *Breakthrough: Elizabeth Hughes, the Discovery of Insulin, and the Making of a Medical Miracle.* New York: St. Martin's Press; 2010:190,191.

70. Cooper T, Ainsberg A. *Breakthrough: Elizabeth Hughes, the Discovery of Insulin, and the Making of a Medical Miracle.* New York: St. Martin's Press; 2010:241.

71. Hughes CE. *The Autobiographical Notes of Charles Evans Hughes.* Eds. Danelski DJ, Tulchin JS. Cambridge, MA: Harvard University Press; 1973.

72. Denning DW. Letter to the editor. *N Engl J Med.* 1982;307:127-128. July 8, 1982. http://www.nejm.org/doi/full/10.1056/NEJM198207083070222 Accessed October 1, 2014.

73. Picchi A. The rising cost of insulin: "Horror stories every day." Moneywatch. CBS News. May 9, 2018. https://www.cbsnews.com/news/the-rising-cost-of-insulin-horror-stories-every-day/.

74. Thomas K. Drug makers accused of fixing prices on insulin. *New York Times.* January 30, 2017. https://www.nytimes.com/2017/01/30/health/drugmakers-lawsuit-insulin-drugs.html.

Chapter 3—Government Steps In

1. Sun LH. Compounding pharmacy linked to meningitis outbreak knew of mold, bacteria contamination. *Washington Post.* October 26, 2012. https://www.washingtonpost.com/national/health-science/compounding-pharmacy-linked-to-meningitis-outbreak-knew

-of-mold-bacteria- contamination/2012/10/26/6e3344ee-1fa0-11e2-afca-58c2f5789c5d_ story.html?utm_term=.7edde79e3fe5.

2. Policy brief: regulating compounding pharmacies. *Health Affairs*. May 1, 2014. http:// www.healthaffairs.org/healthpolicybriefs/brief.php?brief_id=114.

3. Current Good Manufacturing Practices. FDA. https://www.fda.gov/food/ guidanceregulation/cgmp/.

4. Tavernise S, Pollack A. F.D.A. details contamination at pharmacy. *New York Times*. October 26, 2012. http://www.nytimes.com/2012/10/27/health/fda-finds-unsanitary -conditions-at-new-england-compounding-center.html.

5. Morgan D, Berkrot B. U.S. Congress takes aim at FDA over meningitis outbreak. Reuters. November 14, 2012. https://www.reuters.com/article/us-usa-health-meningitis-widow/u -s-congress-takes-aim-at-fda-over-meningitis-outbreak-idUSBRE8AD13020121114.

6. Brill S. How baby boomers broke America. *Time*. May 17, 2018. http://www.time .com/5280446/baby-boomer-generation-america-steve-brill/.

7. About FDA: significant dates in U.S. food and drug law history. FDA. https://www.fda .gov/aboutfda/history/forgshistory/evolvingpowers/ucm2007256.htm.

8. Office of Regulatory Affairs (ORA) organization chart. FDA. https://www.fda.gov/ aboutfda/centersoffices/organizationcharts/ucm347891.htm.

9. Eyre E. Drug firms poured 780M painkillers into WV amid rise of overdoses. *Charleston Gazette-Mail*. December 17, 2016. https://www.wvgazettemail.com/news/health/ drug-firms-poured-m-painkillers-into-wv-amid-rise-of/article_78963590-b050-11e7 -8186-f7e8c8a1b804.html.

10. Baker P. Tom Marino, drug czar nominee, withdraws in latest setback for Trump's opioid fight. *New York Times*. October 17, 2017. https://www.nytimes.com/2017/10/17/ us/politics/trump-says-drug-czar-nominee-tom-marino-withdraws-from-consideration. html.

11. Higham S, Bernstein L. Rep. Tom Marino: Drug czar nominee and the opioid industry's advocate in Congress. *Washington Post*. October 15, 2017. https://www.washingtonpost .com/investigations/rep-tom-marino-drug-czar-nominee-and-the-opioid-industrys-advocate-in-congress/2017/10/15/555211a0-b03a-11e7-9e58-e6288544af98_story.html ?utm_term=.d560b031e79a.

12. Tom Marino out as Trump's drug czar nominee after "60 Minutes"/*Washington Post* report. CBS News. October 17, 2017. https://www.cbsnews.com/news/tom-marino-out -trump-drug-czar-nominee-60- minutes-report-live-updates/.

13. A history of the FDA and drug regulation in the United States. FDA. https://www .fda.gov/downloads/Drugs/ResourcesForYou/ Consumers/BuyingUsingMedicineSafely/ UnderstandingOver-the- CounterMedicines/UCM093550.pdf.

14. Janssen WF. The story of the laws behind the labels. *FDA Consumer* magazine. June 1981. https://www.fda.gov/downloads/AboutFDA/WhatWe Do/History/FOrgsHistory/ EvolvingPowers/UCM593437.pdf.

15. U.S. Pharmacopeia. 1902 Biologics Control Act. October 7, 2010. http://www.usp .org/sites/default/files/fda-exhibit/legislation/1902.html.

16. DeHovitz RE. The 1901 St Louis incident: the first modern medical disaster. *Pediatrics.* June 2014;133:6. http://pediatrics.aappublications.org/content/133/6/964.

17. Piascik A. Ida Tarbell: the woman who took on Standard Oil. Connecticut History. https://connecticuthistory.org/ida-tarbell-the-woman-who-took-on-standard-oil/.

18. The Pure Food and Drug Act [editorial]. June 23, 1906. History, Art, and Archives. US House of Representatives. http://history.house.gov/HistoricalHighlight/Detail/15032393280?ret=True.

19. The Federal Food and Drugs Act: 1906–1931. *JAMA.* 1931;97(1):32. doi:10.1001/jama.1931.02730010036012. http://jama.jamanetwork.com/article.aspx?articleid=259937.

20. United States v. Johnson, 221 U.S. 488 (1911). https://supreme.justia.com/cases/federal/us/221/488/case.html.

21. The Sherley Amendment: false statements regarding the curative properties of proprietary medicines held to be unlawful. JSTOR. December 8, 1916. https://archive.org/details/jstor-4574317.

22. Harrison Narcotics Tax Act 1914. http://www.druglibrary.org/Schaffer/history/e1910/harrisonact.htm.

23. King RB. The Narcotics Bureau and the Harrison Act: jailing the healers and the sick. *Yale Law Journal.* 1953; 62:784-787. http://www.druglibrary.org/special/king/king1.htm.

24. Amadeo K. Great depression timeline: 1929–1941. The Balance. April 30, 2018. https://www.thebalance.com/great-depression-timeline-1929-1941-4048064.

25. Cavers DF. The Food, Drug and Cosmetic Act of 1938: its legislative history and its substantive provisions. *Law and Contemporary Problems.* Winter 1939;6:2-42. https://scholarship.law.duke.edu/lcp/vol6/iss1/2/.

26. Akst J. The Elixir tragedy, 1937. *Scientist Magazine.* June 1, 2013. https://www.the-scientist.com/foundations/the-elixir-tragedy-1937-39231.

27. Ballentine C. Taste of raspberries, taste of death: the 1937 Elixir Sulfanilamide incident. *FDA Consumer* magazine. June 1981. https://www.fda.gov/AboutFDA/History/ProductRegulation/ucm2007257.htm.

28. Medicine post-mortem. *Time.* December 20, 1937. http://content.time.com/time/subscriber/article/0,33009,758704-2,00.html.

29. Akst J. The Elixir tragedy, 1937. *Scientist Magazine.* June 1, 2013. http://www.the-scientist.com/?articles.view/articleNo/35714/title/The-Elixir-Tragedy—1937/.

30. American Medical Association Clinical Laboratory. Elixir of sulfanilamide—Massengill. *JAMA.* November 6, 1937;109:19:1531. http://jama.jamanetwork.com/article.aspx?articleid=279102.

31. Martin B. Elixir Sufanilamide: deaths of 1937. Pathophilia. http://bmartinmd.com/elixir-sulfanilamide-deaths/.

32. Karst KR. Diamond jubilee: the federal Food, Drug and Cosmetic Act turns 75! FDA Law Blog. June 25, 2013. http://www.fdalawblog.net/fda_law_blog_hyman_phelps/2013/06/diamond-jubilee-the-federal-food-drug-and-cosmetic-act-turns-75.html.

33. Cavers DF. The Food, Drug and Cosmetic Act of 1938: its legislative history and its substantive provisions. *Duke Law Journal.* 1939: 1-41. http://scholarship.law.duke.edu/cgi/viewcontent.cgi?article=1937&context=lcp.

34. Copeland RS. Protection for the public. *Scientific American.* February 1, 1938;158(2). http://www.scientificamerican.com/magazine/sa/1938/02-01/.

35. History: the 1938 Food, Drug, and Cosmetic Act. FDA. https://www.fda.gov/regulatoryinformation/lawsenforcedbyfda/federalfooddrugandcosmeticactfdcact/default.htm.

36. Tabler D. My chemists and I deeply regret the fatal results. Appalachian History. October 29, 2012. http://www.appalachianhistory.net/2016/10/my-chemists-and-i-deeply-regret-fatal.html

37. Hamowy R. Medical disasters and the growth of the FDA: the sulfanilamide crisis of 1937. February 2010:17. Independent Institute. http://www.independent.org/pdf/policy_reports/2010-02-10-fda.pdf.

38. Lesney MS. The ghosts of pharma past: the timeline. January 2004: 26. http://pubs.acs.org/subscribe/archive/mdd/v07/i01/pdf/104timeline.pdf.

39. Martin B. Pfizer cuts jobs at Bristol plant, former site of Massengill headquarters. Pathophilia. August 11, 2011. http://bmartinmd.com/2011/08/pfizer-cuts-jobs-bristol/.

40. Milestones in food and drug law history. About FDA. FDA. https://www.fda.gov/downloads/AboutFDA/WhatWeDo/History/FOrgs History/HistoryofFDAsCentersandOffices/UCM586461.pdf.

41. Public Health Service Act, 1944 [editorial]. *Public Health Rep.* July–August 1994; 109(4):468. https://www.ncbi.nlm.nih.gov/pmc/articles/PMC1403520/?page=1.

42. Swann JP. The race to bring penicillin to the troops in WWII. *FDA Voice.* November 7, 2016. https://blogs.fda.gov/fdavoice/index.php/2016/11/the-race-to-bring-penicillin-to-the-troops-in-wwii/.

43. Alberty Food Products et al. v. United States, 194 F.2d 463 (9th Cir. 1952). Justia US Law. February 15, 1952. https://law.justia.com/cases/federal/appellate-courts/F2/194/463/460503/.

44. The Durham-Humphrey Amendment. *JAMA.* May 24, 1952;149(4):371. https://jamanetwork.com/journals/jama/article-abstract/314797.

45. Famous people who have had polio. Disabled World Towards Tomorrow. https://www.disabled-world.com/artman/publish/famous-polio.shtml.

46. Fitzpatrick M. The Cutter incident: how America's first polio vaccine led to a growing vaccine crisis. *J R Soc Med.* March 2006;99(3):156. https://www.ncbi.nlm.nih.gov/pmc/articles/PMC1383764/.

47. Senator Morse and Senator Humphrey, "The Salk Vaccine." *Congressional Record* 101, pt.6. 1955: 7115-7119. Tobbell DA. *Pills, Power, and Policy: The Struggle for Drug Reform in Cold War America and Its Consequences.* Berkeley: University of California Press; 2012:69.

48. Tobbell DA. *Pills, Power, and Policy: The Struggle for Drug Reform in Cold War America and Its Consequences.* Berkeley: University of California Press; 2012:71.

49. Special Committee on Organized Crime in Interstate Commerce (The Kefauver Committee). May 2, 1950. United States Senate: Senate History. Accessed October 22, 2014. http://www.senate.gov/artandhistory/history/common/investigations/Kefauver .htm.

50. Tobbell DA. *Pills, Power, and Policy: The Struggle for Drug Reform in Cold War America and Its Consequences.* Berkeley: University of California Press; 2012:59.

51. 50th anniversary of the Kefauver-Harris Drug Amendments of 1962: interview with FDA historian John Swann. FDA. Accessed October 23, 2014. http://regulatorydoctor.us/ wp-content/uploads/2014/12/FDA-Information-on-The-Kefauver-Harris-Amendments .pdf.

52. Tobbell DA. *Pills, Power, and Policy: The Struggle for Drug Reform in Cold War America and Its Consequences.* Berkeley: University of California Press; 2012:76.

53. Barmash I. Judge clears Pfizer, Cyanamid and Bristol-Myers in trust suit. *New York Times.* December 1, 1973. https://www.nytimes.com/1973/12/01/archives/judge-clears -pfizer-cyanamid-and-bristolmyers-in-trust-suit-judge.html.

54. Squires S. The other side of thalidomide. *Washington Post.* June 20, 1989. Accessed October 23, 2014. http://www.washingtonpost.com/wp-srv/washtech/longterm/ thalidomide/keystories/patient062089.htm.

55. Rice E. Dr. Francis Kelsey: turning the thalidomide tragedy into Food and Drug Administration reform. FDA Research Paper Division. Accessed October 23, 2014. http:// www.section216.com/history/Kelsey.pdf.

56. Wadman M. Lawsuit blames thalidomide for more birth defects. *Scientific American.* November 7, 2011. https://www.scientificamerican.com/article/lawsuit-blames -thalidomide-for-more/.

57. Fintel B, Samaras AT, Carias E. The thalidomide tragedy: lessons for drug safety and regulation. *Helix Magazine.* Northwestern University. July 28, 2009. Accessed October 23, 2014. https://helix.northwestern.edu/article/thalidomide-tragedy-lessons-drug-safety -and-regulation.

58. Podolsky SH. *The Antibiotic Era: Reform, Resistance and the Pursuit of Rational Therapeutics.* Baltimore, MD: Johns Hopkins University Press; 2015:84-94.

59. Leslie FA. Is thalidomide to blame? *Bri Med J.* December 31, 1960;2:1954. http:// www.bmj.com/content/2/5217/1954.1.

60. Mintz M. Heroine of FDA keeps bad drug off market. *Washington Post.* July 15, 1962. Accessed October 23, 2014. http://www.washingtonpost.com/wp-srv/washtech/longterm/ thalidomide/keystories/071598drug.htm.

61. Tausig HB. A study of the German outbreak of phocomelia: the thalidomide syndrome. *JAMA.* June 30, 1962;180:1106-1114. https://www.ncbi.nlm.nih.gov/pubmed/13919869.

62. President John F. Kennedy's 40th news conference, August 1, 1962. YouTube video. Accessed October 23, 2014. https://www.youtube.com/watch?v=g64NiKCL6yA.

63. US National Library of Medicine. Dr. Frances Kathleen Oldham Kelsey: biography. NIH. Changing the Face of Medicine. Accessed October 23, 2014. http://www.nlm.nih .gov/changingthefaceofmedicine/physicians/biography_182.html.

64. The full story of the drug thalidomide. *Life.* August 1, 1962. Accessed October 23, 2014. https://www.bing.com/images/search?view=detailV2&ccid=%2fQ9YPVq6&id=AA 040049A403A39A60B4EB8D66B0A8764C758099&thid=OIP._Q9YPVq6cq4dgBM8kv8 kkgHaJy&mediaurl=http%3a%2f%2f4.bp.blogspot.com%2f-Tmqgmimtltw% 2fUJkewScB9aI%2fAAAAAAAAAJc%2f2QTcI1kzH38%2fs1600%2fLife%2b1.jpg&ex ph=1600&expw=1210&q=thalidomide+life.+august+1%2c+1962.& simid=6080076719 05324234&selectedIndex=2&ajaxhist=0.

65. Taussig HB. The thalidomide syndrome. *Scientific American.* August 1962; 207(2):29-35. http://www.scientificamerican.com/magazine/sa/1962/08-01/.

66. Gaffney A. FDA marks half-century of regulation based on safety, efficacy. October 10, 2012. Regulatory Affairs Professional Society. Accessed October 23, 2014. https:// www.raps.org/regulatory-focus%E2%84%A2/news-articles/2012/10/fda-marks-half -century-of-regulation-based-on-safety,-efficacy.

67. Greene JA, Podolsky SH. Reform, regulation, and pharmaceuticals—the Kefauver-Harris amendments at 50. *N Engl J Med.* 2012;367:1481-1483. http://www.nejm.org/doi/ full/10.1056/NEJMp1210007#t=article.

68. Ethical drugs—reflections on the inquiry. *N Engl J Med.* 1961;265:1015-1016. http:// www.nejm.org/doi/10.1056/NEJM196111162652013.

69. Drews G. Federal Drug Regulation Act. *Brook L Rev.* 1962-1963; 29:91. HeinOnline. http://heinonline.org/HOL/LandingPage?handle=hein.journals/brklr29&div =15&id=&page=.

70. Tobbell DA. *Pills, Power, and Policy: The Struggle for Drug Reform in Cold War America and Its Consequences.* Berkeley: University of California Press; 2012:118,119.

Chapter 4—The War of Science against Disease

1. Stolberg SG. The biotech death of Jesse Gelsinger. *New York Times.* November 28, 1999. http://www.nytimes.com/1999/11/28/magazine/the-biotech-death-of-jesse-gelsinger .html.

2. Wilson RF. The death of Jesse Gelsinger: new evidence of the influence of money and prestige in human research. *Washington and Lee University School of Law Scholarly Commons.* 2010. https://scholarlycommons.law.wlu.edu/cgi/viewcontent.cgi?referer=https://www .bing.com/&httpsredir=1&article=1125&context=wlufac.

3. Barlow D. Trial and error. BBC Two. February 27, 2014. http://www.bbc.co.uk/science/ horizon/2003/trialerrortrans.shtml.

4. Strong medicine: health system cuts 1700 after record deficit [editorial]. *Pennsylvania Gazette.* January–February 2000. http://www.upenn.edu/gazette/0100/0100gaz1.html.

5. Medical Roundtable. Antonio M. Gotto, Jr., MD, DPhil. Biography. Weill-Cornell Medicine-Qatar. https://themedicalroundtable.com/users/antonio-gotto-jr.

6. Merck. Timeline (1925). https://www.merck.com/about/our-history/home.html.

7. Ginzberg E. *The Medical Triangle.* Cambridge, MA: Harvard University Press; 1990:79,80,177.

8. Vannevar Bush to Franklin D. Roosevelt—NARA. *Time*. April 3, 1944. http://content.time.com/time/covers/0,16641,19440403,00.html.

9. Science: Yankee scientist. *Time*. April 3, 1944. http://content.time.com/time/subscriber/article/0,33009,850430-1,00.html.

10. Sensata. History of our company. https://www.sensata.com/about.

11. Dalakov G. History of computers: biography of Vannevar Bush. Accessed January 14, 2015. http://history-computer.com/People/BushBio.html.

12. Zachary GP. The godfather. *Wired*. Accessed January 15, 2015. http://archive.wired.com/wired/archive/5.11/es_bush_pr.html.

13. OSRD atomic bomb: Vannevar Bush–James Conant papers. Paperless Archives. http://www.paperlessarchives.com/wwii-vannevar-bush-atomic-bomb.html.

14. Franklin D. Roosevelt to Vannevar Bush. November 17, 1944. http://delong.typepad.com/sdj/2014/11/liveblogging-world-war-ii-november-17-1944-fdr-to-vannevar-bush.html#more.

15. US Department of Energy. Letter to FDR from Vannevar Bush, returned with "OK—FDR." Manhattan Project interactive history. https://www.osti.gov/opennet/manhattan-project-history/images/vbok_image.htm.

16. Long AP. The Army immunization program. In: Coates JB, ed. *Preventive Medicine in World War II. Vol III—Personal Health Measures and Immunization*. U.S. Army Medical Department. Office of Medical History. http://history.amedd.army.mil/booksdocs/wwii/PrsnlHlthMsrs/chapter8.htm.

17. Hoyt K. How World War II spurred vaccine innovation. The Conversation. March 8, 2015. http://theconversation.com/how-world-war-ii-spurred-vaccine-innovation-39903.

18. NurseGroups. Nursing history: the history of WWII medicine for schools—the use of sulfanilamide in World War II. 2018. http://www.nursegroups.com/article/history-of-wwii-medicine-for-schools.html.

19. Dole B. *One Soldier's Story*. New York: HarperCollins; 2005:32.

20. Biography.com. Dr. Charles Drew biography: surgeon, doctor, educator (1905–1950). https://www.biography.com/people/charles-drew-9279094.

21. Krensky P. Dr. Charles Drew, father of the blood bank. American Red Cross. October 26, 2015. http://www.redcross.org/news/article/Dr-Charles-Drew-father-of-the-blood-bank.

22. Red Cross. Red Cross Blood Services History. 1945. http://www.redcross.org/news/article/RedCrossMonth-Supporting-Our-Military-For-More-Than-A-Century.

23. Venereal disease and treatment in WWII. WW2 U.S. Medical Research Centre. http://www.med-dept.com/articles/venereal-disease-and-treatment-during-ww2/.

24. Appel JW, Beebe G, Hilger DW. Comparative incidence of neuropsychiatric casualties in World War I and World War II. *Am J Psychiatry*. 1946;103(2):196-199. http://www.ncbi.nlm.nih.gov/pubmed/21001991.

25. Salmon TW. *The Care and Treatment of Mental Diseases and War Neuroses ("Shell Shock") in the British Army*. New York: War Work Committee of the National Committee for Mental Hygiene; 1917:47.

26. Leese P. *Shell Shock: Traumatic Neurosis and the British Soldiers of the First World War.* New York: Palgrave Macmillan; 2002.

27. Pols H, Oak S. War and military mental health: the U.S. psychiatric response in the 20th century. *Am. J Public Health.* December 2007;97(12):2132-2142. http://www.ncbi .nlm.nih.gov/pmc/articles/PMC2089086/.

28. Strecker EA. Experiences in the immediate treatment of war neuroses. *American Journal of Insanity.* 1919;76:45-69.

29. Sullivan HS. Mental hygiene and national defense: a year of selective-service psychiatry. *Mental Hygiene.* 1942;26(1):7-14; Sullivan HS. Psychiatry and the national defense. *Psychiatry.* 1941; 4:201-217.

30. Rioch DM. Recollections of Harry Stack Sullivan and the development of his interpersonal psychiatry. *Psychiatry.* May 1985;48(2):141-158. http://www.ncbi.nlm.nih.gov/ pubmed/3887444.

31. Ginzberg E, Anderson JK, Ginsburg SW, Herma JL. *The Lost Divisions.* New York: Columbia University Press; 1959:6-15.

32. Appel JW, Beebe GW, Hilger DW. Comparative incidence of neuropsychiatric casualties in World War I and World War II. *Am J Psych.* 1946;103(2):196-199. http://www .ncbi.nlm.nih.gov/pubmed/21001991.

33. Jonas CH. Psychiatry has growing pains. *Am J Psychiatry.* 1946;102(6):819-821. http:// www.ncbi.nlm.nih.gov/pubmed/20987746.

34. Jones E, Hyams KC, Wessely C. Screening for vulnerability to psychological disorders in the military: an historical survey. *Journal of Medical Screening.* 2003;10(1):40-46. http:// www.ncbi.nlm.nih.gov/pubmed/12790314.

35. Hanson F, ed. *Combat Psychiatry: Experiences in the North African and Mediterranean Theaters of Operation, American Ground Forces, World War II.* Supplement, *Bulletin of the US Army Medical Department* 9 (Washington, DC, 1949).

36. Ginzberg E, Anderson JK, Ginsburg SW, Herma JL. *The Lost Divisions.* New York: Columbia University Press; 1959:88-103.

37. Grinker RR, Spiegel JP. *War Neurosis in North Africa: The Tunisian Campaign, January–May 1943.* Washington, DC: Josiah Macy Foundation; 1943. https://www.journals .uchicago.edu/doi/10.1086/394854.

38. The World War II Military Hospitals. Types of hospitals. https://www.med-dept .com/articles/ww2-military-hospitals-general-introduction/.

39. Bartemeier LH, Kubie LS, Menninger KA, Romano J, Whitehorn JC. Combat exhaustion. *Journal of Nervous and Mental Disease.* 1946; 104:358-389,489-525.

40. Houts AC. Fifty years of psychiatric nomenclature: reflections on the 1943 War Department Technical Bulletin, Medical 203. *J Clinical Psychol.* 2000;56:935-967. http:// onlinelibrary.wiley.com/doi/10.1002/1097-4679(200007)56:7%3C935:AID-JCLP11 %3E3.0.CO;2-8/abstract.

41. Younkin P. Making the market: how the American pharmaceutical industry transformed itself during the 1940s. University of California at Berkeley; 2008:1-31. http://www.irle .berkeley.edu/culture/papers/Younkin-Mar08.pdf.

42. Discovery and development of penicillin. American Chemical Society. http://www .acs.org/content/acs/en/education/whatischemistry/landmarks/flemingpenicillin.html.

43. Pfizer's work on penicillin for World War II becomes a national historic chemical landmark. American Chemical Society. June 12, 2008. http://www.acs.org/content/ acs/en/pressroom/newsreleases/2008/june/pfizers-work-on-penicillin-for-world-war-ii -becomes-a-national-historic-chemical-landmark.html.

44. Short A. Better than Viagra! Sale of Pfizer plant gives rise to jobs. *Brooklyn Paper.* February 15, 2011. https://www.brooklynpaper.com/stories /34/7/wb_pfizersite_2011_2_18_ bk.html.

45. Tobbell DA. *Pills, Power, and Policy: The Struggle for Drug Reform in Cold War America and Its Consequences.* Berkeley: University of California Press; 2012:22.

46. Wiesner JB. *Vannevar Bush: 1890–1974.* Washington, DC: National Academy of Sciences; 1979:96. http://www.nasonline.org/publications/biographical-memoirs/memoir -pdfs/bush-vannevar.pdf.

47. NIH directors. https://www.nih.gov/about-nih/what-we-do/nih-almanac/nih -directors.

48. Jones S et al. *Securing Health: Lessons from Nation-Building Missions.* Santa Monica, CA: RAND Corporation, MG-321-RC; 2006. https://www.rand.org/pubs/research_briefs/ RB9237/index1.html.

49. CDC. Achievements in public health, 1900-1999: changes in the public health system. MMWR. December 24, 1999. https://www.cdc.gov/mmwr/preview/mmwrhtml/ mm4850a1.htm.

50. Announcement of the CDC name change. CDC MMWR Weekly. October 30, 1992; 41(43):829. https://www.cdc.gov/mmwr/preview/mmwrhtml/00017962.htm.

51. Tobbell DA. *Pills, Power, and Policy: The Struggle for Drug Reform in Cold War America and Its Consequences.* Berkeley: University of California Press; 2012:17, 27.

52. Tobbell DA. *Pills, Power, and Policy: The Struggle for Drug Reform in Cold War America and Its Consequences.* Berkeley: University of California Press; 2012:27, 28.

53. Tobbell DA. *Pills, Power, and Policy: The Struggle for Drug Reform in Cold War America and Its Consequences.* Berkeley: University of California Press; 2012:20-23.

54. Tobbell DA. *Pills, Power, and Policy: The Struggle for Drug Reform in Cold War America and Its Consequences.* Berkeley: University of California Press; 2012:19.

55. Tobbell DA. *Pills, Power, and Policy: The Struggle for Drug Reform in Cold War America and Its Consequences.* Berkeley: University of California Press; 2012:17-20.

56. Tobbell DA *Pills, Power, and Policy: The Struggle for Drug Reform in Cold War America and Its Consequences.* Berkeley: University of California Press; 2012:23-34.

57. Tobbell DA. *Pills, Power, and Policy: The Struggle for Drug Reform in Cold War America and Its Consequences.* Berkeley: University of California Press; 2012:46-54.

58. Tobbell DA. *Pills, Power, and Policy: The Struggle for Drug Reform in Cold War America and Its Consequences.* Berkeley: University of California Press; 2012:35.

59. Tobbell DA. *Pills, Power, and Policy: The Struggle for Drug Reform in Cold War America and Its Consequences.* Berkeley: University of California Press; 2012:35-37.

60. Graduate medical education and public policy: a primer. HRSA, December 2000. http://docplayer.net/2554780-Graduate-medical- education-and-public-policy.html.

61. Starr P. *The Social Transformation of American Medicine*. New York: Basic Books; 1982:358.

62. Gill CJ, Gill GC. Nightingale in Scutari: her legacy reexamined. *Clinical Infectious Diseases*. June 2005;40(12):1799-1805. doi:10.1086/430380. ISSN 1058-4838. PMID 15909269.

63. Nightingale F. *Notes on Nursing: What It Is and What It Is Not*. Blackie & Son Ltd; 1974 (1st published 1859). ISBN 9780216899742.

64. US Army Center of Military History. *The Army Nurse Corps*. December 18, 2014; 3, 6. http://www.history.army.mil/books/wwii/72-14/72-14.HTM.

65. US Army Center of Military History. *The Army Nurse Corps*. December 18, 2014; 7. http://www.history.army.mil/books/wwii/72-14/72-14.HTM.

66. US Army Center of Military History. *The Army Nurse Corps*. December 18, 2014; 6. http://www.history.army.mil/books/wwii/72-14/72-14.HTM.

67. US Army Center of Military History. *The Army Nurse Corps*. December 18, 2014. 8. http://www.history.army.mil/books/wwii/72-14/72-14.HTM.

68. Hill-Burton Act (1946). Encyclopedia.com (2006). http://www.encyclopedia.com/ history/encyclopedias-almanacs-transcripts-and-maps/hill-burton-act-1946.

69. Cooper T, Ainsberg A. *Breakthrough*. New York: St. Martins; 2010.

70. Goodwin DK. *No Ordinary Time*. New York: Simon and Schuster; 1994:622-625.

Chapter 5—Advocates

1. Kopp E, Lupkin S, Lucas E. KHN launches "Pre$cription for Power," a groundbreaking database to expose Big Pharma's ties to patient groups. KHN. April 6, 2018. https:// khn.org/news/patient-advocacy-groups-take-in-millions-from-drugmakers-is-there-a -payback/?utm_source=STAT+Newsletters&utm_campaign=32da8bc99a-MR&utm_ medium=email&utm_term=0_8cab1d7961-32da8bc99a-150335297.

2. Susan G. Komen Foundation. Think Pink. https://ww5.komen.org/.

3. Orenstein P. Our feel-good war on breast cancer. *New York Times*. April 25, 2013. http://www.nytimes.com/2013/04/28/magazine/our-feel-good-war-on-breast-cancer .html?pagewanted=all.

4. Think before You Pink. 4 questions before you buy pink. Breast Cancer Action. http:// thinkbeforeyoupink.org/resources/before-you-buy/.

5. National Cancer Institute. Milestone: National Cancer Act of 1971. https://dtp.cancer .gov/timeline/noflash/milestones/M4_Nixon.htm.

6. Von Eschenbach A. Eliminating the suffering and death due to cancer by 2015. MI Report. September 1, 2005. https://www.manhattan- institute.org/html/eliminating -suffering-and-death-due-cancer- 2015-5951.html.

7. Charles D. Obama announces $5 billion for new medical research. Reuters. September 30, 2009. https://www.reuters.com/article/us-usa-healthcare-obama/obama-announces -5-billion-for-new-medical-research-idUSTRE58T43G20090930.

8. Begley S. A serious new hurdle for CRISPR: edited cells might cause cancer find two studies. STAT. June 11, 2018. https://www.statnews.com/2018/06/11/crispr-hurdle -edited-cells-might-cause-cancer/?utm_source=STAT+Newsletters&utm_ campaign=b01fef7a77-MR_COPY_09&utm_medium=email&utm_term=0_ 8cab1d7961-b01fef7a77-150335297.

9. National Cancer Institute. Cancer statistics. 2018. https://www.cancer.gov/about -cancer/understanding/statistics.

10. Kaplan K. A plan to prevent more than 1 in 5 cancer deaths, without having to invent any new treatments. *Los Angeles Times.* July 10, 2018. http://www.latimes.com/science/ sciencenow/la-sci-sn-cancer-health-disparities-20180710-story.html.

11. National Institutes of Health. Budget. 2018. https://www.nih.gov/about-nih/what -we-do/budget.

12. Squires D. U.S. health care from a global perspective. Commonwealth Fund. October 8, 2015. https://www.commonwealthfund.org/publications/issue-briefs/2015/oct/ us-health-care-global-perspective.

13. Blumenthal D, Seervai S. Rising obesity in the United States: a public health crisis. Commonwealth Fund. April 24, 2018. https://www.commonwealthfund.org/blog/2018/rising -obesity-united-states-public-health-crisis?redirect_source=/publications/blog/2018/apr/ rising-obesity-public-health-crisis.

14. Rank MR, Hirschi TA. The likelihood of experiencing poverty over the life course. *PLOS One.* July 22, 2015. http://journals.plos.org/plosone/article/file?id=10.1371/journal .pone.0133513&type=printable.

15. Weissmann J. 5 percent of Americans made up 50 percent of U.S. spending. *Atlantic.* January 13, 2012. https://www.theatlantic.com/business/archive/2012/01/5-of-americans -made-up-50-of-us-health-care-spending/251402/.

16. Yarrow A. What no one tells new moms about what childbirth can do to their bodies. Vox. May 4, 2018. https://www.vox.com/science-and-health/2017/6/26/15872734/ postnatal-care-america.

17. Bayer R, Galea S. Public health in the precision medicine era. *New Engl. J. Med.* 2015;373:499-501. https://www.nejm.org/doi/full/10.1056/NEJMp1506241.

18. Rose SL. Patient advocacy organizations: institutional conflicts of interest, trust, and trustworthiness. *J Law Med Ethics.* Fall 2013; 41(3):680-687. https://www.ncbi.nlm.nih .gov/pmc/articles/PMC4107906/?_escaped_fragment_=po=0.632911.

19. Mary Lasker Papers: biographical information. National Library of Medicine. NIH. https://profiles.nlm.nih.gov/ps/retrieve/Narrative/TL/ p-nid/199.

20. Cavallo J. A leading light in cancer advances, Mary Lasker used wealth and connections to increase funding for medical research. *ASCO Post.* September 15, 2012. www.ascopost .com/issues/september-15-2012/a-leading-light-in-cancer-advances-mary-lasker-used -wealth-and- connections-to-increase-funding-for-medical-research/.

21. Mary Woodward Lasker: The Eleanor Roosevelt Papers. https/www2.gwu.edu/ ~erpapers/mep/displaydoc.cfm?docid=erpn-marlas.

352 NOTES

22. Notable New Yorkers: Mary Lasker. Audio transcript. Columbia University Libraries. http://www.columbia.edu/cu/lweb/digital/collections/nny/laskerm/transcripts/laskerm_1_1_28.html.

23. Notable New Yorkers: Mary Lasker. Audio transcript. Columbia University Libraries.
http://www.columbia.edu/cu/lweb/digital/collections/nny/laskerm/transcripts/laskerm_1_15_454.html.

24. Mary Lasker Papers: biographical information. National Library of Medicine. NIH. http://www.columbia.edu/cu/lweb/digital/collections/nny/laskerm/transcripts/laskerm_1_4_115.html.

25. Mary Lasker Papers: biographical information. National Library of Medicine. NIH. http://www.columbia.edu/cu/lweb/digital/collections/nny/laskerm/transcripts/laskerm_1_4_114.html.

26. Notable New Yorkers: Mary Lasker. Audio transcript. Columbia University Libraries. http://www.columbia.edu/cu/lweb/digital/collections/nny/laskerm/transcripts/laskerm_1_4_103.html.

27. Notable New Yorkers: Mary Lasker. Audio transcript. Columbia University Libraries. http://www.columbia.edu/cu/lweb/digital/collections/nny/laskerm/transcripts/laskerm_1_9_253.html.

28. American Society for the Control of Cancer. History. December 20, 2015. http://www.smokershistory.com/ASCC.htm.

29. Free Dictionary. Lasker Awards. http://encyclopedia2.thefreedictionary.com/Lasker+Award. Immigrant Entrepreneurship. Albert Lasker (1880–1952). http://www.immigrantentrepreneurship.org/entry.php?rec=57.

30. Notable New Yorkers: Mary Lasker. Audio transcript. Columbia University Libraries. http://www.columbia.edu/cu/lweb/digital/collections/nny/laskerm/transcripts/laskerm_1_16_482.html.

31. Meyer HS, Morse DH, Hogan R. Noble conspirator: Florence S. Mahoney and the rise of the National Institutes of Health. *JAMA*. 2002;287(13):1732-1733. http://jama.jamanetwork.com/article.aspx?articleid=1844693.

32. Obituaries: Florence Mahoney, advocate of NIH and NIA, dies at 103. NIH Record. https://nihrecord.nih.gov/newsletters/01_07_2003/obits.htm.

33. Dougherty J. Age sage. *Phoenix New Times*. October 4, 2001. http://www.phoenixnewtimes.com/news/age-sage-6414303.

34. Notable New Yorkers: Mary Lasker. Audio transcript. Columbia University Libraries. http://www.columbia.edu/cu/lweb/digital/collections/nny/laskerm/transcripts/laskerm_1_22_667.html.

35. This Day in Truman History: November 19, 1945. President Truman's proposed health care program. Harry S. Truman Presidential Library and Museum. https://trumanlibrary.org/anniversaries/healthprogram.htm.

36. Markel H. 69 years ago a president pitches his idea for national health care. PBS.

November 19, 2014. https://www.pbs.org/newshour/health/november-19-1945-harry -truman-calls-national-health-insurance-program.

37. What is basic research? 1953. National Science Foundation. https://www.nsf.gov/ pubs/1953/annualreports/ar_1953_sec6.pdf.

38. Baranauckas C. Florence S. Mahoney, 103, health advocate. *New York Times*. December 16, 2002. http://www.nytimes.com/2002/12/16/us/florence-s-mahoney-103-health -advocate.html.

39. Notable New Yorkers: Mary Lasker. Audio transcript. Columbia University Libraries. http://www.columbia.edu/cu/lweb/digital/collections/nny/laskerm/transcripts/laskerm _1_5_136.html.

40. Notable New Yorkers: Mary Lasker. Audio transcript. Columbia University Libraries. http://www.columbia.edu/cu/lweb/digital/collections/nny/laskerm/transcripts/laskerm _1_5_131.html.

41. Notable New Yorkers: Mary Lasker. Audio transcript. Columbia University Libraries. http://www.columbia.edu/cu/lweb/digital/collections/nny/laskerm/transcripts/laskerm _1_5_133.html.

42. Notable New Yorkers: Mary Lasker. Audio transcript. Columbia University Libraries. http://www.columbia.edu/cu/lweb/digital/collections/nny/laskerm/transcripts/laskerm _1_5_135.html.

43. Notable New Yorkers: Mary Lasker. Audio transcript. Columbia University Libraries. http://www.columbia.edu/cu/lweb/digital/collections/nny/laskerm/transcripts/laskerm _1_9_254.html.

44. Notable New Yorkers: Mary Lasker. Audio transcript. Columbia University Libraries. http://www.columbia.edu/cu/lweb/digital/collections/nny/laskerm/transcripts/laskerm _1_8_222.html.

45. Legislative history of the National Science Foundation Act of 1950. National Science Foundation. http://www.nsf.gov/pubs/1952/b_1952_8.pdf.

46. Mike Gorman: Biographical notes. SNAC. http://snaccooperative.org/ark:/99166/ w6fz1b58.

47. Bishop JM. Mary Lasker and her prizes: an appreciation. *JAMA*. September 2005;294(11):1418-1419. https://jamanetwork.com/journals/jama/article -abstract/201532.

48. Robinson J. *Noble Conspirator: Florence S. Mahoney and the Rise of the National Institutes of Health*. Washington, DC: Francis Press; 2001:21.

49. Mary Lasker Papers: biographical information. National Library of Medicine. NIH. https://profiles.nlm.nih.gov/ps/retrieve/Narrative/TL/ p-nid/199.

50. Pomeroy C. Empress of all maladies: Mary Lasker. The Hill. March 20, 2015. thehill .com/blogs/congress-blog/healthcare/236121-3mpress-of-all-maladies-mary-laskar.

51. Mary Lasker Papers: biographical information. National Library of Medicine. NIH. https://profiles.nlm.nih.gov/ps/retrieve/Narrative/TL/ p-nid/200.

52. Heightening the worldwide prestige of "America's Nobels." Geto and de Milly Case

Study/Press Release. www.getodemilly.com/case-studies/the-albert-mary-lasker-founda
tion-the-mary-woodward-lasker- charitable-trust.

53. Drew E. The health syndicate: Washington's noble conspirators. *Atlantic Monthly.*
1967;220:75-82.

54. Bush V. Science, the endless frontier. National Science Foundation. July 1945. https://
www.nsf.gov/about/history/nsf50/vbush1945.jsp.

55. Healey B. Shattuck Lecture: NIH and the bodies politic. *New Engl J Med.*
1994;330(21):1493-1498. https://www.researchgate.net/publication/15033960_
Shattuck_Lecture--NIH_and_the_bodies_politic.

56. End Duchenne. Parent Project Muscular Dystrophy. http://www.parentprojectmd
.org/site/PageServer?pagename=nws_index.

57. Muscular Dystrophy Association. Partners. https://www.mda.org/get-involved/meet
-our-partners.

58. Parent Project Muscular Dystrophy. History. https://www.parentprojectmd.org/about
-ppmd/history/.

59. Parent Project Muscular Dystrophy. 2015 IRS Form 990. http://990s.foundationcenter
.org/990_pdf_archive/311/311405490/311405490 _201512_990.pdf?_ga=1.245628162
.721333527.1471133769.

60. Furlong P. A community united to end Duchenne: FDA grants accelerated approval
to first drug for Duchenne muscular dystrophy. September 19, 2016. http://community
.parentprojectmd.org/profiles/blogs/fda-grants-accelerated-approval-to-first-drug-for
-duchenne.

61. Tavernise S. F.D.A. approves muscular dystrophy drug that patients lobbied
for. *New York Times.* September 19, 2016. http://www.nytimes.com/2016/09/20/
business/fda-approves-muscular-dystrophy-drug-that-patients-lobbied-for.html?ref=
todayspaper.

62. Tribble SJ. A golden ticket that fast-tracks a drug through the FDA. Kaiser Health
News. September 29, 2016. http://khn.org/news/a-golden-ticket-that-fast-tracks-a-drug
-through-the-fda/.

63. Thomas K. Australian drug maker has low profile but powerful backers in Washington.
New York Times. January 13, 2017. https://www.nytimes.com/2017/01/13/health/innate
-immunotherapeutics-tom-price.html.

64. Baker P, Thrush G, Haberman M. Health secretary Tom Price resigns after drawing ire for chartered flights. *New York Times.* September 29, 2017. https://www.nytimes
.com/2017/09/29/us/politics/tom-price-trump-hhs.html.

65. Foderaro LW. Who will replace Chris Collins, the indicted congressman, on the
ballot? Perhaps no one. *New York Times.* September 10, 2018. https://www.nytimes
.com/2018/09/10/nyregion/chris-collins-congress-replacement.html.

66. Begley S. NIH rejected a study of alcohol advertising while pursuing industry funding for other research. STAT. April 2, 2018. https://www.statnews.com/2018/04/02/nih
-rejected-alcohol-advertising-study/.

67. Facher L. NIH director: agency is looking at alcohol industry influence "in a very

aggressive way." STAT. April 11, 2018. https://www.statnews.com/2018/04/11/nih-alcohol-industry-influence-research/.

68. Hartocollis A. New dean of Weill Cornell Medical College. *New York Times*. September 7, 2011. http://www.nytimes.com/2011/09/08/ nyregion/laurie-h-glimcher-named-dean-of-weill-cornell-medical- college.html?_r=1.

69. McCluskey PD. Dana-Farber recruits Cornell medical dean as CEO. *Boston Globe*. February 23, 2016. https://www.bostonglobe.com/business/2016/02/23/dana-farber-recruits-cornell-medical-dean-ceo/ HuSs5jM80CAJnPoOhrM5eP/story.html.

Chapter 6—The House of God

1. Schmidt S. A hospital threw a stillborn baby out with dirty laundry. Now the family is suing. *Washington Post*. October 10, 2017. https://www.washingtonpost.com/news/morning-mix/wp/2017/10/10/a- hospital-threw-a-stillborn-baby-out-with-dirty-laundry-now-the-family-is-suing/?utm_term=.17b98c128383.

2. Schulte F. Pain hits after surgery when a doctor's daughter is stunned by $17,850 urine test. Kaiser Health News. February 16, 2018. https://khn.org/news/pain-hits-long-after-surgery-when-a-doctors-daughter-is-stunned-by-17850-urine-test/.

3. To err is human: building a safer health system. Institute of Medicine. NAS. October 1999. http://www.nationalacademies.org/hmd/~/media/Files/Report%20Files/1999/To-Err-is-Human/To%20Err%20is%20Human%201999%20%20report%20brief.pdf.

4. James JT. A new evidence-based estimate of patient harms associated with hospital care. *J Patient Saf*. September 2013;9(3):122-128. http://journals.lww.com/journalpatientsafety/Abstract/ 2013/09000/A_New,_Evidence_based_Estimate_of_Patient_Harms.2.aspx.

5. Robeznieks A. U.S. has highest maternal death rates among developed countries. Modern Healthcare. May 6, 2015. http://www.modernhealthcare.com/article/20150506/NEWS/150509941.

6. Montagne R. For every woman who dies in childbirth in the U.S., 70 more come close. NPR. May 10, 2018. https://www.npr.org/ 2018/05/10/607782992/for-every-woman-who-dies-in-childbirth- in-the-u-s-70-more-come-close?utm_source=STAT+Newsletters&utm_campaign=b5df7c09fd-MR&utm_medium=email&utm_term=0_8cab1d7961-b5df-7c09fd-150335297.

7. Healy J. It's 4 a.m. The baby's coming. But the nearest hospital is 100 miles away. *New York Times*. June 17, 2018. https://www.nytimes.com/2018/07/17/us/hospital-closing-missouri-pregnant.html?smid=nytcore-ipad-share&smprod=nytcore-ipad.

8. Barrasso J, Thune J. Government hospitals are failing Native Americans. *Wall Street Journal*. July 1, 2016. https://www.wsj.com/articles/government-hospitals-are-failing-native-americans-1467412690.

9. Burke LG, Frakt AB, Khullar D, et al. Association between teaching status and mortality in US hospitals. *JAMA*. 2017;317(20):2105-2113. https://jamanetwork.com/journals/jama/fullarticle/2627971.

10. Armour S. Hospital watchdog gives seal of approval, even after problems emerge.

Wall Street Journal. September 8, 2017. https://www.wsj.com/articles/watchdog-awards -hospitals-seal-of-approval-even-after-problems-emerge-1504889146.

11. About the Joint Commission. Joint Commission. https://www.jointcommission.org/ about_us/about_the_joint_commission_main.aspx.

12. Gold Seal of Approval downloads. Joint Commission. https://www.jointcommission .org/accreditation/goldseal_downloads.aspx.

13. Governing board. Joint Commission. https://www.jointcommission.org/facts_about_ the_board_of_commissioners/.

14. WSJ casts doubt on value of TJC accreditation. Relias Media. November 1, 2017. https://www.ahcmedia.com/articles/141601-wsj-casts-doubt-on-value-of-tjc-accreditation.

15. Consultative technical assistance services. Joint Commission Resources. https://www .jcrinc.com/consulting/.

16. Quality Check. Joint Commission. https://www.qualitycheck.org/.

17. History of the Joint Commission. Joint Commission. https://www.jointcommission .org/about_us/history.aspx.

18. Ernest A. Codman, MD, FACS (1869–1940). American College of Surgeons Archives. https://www.facs.org/about%20acs/archives/ pasthighlights/codmanhighlight. The 1919 "Minimum Standard" document. https://www.facs.org/about-acs/archives/pasthighlights/ minimumhighlight.

19. U.S. Army Medical Department. Office of Medical History. History of the Army Medical Corps: Table of Personnel. Washington, DC, 1963. http://history.amedd.army .mil/booksdocs/wwii/personnel/ch01tbl01.pdf.

20. Office for Civil Rights. Medical treatment in Hill-Burton funded medical facilities. HHS. https://www.hhs.gov/civil-rights/for-individuals/hill-burton/index.html.

21. Allen AW. The hospital standardization program of the American College of Surgeons. *Bull Am Coll Surg.* January 1951;36(1):22-23. https://www.ncbi.nlm.nih.gov/ pubmed/14792115.

22. Understanding the basics. Joint Commission. http://www.hcpro.com/content/203861 .pdf.

23. Over a century of quality and safety. Joint Commission. https://www.jointcommission .org/assets/1/6/TJC-history-timeline_through_20161.PDF.

24. Letter to Mark Chassin, MD, MHP, from Physicians for Responsible Opioid Prescribing. April 13, 2016. https://www.citizen.org/sites/default/files/2314b.pdf.

25. Fast facts on U.S. hospitals. American Hospital Association. http://www.aha.org/ research/rc/stat-studies/fast-facts.shtml#community.

26. About us. New York–Presbyterian Hospital. http://www.nyp.org/about-us, https:// healthmatters.nyp.org/newyork-presbyterian-timeline/.

27. Craig S. Columbia University Medical Center receives the most NIH funding among academic medical centers in New York City and state. Press release. May 22, 2008. http:// www.cumc.columbia.edu/publications/press_releases/nih-funding-cumc.html.

28. Highest research and development funding. Best Colleges. 2017. http://www.bestcolleges.com/features/colleges-with-highest-research-and-development-expenditures/.

29. Brill S. *America's Bitter Pill.* New York: Random House; 2015:424-430.

30. Gunderman R. Why are hospital CEOs paid so well? *Atlantic.* October 16, 2013. https://www.theatlantic.com/health/archive/2013/10/why-are-hospital-ceos-paid-so-well/280604/.

31. Brill S. *America's Bitter Pill.* New York: Random House; 2015: 23.

32. Brill S. *America's Bitter Pill.* New York: Random House; 2015:21-23.

33. Ginzberg E. *The Medical Triangle.* Cambridge, MA: Harvard University Press;1990:23.

34. Health plans and benefits: Employment Retirement Security Act (ERISA). US Department of Labor. https://www.dol.gov/general/topic/health-plans/erisa.

35 Altman SH. The lessons of Medicare's prospective payment system show that the bundled payment system faces challenges. Health Affairs. September 1, 2012; 31(9). https://doi.org/10.1377/hlthaff.2012.0323.

36. Mistichelli J. Diagnosis related groups (DRGs). Georgetown University Library. 2009. https://repository.library.georgetown.edu/handle/10822/556896.

37. Magee M. The 3 pillars of the Medical Industrial Complex. Part 2: Evolution of the hospitals and insurers. Health Commentary. June 27, 2016. http://www.healthcommentary.org/2016/06/27/the-3-pillars-of-the-medical-industrial-complex-and-the-physician-part-2/.

38. Levit KR, Lazenby H, Waldo DR, Dabvidoff LM. National health expenditures, 1984. *Health Care Financ Rev.* 1985;7(1):1-35. https://www.cms.gov/Research-Statistics-Data-and-Systems/Research/Health CareFinancingReview/Downloads/CMS1191930dl.pdf.

39. Moon M, Gage B, Evans A. An examination of the key Medicare provisions in the Balanced Budget Act of 1997. Commonwealth Fund. September 1, 1997. http://www.commonwealthfund.org/publications/fund-reports/1997/sep/an-examination-of-key-medicare-provisions-in-the-balanced-budget-act-of-1997.

40. Whiteis DG. Hospital and community characteristics in closures of urban hospitals, 1980–1987. *Public Health Rep.* July-August 1992;107(4):409-416. https://www.ncbi.nlm.nih.gov/pmc/articles/PMC1403671/?page=1.

41. Chen DW. Where halls of ivy meet silicon dreams, a new city rises. *New York Times.* March 22, 2017. https://www.nytimes.com/2017/03/22/nyregion/nyc-cornell-columbia-nyu-campuses.html.

42. Hancock J. How below-the-radar mergers fuel health care monopolies. Kaiser Health News. September 5, 2017. http://khn.org/news/how-below-the-radar-mergers-fuel-health-care-monopolies/.

43. History of Pennsylvania Hospital: historical timeline. Penn Medicine. http://www.uphs.upenn.edu/paharc/timeline/.

44. Personal records.

45. Mello MM, Livingston EH. The evolving story of overlapping surgery. *JAMA.* 2017;318(3):233-234. http://jamanetwork.com/journals/jama/fullarticle/2636711?amp;utm_source=JAMALatestIssue&utm_ campaign=18-07-2017.

46. Uhlman M. Hospital's CEO says he will resign. November 15, 1995. Philly.com. http://articles.philly.com/1995-11-15/business/25684141_1_physician-practices-hospital -administrator-pennsylvania-hospital.

47. Internal marketing reports, 2006. Pennsylvania Hospital.

48. Holmes EW. Of rice and men: Bill Kelley's next generation. *J Clin Invest.* October 1, 2005;115(10):2948-2952. http://www.ncbi.nlm.nih.gov/pmc/articles/PMC1240120/ pdf/JCI0526871.pdf.

49. Goldstein J. Jefferson's president announces his retirement: Paul C. Brucker, 71, said he would step down in June 2004. July 23, 2003. http://articles.philly.com/2003-07-29/ business/25451723_1_health-care- system-philadelphia-health-care-paul-c-brucker.

50. Stark K, Uhlman M. Jefferson's medical dean will step down. June 13, 2000. Philly .com. http://articles.philly.com/2000-06-13/business/25602087_1_dean-for-academic -affairs-sidney-kimmel-trustees.

51. Burling S. Rothman Institute founder on the cusp of 80 and still in the OR. *Inquirer.* November 28, 2016. http://www.philly.com/philly/health/20161127_Rothman_ Institute_founder_on_the_cusp_of_80_and_still_in_the_OR.html.

52. Rosenthal E. Those indecipherable medical bills? They're one reason health care costs so much. *New York Times.* March 29, 2017, https://www.nytimes.com/2017/03/29/ magazine/those-indecipherable-medical-bills-theyre-one-reason-health-care-costs-so -much.html?smid=nytcore-ipad-share&smprod=nytcore-ipad.

53. Bertillon classification. Statistics. *Encyclopaedia Britannica.* https://www.britannica .com/topic/Bertillon-classification.

54. History of ICD. WHO. http://www.who.int/classifications/icd/en/.

55. International classification of diseases (ICD-10/PCS) transition—background. CDC. https://www.cdc.gov/nchs/icd/icd10cm_pcs_background.htm.

56. American Academy of Professional Coders. https://www.aapc.com.

57. CPT code applications and criteria. AMA. https://www.ama-assn.org/practice -management/cpt-code-applications-criteria; http://www.guidestar.org/FinDocuments/ 2014/360/727/2014-360727175-0bb01fe9-90.pdf.

58. Sanger-Katz M. Even insured can face crushing medical debt, study finds. *New York Times.* January 6, 2016. https://www.nytimes.com/2016/01/06/upshot/lost-jobs-houses -savings-even-insured-often-face-crushing-medical-debt.html.

59. Mattioli D, Evans M. UnitedHealth is among suitors circling Tenet's Conifer business. *Wall Street Journal.* July 18, 2018. https://www.wsj.com/articles/unitedhealth-is-among -suitors-circling-tenets-conifer- business-1531950854.

60. Fritz V. No margin, no mission: flying nuns and sister Irene Kraus. TeleTracking. March 20, 2012. http://blog.teletracking.com/2012/03/20/margin-mission-flying-nuns -sister-irene-kraus/.

61. Commins J. Healthcare job growth slows in 2017. MedPage. May 14, 2017. https://www .medpagetoday.com/PublicHealthPolicy/WorkForce/ 65273?xid=nl_mpt_DHE_2017 -05-15&eun=g1002037d0r&pos=4.

62. Haught R, Dobson A, DaVanzo J, Abrams MK. How the American Health Care Act's changes to Medicaid will affect hospital finances in every state. Commonwealth Fund. June 23, 2017. http://www.commonwealthfund.org/publications/blog/2017/jun/how -changes-to-medicaid-will-affect-hospital-finances-in-every-state.

63. Abelson R. Go to the wrong hospital and you're 3 times more likely to die. *New York Times*. December 14, 2016. https://www.nytimes.com/2016/12/14/business/hospitals -death-rates-quality-vary-widely.html?smid=nytcore-ipad-share&smprod=nytcore-ipad.

64. Wennberg JE. Dealing with medical practice variations: a proposal for action. *Health Affairs*. Summer 1984;3(2). https://www.healthaffairs.org/doi/abs/10.1377/hlthaff.3.2.6.

65. Wennberg JE et al. Use of Medicare claims data to monitor provider specific performance among patients with severe chronic illness. *Health Aff* (Millwood). 2004;Suppl Variation:VAR5-18. https://www.ncbi.nlm.nih.gov/pubmed/15471771.

66. Fleming C. Don Berwick's vision: the triple aim. *Health Affairs*. April 20, 2010. https://www.healthaffairs.org/do/10.1377/hblog20100420.004794/full/.

67. Winslow R. Not even the mattress pads were spared: an inside look at a top hospital's struggle to cut costs. STAT. September 28, 2017. https://www.statnews.com/2017/09/28/ brigham-and-womens-hospital-budget/?utm_source=STAT+Newsletters&utm_ campaign=b9dd23efbd-MR&utm_medium=email&utm_term=0_8cab1d7961 -b9dd23efbd-150335297.

68. Destination Medical Center Corporation. https://dmc.mn/dmc- corporation.

69. Iglehart J. An interview with AHA president Rich Umbdenstock. *Health Affairs*. October 21, 2009. https://www.healthaffairs.org/do/10.1377/hblog20091021.002465/full/.

Chapter 7—Insuring Complexity

1. Walsh MW. UnitedHealth overbilled Medicare by billions, U.S. says in suit. *New York Times*. May 19, 2017. https://www.nytimes.com/2017/05/19/business/dealbook/ unitedhealth-sued-medicare-overbilling.html?_r=0.

2. Facts and statistics: industry overview. Insurance Information Institute. September 7, 2017. https://www.iii.org/fact-statistic/facts-statistics-industry-overview.

3. Grant C. A healthy dose of profits at Cigna. *Wall Street Journal*. https://www.wsj.com/ articles/a-healthy-dose-of-profits-at-cigna-1504792302.

4. Collins SR, Gunja MZ, Doty MM. How well does insurance coverage protect consumers from health care costs? Commonwealth Fund Report. 2016. http://www.common wealthfund.org/publications/issue-briefs/2017/oct/insurance-coverage-consumers -health-care-costs.

5. Krugman P. Conservative origins of Obamacare. *New York Times*. July 27, 2011. https:// krugman.blogs.nytimes.com/2011/07/27/conservative-origins-of-obamacare/.

6. Kessler G. When did McConnell say he wanted to make Obama a "one-term president"? *Washington Post*. September 25, 2012. https://www.washingtonpost.com/ blogs/fact-checker/post/when-did-mcconnell-say-he-wanted-to-make-obama-a-one

-term-president/2012/09/24/79fd5cd8-0696-11e2-afff-d6c7f20a83bf_blog.html?utm_term=.96ddb7000401.

7. Historica Canada. Peace, order and good government. http:// thecanadianencyclopedia.ca/en/article/peace-order-and-good-government/.

8. Underwood A. Health care abroad: Germany—interview of Uwe Reinhardt. *New York Times*. September 29, 2009. https://prescriptions.blogs.nytimes.com/2009/09/29/health-care-abroad-germany/?_r=0.

9. Fahs MC. Japan's universal and affordable health care. Japan Society. April 30, 1993. https://www.nyu.edu/projects/rodwin/lessons.html.

10. Jones SG, Hilborne LH, et al. Health system reconstruction and nation-building. RAND. 2007. https://www.rand.org/pubs/research_briefs/RB9237/index1.html.

11. Blumberg A, Davidson A. Accidents of history created U.S. healthcare system. October 22, 2009. NPR. http://www.npr.org/templates/story/story.php?storyId=114045132. Accessed October 10, 2014.

12. Health insurance from invention to innovation: a history of the Blue Cross and Blue Shield plans. Blue Cross/Blue Shield. November 11, 2012. http://www.bcbs.com/the-health-of-america/articles/health-insurance-invention-innovation-history-of-the-blue-cross-and.

13. Our history. Kaiser Permanente. https://share.kaiserpermanente.org/article/history-of-kaiser-permanente/.

14. Byellin J. Today in 1943: FDR freezes prices, wages and employment. Reuters/Legal Solutions Blog. April 8, 2011. http://blog.legalsolutions.thomsonreuters.com/top-legal-news/today-in-1943-fdr-freezes-prices-wages-and-employment/.

15. Blumenthal, D. Employer-sponsored health insurance in the United States—origins and implications. *N Engl J Med*. July 6, 2006;355:1. http://people.umass.edu/econ340/nejm-ebhi.pdf Accessed October 10, 2014.

16. Gladwell, M. The risk pool. *New Yorker*. August 28, 2006. http://www.newyorker.com/magazine/2006/08/28/the-risk-pool.

17. Blumenthal D, Morone JA. *The Heart of Power: Health and Politics in the Oval Office*. Berkeley: University of California Press; 2009:99-110.

18. Blumenthal D, Morone JA. *The Heart of Power: Health and Politics in the Oval Office*. Berkeley: University of California Press; 2009:103.

19. Cohen WJ. The Forand Bill: health insurance for the aged. *Am J Nurs*. May 1958;58(5):698-702. Accessed November 3, 2014. http://www.jstor.org/discover/10.2307/3461578?uid=3739576&uid=2&uid=4&uid=3739256&sid=21104453266991.

20. Corning, PA. Social Security history: chapter 4—the fourth round, 1957 to 1965. Accessed November 3, 2014. http://www.ssa.gov/history/corningchap4.html.

21. Blumenthal D, Morone JA. *The Heart of Power: Health and Politics in the Oval Office*. Berkeley: University of California Press; 2009:122-126.

22. Medical assistance for the aged: the Kerr Mills Program—1960–1963. 88th Congress, 1st session. Accessed November 3, 2014. http://www.aging.senate.gov/imo/media/doc/reports/rpt263.pdf/.

23. Rapaport R. How AMA "Coffeecup" gave Reagan a boost. June 21, 2009. Accessed November 3, 2014. http://www.sfgate.com/opinion/article/How-AMA-Coffeecup-gave-Reagan-a-boost-3228367.php.

24. Ronald Reagan—corporate spokesman and rising conservative. Profiles of U.S. Presidents. Accessed November 3, 2014. http://www.presidentprofiles.com/Kennedy-Bush/Ronald-Reagan-Corporate-spokesman-and-rising-conservative.html.

25. Lemuel R. Boulware Papers. Biography/History. University of Pennsylvania. Accessed November 3, 2014. http://dla.library.upenn.edu/dla/ead/ead.html?id=EAD_upenn_rbml_MsColl52.

26. Brecher J. The World War II and post-war strike wave. Libcom.org. December 17, 2009. http://libcom.org/history/world-war-ii-post-war-strike-wave.

27. Evans TW. *The Education of Ronald Reagan: The General Electric Years and the Untold Story of His Conversion to Conservatism.* New York: Columbia University Press; 2006: 37-56.

28. Peterson WH. Boulwarism: ideas have consequences. Foundation for Economic Freedom. April 1, 1991. Accessed November 3, 2014. http://fee.org/the_freeman/detail/boulwarism-ideas-have-consequences.

29. Evans TW. *The Education of Ronald Reagan: The General Electric Years and the Untold Story of His Conversion to Conservatism.* New York: Columbia University Press; 2006: 69-82.

30. Evans TW. The GE years: what made Reagan Reagan? History News Network. January 8, 2007. Accessed November 3, 2014. http:// historynewsnetwork.org/article/32681.

31. AMA Alliance: 1963. Operation Hometown. https://www.amaalliance.org/legislative-history.

32. Ronald Reagan speaks out against socialized medicine. 1961. Operation Coffee Cup Sponsored by AMA. YouTube. https://www.youtube.com/watch?v=kDnxxsjVr20.

33. Profile: Operation Coffeecup. 1962. History Commons. Accessed November 3, 2014. http://www.historycommons.org/entity.jsp?entity= operation_coffeecup_1.

34. Pearson D. On the Washington merry-go-round. June 17, 1961. Bell Syndicates. Accessed November 3, 2014. https://www.democraticunder ground.com/discuss/duboard.php?az=view_all&address=389x8141205.

35. Canada Health Insurance. The history of Medicare in Canada. http://www.canada-health-insurance.com/history-medicare.html.

36. Knox R. History of tinkering helps German system endure. NPR. July 3, 2008. https://www.npr.org/templates/story/story.php?storyId=92189596.

37. Reich MR, Shibuya K. The future of Japan's health system—sustaining good health with equity at low cost. *N Engl J Med.* November 5, 2015;373:1793-1797. http://www.nejm.org/doi/full/10.1056/NEJMp1410676.

38. AAPS interview with J. Bruce Henriksen MD. http://www.aapsonline.org/brochures/persuasi.htm.

39. JFK speech. May 20, 1962. https://www.youtube.com/watch?v= VXUJErr_vfo

40. Arnett JC. Book review: Code Blue. Health Care in Crisis by Edward R. Annis M.D. *JAMA*. July 6, 1994; 272(1):74-75. http://www.jpands.org/hacienda/codeblue.html.

41. Eck A. JFK-Annis 1962 Medicare debate, part 1. YouTube. https://www.bing.com/videos/search?q=Dr.+Joseph+Annis+1962+speech+at+Madison+Square+Garden+YouTube&view=detail&mid=ABB5D3AB8B0D4C836645ABB5D3AB8B0D4C836645&FORM=VIRE.

42. American Presidency Project. John F. Kennedy: 374—remarks upon signing the Health Professions Educational Assistance Act. September 24, 1963. Accessed November 4, 2014. http://www.presidency.ucsb.edu/ws/?pid=9425.

43. Ginzberg E. *The Medical Triangle: Physicians, Politicians, and the Public.* Cambridge, MA: Harvard University Press; 1990:24.

44. Berkowitz E. Medicare and Medicaid: past is prologue. Centers for Medicaid and Medicare Services. 2008. Accessed November 4, 2014. http://www.cms.gov/Research-Statistics-Data-and-Systems/Research/HealthCareFinancingReview/downloads/08Springpg81.pdf.

45. Blumenthal D, Morone JA. *The Heart of Power: Health and Politics in the Oval Office.* Berkeley: University of California Press; 2009:177.

46. Blumenthal D, Morone JA. *The Heart of Power: Health and Politics in the Oval Office.* Berkeley: University of California Press; 2009:163.

47. Blumenthal D, Morone JA. *The Heart of Power: Health and Politics in the Oval Office.* Berkeley: University of California Press; 2009:170,171,198.

48. Blumenthal D, Morone JA. *The Heart of Power: Health and Politics in the Oval Office.* Berkeley: University of California Press; 2009:166,169.

49. Blumenthal D, Morone JA. *The Heart of Power: Health and Politics in the Oval Office.* Berkeley: University of California Press; 2009:166.

50. Johnson LB. The great society speech. Commencement address, May 22, 1964. University of Michigan, Ann Arbor. http://www.c-span.org/video/?153610-1/great-society-speech.

51. Civil Rights Act of 1964. July 2, 1964. Our Documents Initiative. http://www.ourdocuments.gov/doc.php?flash=true&doc=97.

52. Blumenthal D, Morone JA. *The Heart of Power: Health and Politics in the Oval Office.* Berkeley: University of California Press; 2009:165,178,187-189.

53. Blumenthal D, Morone JA. *The Heart of Power: Health and Politics in the Oval Office.* Berkeley: University of California Press; 2009:178-180.

54. Blumenthal D, Morone JA. *The Heart of Power: Health and Politics in the Oval Office.* Berkeley: University of California Press; 2009:148,156,160.

55. Blumenthal D, Morone JA. *The Heart of Power: Health and Politics in the Oval Office.* Berkeley: University of California Press; 2009:188.

56. Blumenthal D, Morone JA. *The Heart of Power: Health and Politics in the Oval Office.* Berkeley: University of California Press; 2009:183,184.

57. 1964 presidential election results. http://uselectionatlas.org/RESULTS/national .php?year=1964.

58. Anderson J. Doctors for Goldwater, like Medicare stand. July 5, 1964. Washington merry-go-round. Around the World Syndicate. *Winona Daily News.* Accessed November 4, 2014. http://newspaperarchive.com/us/minnesota/winona/winona-daily -news/1964/07-05/page-6.

59. Blumenthal D, Morone JA. *The Heart of Power: Health and Politics in the Oval Office.* Berkeley: University of California Press; 2009:185.

60. Blumenthal D, Morone JA. *The Heart of Power: Health and Politics in the Oval Office.* Berkeley: University of California Press; 2009:189.

61. Blumenthal D, Morone JA. *The Heart of Power: Health and Politics in the Oval Office.* Berkeley: University of California Press; 2009:192.

62. Blumenthal D, Morone JA. *The Heart of Power: Health and Politics in the Oval Office.* Berkeley: University of California Press; 2009:193,194.

63. Social Security History. President Lyndon B. Johnson, 6: remarks with President Truman at the signing in Independence of the Medicare Bill. July 30, 1965. Social Security Administration. http://www.ssa.gov/history/lbjstmts.html#medicare.

64. Blumenthal D, Morone JA. *The Heart of Power: Health and Politics in the Oval Office.* Berkeley: University of California Press; 2009:195.

65. Overview of Title VI of the Civil Rights Act of 1964. United States Department of Justice. http://www.justice.gov/crt/about/cor/coord/titlevi.php.

66. Smith DG, Moore JD. *Medicaid Politics and Policy.* New Brunswick, NJ: Transaction Publishers; 2010:84-88.

67. Blumenthal D, Morone JA. *The Heart of Power: Health and Politics in the Oval Office.* Berkeley: University of California Press; 2009:197.

68. Blumenthal D, Morone JA. *The Heart of Power: Health and Politics in the Oval Office.* Berkeley: University of California Press; 2009:198.

69. Blumenthal D, Morone JA. *The Heart of Power: Health and Politics in the Oval Office.* Berkeley: University of California Press; 2009:199.

70. Blumenthal D, Morone JA. *The Heart of Power: Health and Politics in the Oval Office.* Berkeley: University of California Press; 2009:200.

71. Blumenthal D, Morone JA. *The Heart of Power: Health and Politics in the Oval Office.* Berkeley: University of California Press; 2009:202.

72. Richard Nixon and health care. On the Issues. http://www.ontheissues.org/Celeb/ Richard_Nixon_Health_Care.htm.

73. Gerald Ford and health care. On the Issues. http://www.ontheissues.org/Celeb/ Gerald_Ford_Health_Care.htm.

74. Harry and Louise on Clinton's health plan. YouTube. https://www.youtube.com/ watch?v=Dt31nhleeCg.

75. Oberlander J. Long time coming: why Obamacare finally passed. *Health Affairs*. June 1, 2010;29(6). https://www.healthaffairs.org/doi/abs/10.1377/hlthaff.2010.0447.

76. Shelbourne M. CVS agrees to buy Aetna for $69B: report. The Hill. December 3, 2017. http://thehill.com/policy/healthcare/363021-cvs-agrees-to-buy-aetna-for-69b-report.

77. Farr C. As Amazon moves into health care, here's what we know—and what we suspect—about its plans. CNBC. March 27, 2018. https://www.cnbc.com/2018/03/27/amazons-moves-into-health-what-we-know.html.

78. Hensley S. Atul Gawande named CEO of health venture by Amazon, Berkshire Hathaway and JP Morgan. NPR. June 20, 2018. https://www.npr.org/sections/health-shots/2018/06/20/621808003/atul-gawande-named-ceo-of-health-venture-by-amazon-berkshire-hathaway-and-jpmorg.

79. Jiwani A, Himmelstein D, Woolhandler S, Kahn JG. Billing and insurance related administrative costs in United States' health care: synthesis of micro-costing evidence. *BMC Health Services Research*. November 13, 2014;14(556). https://bmchealthservres.biomedcentral.com/articles/10.1186/s12913-014-0556-7.

Chapter 8—Masters of Manipulation

1. The Temple of Dendur in the Sackler Wing. Metropolitan Museum of Art. http://maps.metmuseum.org.

2. Dr. Arthur M. Sackler biography. http://www.sackler.org/about.

3. Keefe PR. The family that built an empire of pain. *New Yorker*. October 30, 2017. https://www.newyorker.com/magazine/2017/10/30/the-family-that-built-an-empire-of-pain.

4. Smith JY. Arthur Sackler dies at 73. *Washington Post*. May 27, 1987. https://www.washingtonpost.com/archive/local/1987/05/27/arthur- sackler-dies-at-73/2f9b0440-d6b3-43be-a46c-55b41a98736e/?utm_term=.d4b4cb61d5c3.

5. Arthur M. Sackler Collections. Arthur M. Sackler Foundation. http://arthurmsacklerfdn.org/the-sackler-collection.

6. *Sex Endocrinology: A Handbook for the Medical and Allied Professions*. Schering Corp.: Medical Research Division; 1944. https://searchworks.stanford.edu/?q=%22Schering+Corporation.+Medical+Research+Division.%22&search_field=search_author.

7. The Schering Award. 1941. http://www.healthcommentary.org/the-schering-award-1941.

8. United States Senate. *Elimination of German Resources for War: Hearings before a Subcommittee on Military Affairs*. 79th Congress, first session, S. Res. 107 and S. Res. 146. p. 592. https://books.google.com/ books?id=5XnsAAAAMAAJ&pg=PA592&lpg=PA592&dq=schering +corp+parent+organization&source=bl&ots=hzKQw5lUoK&sig=aGec5vYLB6cIdQLUgPlLR8DbFjE&hl=en&sa=X&ved= 0ahUKEwjjx8KIkbvJAhVJjz4KHYFmCZUQ6AEIKDAC#v= onepage&q=schering%20corp%20parent%20organization&f=false.

9. Glueck G. Dr. Arthur Sackler dies at 73; philanthropist and art patron. *New York Times*. May 27, 1987. https://www.nytimes.com/1987/05/27/obituaries/dr-arthur-sackler-dies-at-73-philanthropist-and-art-patron.html.

10. Creedmore Psychiatric Center training program. Psychiatric residency and training education program. New York State Office of Mental Health. https://www.omh.ny.gov/omhweb/facilities/crpc/docs/residencyprogram.pdf.

11. Company history of Dr. Kade Pharmaceuticals. 1949. Marietta Lutz. https://www.kade.com/company/history.

12. Arthur M. Sackler. Medical Advertising Hall of Fame. Inducted 1997. https://www.mahf.com/mahf-inductees.

13. Podolsky SH. *The Antibiotic Era: Reform, Resistance and the Pursuit of Rational Therapeutics.* Baltimore, MD: Johns Hopkins University Press; 2015:25-27.

14. Podolsky SH. *The Antibiotic Era: Reform, Resistance and the Pursuit of Rational Therapeutics.* Baltimore, MD: Johns Hopkins University Press; 2015:27.

15. Podolsky SH. *The Antibiotic Era: Reform, Resistance and the Pursuit of Rational Therapeutics.* Baltimore, MD: Johns Hopkins University Press; 2015:27,30.

16. Pfizer Inc.: exploring our history. 1951–1999. http://www.pfizer.com/about/history/1951-1999.

17. Roerig sales force. Pfizer Inc: exploring our history. 1952. http://www.pfizer.com/about/history/1951-1999.

18. Lopez-Munoz F, Ucha-Udabe R, Alamo C. The history of barbiturates a century after their clinical introduction. *Neuropsychiatr Dis Treat.* December 2005;1(4):329-343. https://www.ncbi.nlm.nih.gov/pmc/ articles/PMC2424120.

19. FDA approves Pfizer's Atarax. April 12, 1956. World History Project. https://worldhistoryproject.org/1956/4/12/fda-approves-pfizers-atarax.

20. Quitney J. Tranquilizers: "The Relaxed Wife." 1957 Roerig-Pfizer. https://www.youtube.com/watch?v=Y3DIBH8Plgo.

21. Stauber J, Rampton S. Smokin'! How Hill & Knowlton helped sell smoking to the public. November 22, 1995. http://whatreallyhappened.com/RANCHO/LIE/HK/SMOKE.html.

22. Snegireff LS, Lombard OM. Survey of smoking habits of Massachusetts Physicians. *N Engl J Med.* 1954;250(24):1042-1045. http://www.nejm.org/doi/full/10.1056/NEJM195406172502408.

23. Wolinsky H, Brune T. *The Serpent on the Staff: The Unhealthy Politics of the American Medical Association* New York: Jeremy P. Tarcher/Putnam; 1994:145-147.

24. Philip Morris. At the AMA convention. June 6, 1942. Bates No. 1003071327. http://legacy.library.ucsf.edu/tid/fvm02a00 and http://legacy.library.ucsf.edu/tid/fvm02a00/pdf.

25. American Tobacco Company. United States of America, Federal Trade Commission: memorandum submitted by the American Tobacco Company, 1976:18-22,80-89. Bates No. 980306396/6603. http://legacy.library.ucsf.edu/tid/rum85f00, http://legacy.library.ucsf.edu/tid/rum85f00/pdf.

26. Just what the doctor ordered. February 22, 1954. Tobacco Documents. Bates No. 2021368933. https://www.industrydocumentslibrary.ucsf.edu/tobacco/docs/#id=kkkw0131.

27. Blum A. When "More Doctors Smoked Camels": cigarette advertising in the Journal. *New York State Journal of Medicine*. 1983;83:1347-1352. http://www.ncbi.nlm.nih.gov/pubmed/6582393. Mulinos MG, Osborne RL. Irritating properties of cigarette smoke as influenced by hygroscopic agents. *New York State Journal of Medicine*. 1935;35:1-3. https://www.industrydocumentslibrary.ucsf.edu/tobacco/docs/#id=gmcj0020.

28. UCSF Truth Tobacco Industry Documents. Truth Initiative. Report on the findings of a group of doctors: call for Philip Morris. October 16, 1937. Bates No. 2061014890. https://www.industrydocumentslibrary.ucsf.edu/tobacco/docs/#id=zycm0125.

29. RJ Reynolds. The medical relations division of Camel cigarettes believes that. September 1942 advertisement. https://ajph.aphapublications.org/doi/full/10.2105/AJPH.2005.066654.

30. Tiemann, Helen, secretary to William Esty, to the RJR Advertising Department dated January 9, 1946. Bates No. 502597537. http://legacy.library.ucsf.edu/tid/ijs78d00. December 26, 1945. Bates No. 502597519. http://legacy.library.ucsf.edu/tid/qis78d00.

31. RJ Reynolds. Camels costlier tobaccos advertisement. https://www.industrydocumentslibrary.ucsf.edu/tobacco/docs/#id=rryc0050.

32. Calfee JE. *Cigarette Advertising, Health Information and Regulation before 1970.* Washington, DC: Federal Trade Commission: 25,26. http://www.ftc.gov/sites/default/files/documents/reports/cigarette-advertising-health-information-and-regulation-1970/wp134.pdf.

33. Spiegel A. The secret history behind the science of stress. July 7, 2014. Accessed October 25, 2014. http://www.npr.org/blogs/health/2014/07/07/325946892/the-secret-history-behind-the-science-of-stress.

34. Norr R. Cancer by the carton. *Reader's Digest*. December 1952. http://legacy.library.ucsf.edu/tid/bcm92f00/pdf.

35. Cigarette hucksterism and the AMA. *JAMA*. April 3, 1954:1180. http://jama.jamanetwork.com/article.aspx?articleid=292962.

36. Tobacco Industry Research Committee. Confidential report on meeting March 15, 1954. https://www.industrydocumentslibrary.ucsf.edu/tobacco/docs/#id=lyyx0067.

37. Truth Tobacco Industry Documents. Phillip Morris Records. https://www.industrydocumentslibrary.ucsf.edu/tobacco/docs/#id=tzjy0219.

38. The Frank Statement. January 4, 1954. SourceWatch. http://www.sourcewatch.org/index.php?title=The_Frank_Statement.

39. Spiegel A. The secret history behind the science of stress. July 7, 2014. http://www.npr.org/blogs/health/2014/07/07/325946892/the-secret- history-behind-the-science-of-stress.

40. Hans Selye: Austrian endocrinologist. *Encyclopaedia Britannica*. https://www.britannica.com/biography/Hans-Selye.

41. Selye H. Confusion and controversy in the stress field. *J Human Stress*. June 1975;1(2):37-44. http://www.ncbi.nlm.nih.gov/pubmed/1235113.

42. Spiegel A. The secret history behind the science of stress. July 7, 2014. http://www.npr.org/blogs/health/2014/07/07/325946892/the-secret-history-behind-the-science-of-stress.

43. Friedman M, Rosenman RH. *Type A Behavior and Your Heart.* New York: Alfred A. Knopf; 1974.

44. Petticrew MP, Lee K. The "Father of Stress" meets "Big Tobacco": Hans Selye and the tobacco industry. *Am J Public Health.* March 2011;101(3):411. http://connection .ebscohost.com/c/articles/59438071/the-father-stress-meets-big-tobacco-hans-selye -tobacco-industry.

45. Rothman L. Meet the doctor who changed our understanding of stress. *Time.* March 10, 2016. http://time.com/4243311/hans-selye-stress.

46. Hans Selye. GSC Research Society. http://www.science.ca/scientists/scientistprofile .php?pID=219&-lang=en.

47. Oreskes N, Conway EM. *Merchants of Doubt.* New York: Bloomsbury Press; 2010.

48. Jones, Day, Reavis & Pogue. Tobacco Activity Project, untitled. Bates No. 681879254- 681879715. Accessed October 25, 2014. http://legacy.library.ucsf.edu/tid/vju87h00/pdf.

49. Sackler AM. *One Man and Medicine.* New York: Medical Tribune Inc.; 1983.

50. Meier B. *Pain Killer: A "Wonder" Drug's Trail of Addiction and Death.* New York: Rodale/ St. Martin's Press; 2003:218-222.

51. Podolsky SH, Greene J. A historical perspective of pharmaceutical promotion and physician education, *JAMA.* 2008;300(7):831-833. doi:10.1001/jama.300.7.831. http:// jamanetwork.com/journals/jama/ fullarticle/182395.

52. Meier B. *Pain Killer: A "Wonder" Drug's Trail of Addiction and Death.* New York: Rodale/ St. Martin's Press; 2003:196.

53. Marantz Henig R. Valium's contribution to our new normal. *New York Times.* September 29, 2012. http://www.nytimes.com/2012/09/30/sunday-review/valium-and-the -new-normal.html.

54. Morrell A. The OxyContin clan: the $14 billion newcomer to Forbes 2015 List of Richest U.S. Families. *Forbes.* July 1, 2015. https://www.forbes.com/sites/alexmorrell /2015/07/01/the-oxycontin-clan-the-14-billion-newcomer-to-forbes-2015-list-of -richest-u-s-families/#6de425c975e0.

55. Meier B. *Pain Killer: A "Wonder" Drug's Trail of Addiction and Death.* New York: Rodale/ St. Martin's Press; 2003:202.

56. Meier B. *Pain Killer: A "Wonder" Drug's Trail of Addiction and Death.* New York: Rodale/ St. Martin's Press; 2003:204.

57. Podolsky SH. *The Antibiotic Era: Reform, Resistance and the Pursuit of Rational Therapeutics.* Baltimore, MD: Johns Hopkins University Press; 2015:79. Lear J. Drug makers and the gov't—who makes the decisions? *Saturday Review.* July 2, 1960; 43:37-42. Lear J. The struggle for control of drug prescriptions. *Saturday Review.* March 31, 1962;45:35–39.

58. Podolsky SH. *The Antibiotic Era: Reform, Resistance and the Pursuit of Rational Therapeutics.* Baltimore, MD: Johns Hopkins University Press; 2015:80.

59. Meier B. *Pain Killer: A "Wonder" Drug's Trail of Addiction and Death.* New York: Rodale/ St. Martin's Press; 2003:219,220.

60. Freeman JW, Kaatz B. The physician and the pharmaceutical detail man. *Journal of Medical Humanities and Bioethics*. Spring–Summer 1987;8(1). http://link.springer.com/article/10 .10072FBF01119346#page-1.

61. Statistics Portal. Pharmaceutical corporations by US revenue in 2016. https://www .statista.com/statistics/233971/top-25-pharmaceutical-corporations-by-us-sales.

62. Schwarz A. *ADHD Nation*. New York: Scribner; 2016:2.

63. D'Agostino R. The drugging of the American boy. *Esquire*. March 27, 2014. https:// www.esquire.com/news-politics/a32858/drugging-of-the-american-boy-0414.

64. Schwarz A, Cohen S. A.D.H.D. seen in 11% of U.S. children as diagnoses rise. *New York Times*. March 31, 2013. http://www.nytimes.com/2013/04/01/health/more-diagnoses -of-hyperactivity-causing-concern.html.

65. Visser SN et al. Treatment of attention deficit/hyperactivity disorder among children with special health care needs. *J Pediatr*. June 2015;166(6):1423-1430.e1-2. https://www .ncbi.nlm.nih.gov/pubmed/25841538. Bilbo R, Baifu Xu KL. Demographic and geographic patterns of ADHD prescriptions among Louisiana's Medicaid children. ADHD Symposium. December 9, 2014. http://dhh.louisiana.gov/assets/ADHD/ADHD SymposiumPresentationRyanBilbo20141209.pdf.

66. Honigsbaum M. ADHD Nation: The disorder. the drugs. The inside story of Alan Schwarz—review. *Guardian*. September 4, 2016. http://www.theguardian.com/ boooks/2016/sep/04/adhd-nation-the-disorder-drugs-inside-story-alan-schwarz-review.

67. What I would never trade away: the positives of ADHD are numerous and mighty— creativity, empathy, and tenacity. Here readers share their amazing superpowers. ADDitude. http://www.additudemag.com/slideshow/135/slide-1.html.

68. "Meducation": Colbert on giving poor kids ADHD drugs so they can focus in school. *Washington Post*. October 11, 2012. https://www.washingtonpost.com/news/answer-sheet/ wp/2012/10/11/meducation-colbert-on-giving-poor-kids-adhd-drugs-so-they-can-focus -in-school/?utm_term=.6b603cebaf0e.

69. Charles Bradley, M.D., 1902–1979. *Am J Psychiatry*. July 1998;155(7):968-968. http:// ajp.psychiatryonline.org/doi/full/10.1176/ajp.155.7.968.

70. Strohl MP. Bradley's Benzedrine studies on children with behavioral disorders. *Yale J Biol Med*. March 2011;84(1):27-33. http://europepmc.org/articles/PMC3064242.

71. Schwarz A. *ADHD Nation*. New York: Scribner; 2016:13,14.

72. Bradley C. The behavior of children receiving Benzedrine. *Am J Psychiatry*. 1937;94:577-581. https://ajp.psychiatryonline.org/doi/abs/10.1176/ajp.94.3.577.

73. Medicine: pep pill poisoning. *Time*. May 10, 1937. http://content.time.com/time/ subscriber/article/0,33009,757775,00.html.

74. Dextroamphetamine. Pharmacology. Drug Bank. https://www.drugbank.ca/drugs/ DB01576#pharmacology.

75. Schwarz A. *ADHD Nation*. New York: Scribner; 2016:29.

76. Schwarz A. *ADHD Nation*. New York: Scribner; 2016:30.

77. Eisenberg L et al. A psychopharmacologic experiment in a training school for delinquent boys. *Am J Orthopsychiatry*. 33(3):431-447. http://onlinelibrary.wiley.com/doi/10.1111/j.1939-0025.1963.tb00377.x/ references.

78. Singh I. *Not Just Naughty: 50 Years of Ritalin Drug Advertising*. In: *Medicating Modern America*. Toon A, Watkins E, eds. New York: NYU Press; 2007:131-155. https://www.researchgate.net/publication/280575517_Not_Just_Naughty_50_years_of_Ritalin_drug_advertising.

79. Conners' Teacher Rating Scale—Revised (S). https://www.stevensonwaplak.com/wp-content/uploads/2011/03/connorsteacher.pdf.

80. CIBA Ritalin advertisement, 1971. http://www.bonkersinstitute.org/medshow/fbp.html.

81. Maynard R. Omaha pupils given "behavior" drugs. *Washington Post*. June 29, 1970. http://www.iasc-culture.org/THR/THR_article_2013_ Summer_short_take_youth_prescription_drugs.php.

82. Schwarz A. *ADHD Nation*. New York: Scribner; 2016:41.

83. Schmitt BD. The minimal brain dysfunction myth. *Am J Dis Child*. 1975;129(11):1313-1318. http://archpedi.jamanetwork.com/article.aspx?articleid=506235.

84. ADHD: the diagnostic criteria. PBS Frontline. http://www.pbs.org/wgbh/pages/frontline/shows/medicating/adhd/diagnostic.html.

85. Safer DJ, Krager JM. Effect of media blitz and a threatened law suit on stimulant treatment. *JAMA*. August 26, 1992;268(8):1004-1007. https://www.ncbi.nlm.nih.gov/pubmed/1501304. Biography of psychologist Steven Stein. http://www.stevenstein.ca/Bio.aspx.

86. Portner J. Worried about message, E.D. halts video distribution. *Education Week*. November 8, 1995. http://www.edweek.org/ew/articles/1995/11/08/10add.h15.html.

87. Merrow 1995 report/transcript: the history of CHADD (CH.A.D.D.), Ciba-Geigy (now, Novartis) and Ritalin attention deficit disorder: a dubious diagnosis? http://www.add-adhd.org/ritalin_CHADD_A.D.D.html.

88. Hallowell EM. *Driven to Distraction: Recognizing and Coping with Attention Deficit Disorder*. New York: Random House; 1994.

89. Hales D, Hales RE. Finally I know what's wrong. *Parade*. January 7, 1996: 8; Schwarz A. *ADHD Nation*. New York: Scribner; 2016:62.

90. Schwarz A. *ADHD Nation*. New York: Scribner; 2016:63.

91. NIH Conference on ADHD. November 16, 1998. Bethesda, MD. https://consensus.nih.gov/1998/1998AttentionDeficitHyperactivityDisorder110html.htm. https://www.youtube.com/watch?v=SvdxW_T01lk. Schwarz A. *ADHD Nation*. New York: Scribner; 2016:68.

92. Schwarz A. The selling of attention deficit disorder. *New York Times*. December 14, 2013. http://www.nytimes.com/2013/12/15/health/the-selling-of-attention-deficit-disorder.html?pagewanted=all.

93. History of marketing death via Adderall n/k/a Obetrol. February 10, 2006. News groupsderkeiler.com. http://newsgroups.derkeiler.com/Archive/Misc/misc.health.alternative/2006-02/msg00489.html.

94. Schwarz A. *ADHD Nation*. New York: Scribner; 2016:95-98.

95. Geist J. Focusing in on Adderall. Food and Drug Law. December 7, 2007. http://www
.canr.msu.edu/iflr/uploads/files/Student%20Papers/Geist_Focusing-on-Adderall.pdf.

96. Silver LB. *Dr. Larry Silver's Advice to Parents on Attention-Deficit Hyperactivity Disorder*. Washington, DC: American Psychiatric Press; 1993. http://www.worldcat
.org/title/dr-larry-silvers-advice-to-parents-on-attention-deficit-hyperactivity-disorder/
oclc/25676758.

97. Bloomberg News. Shire Pharmaceuticals buying U.S. drug maker. *New York Times*.
August 5, 1997. http://www.nytimes.com/1997/08/05/business/shire-pharmaceuticals
-buying-us-drug-maker.html.

98. A 14-month randomized clinical trial of treatment strategies for attention-deficit/
hyperactivity disorder. The MTA Cooperative Group. Multimodal Treatment Study of
Children with ADHD. *Arch Gen Psychiatry*. 1999:1073-1086. https://www.ncbi.nlm.nih
.gov/pubmed/10591283.

99. *Time* cover. June 18, 1994. http://www.bing.com/images/search?view=detailV2&ccid
=TuqUjXvy&id=8465CDA88E9D9687B087FD5E8594A062E70B00A1&thid=OIP.Tuq
UjXvyP8v0hRp32xpdLADjEs&q=ADD+cover+TIME+magazine+1994&simid=608001
997270680275&selectedIndex=2&ajaxhist=0.

100. *Journal of Attention Disorders*. http://jad.sagepub.com/content/by/year.

101. Joseph Biederman list of publications. NIH. https://www.ncbi.nlm.nih.gov/
pubmed/?term=joseph+biederman.

102. Harris G, Carey B. Researchers fail to reveal full drug pay. *New York Times*. June 8,
2008. http://www.nytimes.com/2008/06/08/us/08conflict.html.

103. Armstrong W. Shire on the wire. *Pharmaceutical Executive*. February 1, 2010. http://
www.pharmexec.com/shire-wire.

104. Kaufman J. Ransom-note ads about children's health are canceled. *New York Times*.
December 20, 2007. https://www.sott.net/article/146121-Ransom-Note-Ads-About
-Childrens-Health-Are-Canceled.

105. Wender PH. Minimal brain dysfunction: an overview. In: *Psychopharmacology: A
Generation of Progress*. Lipton MA et al., eds. New York: Ravel Press; 1978:1429-1435.

106. Tortora A. It's not just kids: ADHD affects adults, too. *Cincinnati Business Courier*.
June 30, 2003. http://www.bizjournals.com/cincinnati/stories/2003/06/30/story6.html.

107. Frontline interview: Dr. William Dodson. CPTV. 2001. http://www.pbs.org/wgbh/
pages/frontline/shows/medicating/interviews/dodson.html.

108. Schwarz A. *ADHD Nation*. New York: Scribner; 2016:184.

109. Wilens TE, Dodson W. A clinical perspective of attention-deficit/hyperactivity disorder into adulthood. *J Clin Psychiatry*. 2004;65:1301-1313.

110. Porter Novelli press release. May 6, 2004. Survey of adults reveals life-long consequences of ADHD. https://www.eurekalert.org/pub_releases/2004-05/pn-soa050604
.php.

111. Carroll L. ADHD diagnosis may be rising in U.S. Reuters Health. August 31, 2018. https://www.reuters.com/article/us-health-adhd/adhd-diagnoses-may-be-rising-in-u-s -idUSKCN1LG21M.

112. State profile: ADHD—North Carolina. CDC. http://www.cdc.gov/ncbddd/adhd/ stateprofiles/stateprofile_northcarolina.pdf.

113. Schwarz A. *ADHD Nation*. New York: Scribner; 2016:204, 205, 281.

114. Frances A. Keith Conners, father of ADHD, regrets its current misuse. *Huffington Post*. March 28, 2016. http://www.huffingtonpost.com/allen-frances/keith-conners-father -of-adhd_b_9558252.html.

115. Visser SN et al. Treatment of attention deficit/hyperactivity disorder among children with special health care needs. *J Pediatr*. June 2015;166(6):1423-1430.e1-2. https://www .ncbi.nlm.nih.gov/pubmed/25841538.

116. Schwartz C. Generation Adderall. *New York Times*. October 12, 2016. https://www .nytimes.com/2016/10/16/magazine/generation-adderall-addiction.html?_r=0.

117. Insurance News Net. 16M U.S. adults on prescription stimulants. April 17, 2018. https://insurancenewsnet.com/oarticle/16m-u-s-adults-on-prescription-stimulants.

118. Compton WM et al. Use disorders and motivations for misuse among adults in the United States. *Psychiatry Online*. April 16, 2018. https://doi.org/10.1176/appi .ajp.2018.17091048.

119. Wedge M. Why French kids don't have ADHD. *Psychology Today*. March 8, 2012. https://www.psychologytoday.com/blog/suffer-the-children/201203/why-french-kids -dont-have-adhd.

120. History. Purdue Pharma. http://www.purduepharma.com/about.

121. Wong S. Thrust under microscope. *Hartford Courant*. September 2, 2001. http:// articles.courant.com/2001-09-02/business/0109020319_1_purdue-pharma-abuse-of -painkiller-oxycontin-oxycontin-problem.

122. Hedges C, Sacco J. A world of hillbilly heroin: the hollowing out of America, up close and personal. *Nation*. August 21, 2012. https://www.thenation.com/article/world -hillbilly-heroin.

123. US FDA. Timeline of selected FDA activities and significant events addressing opioid misuse and abuse. https://www.fda.gov/Drugs/DrugSafety/InformationbyDrugClass/ ucm338566.htm.

124. Ryan H, Girion L, Glover S. "You want a description of hell?" OxyContin's 12-hour problem. *Los Angeles Times*. May 6, 2016. http://www.latimes.com/projects/oxycontin -part1/.

125. Mariani M. How the American opiate epidemic was started by one pharmaceutical company. The Week. March 4, 2015. http://theweek.com/articles/541564/how-american -opiate-epidemic-started-by-pharmaceutical-company.

126. Dubb S. Philanthropy on OxyContin: does charity cleanse this family's complicity in the opioid crisis? *NPQ*, October 26, 2017, https://nonprofitquarterly.org/2017/10/26/ philanthropy-oxycontin-charity-cleanse-familys-complicity-opioid-crisis.

127. Keefe PR. The family that built an empire of pain. *New Yorker*. October 30, 2017. https://www.newyorker.com/magazine/2017/10/30/the-family-that-built-an-empire -of-pain.

128. Meier B, Lipton E. Under attack, drug maker turned to Giuliani for help. *New York Times*. December 28, 2007. http://www.nytimes.com/2007/12/28/us/politics/28oxycontin .html.

129. Purdue Pharma. Safeguard my meds medicine cabinet. Public service announcement. https://www.youtube.com/watch?v=FU5TqCBeoSE.

130. Quinn M. The opioid files: hundreds of states and cities are suing drug compa- nies. Governing. November 13, 2017. http://www.governing.com/gov-opioid-lawsuits -companies-states-cities.html.

131. Radelat A. Growing number of states press opioid suits against Stamford's Purdue Pharma. July 6, 2017. https://ctmirror.org/2017/07/06/growing-number-of-states-press -opioid-suits-against-stamfords-purdue-pharma.

132. Burke J. The OxyContin reformulation: is it working? *Pharmacy Times*. May 16, 2011, http://www.pharmacytimes.com/publications/issue/2011/may2011/drugdiversion -0511.

133. Szabo L. FDA approves OxyContin for kids 11 to 16. *USA Today*. August 14, 2015. https://www.usatoday.com/story/news/2015/08/14/fda-approves-oxycontin -kids/31711929.

Chapter 9—Equal Parts Politics and Science

1. Davidson A. Why is Allergan partnering with the St. Regis Mohawk tribe? *New Yorker*. November 20, 2017.https://www.newyorker.com/magazine/2017/11/20/why-is-allergan -partnering-with-the-st-regis-mohawk-tribe.

2. Thomas K. How to protect a drug patent? Give it to a Native American tribe. *New York Times*. September 8, 2017. https://www.nytimes.com/2017/09/08/health/allergan -patent-tribe.html?_r=0.

3. Thomas K. 20 states accuse generic drug companies of price fixing. *New York Times*. December 15, 2016. https://www.nytimes.com/2016/12/15/business/generic-drug-price -lawsuit-teva-mylan.html?smid=nytcore-ipad-share&smprod=nytcore-ipad&_r=0.

4. Tribble SJ. Flurry of federal and state probes target insulin drugmakers and pharma middlemen. Kaiser Health News. October 30, 2017. https://khn.org/news/flurry-of -federal-and-state-probes-target-insulin-drugmakers- and-pharma-middlemen.

5. Relman AS. The new medical-industrial complex. *N Engl J Med*. 1980;303:963-970. https://www.nejm.org/doi/full/10.1056/NEJM198010233031703.

6. CVS company history. https://cvshealth.com/about/company-history.

7. De la Merced MJ, Abelson R. CVS to buy Aetna for $67 billion in a deal that may reshape the health industry. *New York Times*. December 3, 2017. https://www.nytimes .com/2017/12/03/business/dealbook/cvs-is-said-to-agree-to-buy-aetna-reshaping-health -care-industry.html.

8. Sundin S. Pharmacy in WW II—the pharmacist. The profession of pharmacy in the 1940s. http://www.sarahsundin.com/pharmacy-in-world-war-ii-the-pharmacist. US Army Center of Military History. *The Army Nurse Corps*: 8. http://www.history.army.mil/books/wwii/72-14/72-14.HTM. Accessed October 10, 2014.

9. Ginn RVN. WWII: the scientific specialties. In: *History of the U.S. Army Medical Service Corps*. US Army Medical Department, Office of Medical History: 181. http://history .amedd.army.mil/booksdocs/HistoryofUSArmyMSC/chapter6.html. Accessed October 10, 2014.

10. Worthen DB. *Pharmacy in World War II*. New York: Pharmaceutical Products Press; 2004:121-148. http://www.amazon.com/Pharmacy-World-War-Dennis-Worthen/dp/1481054422 Accessed October 10, 2014.

11. Lupkin S. Big pharma greets hundreds of ex-federal workers at the "revolving door." STAT. January 25, 2018. https://www.statnews.com/2018/01/25/pharma-federal-workers -revolving-door/?wpisrc=nl_health202&wpmm=1.

12. Healy D. The tragedy of Lou Lasagna. April 9, 2013. http://davidhealy.org/the -tragedy-of-lou-lasagna/.

13. Cohen JS, Insel PA. *The Physicians' Desk Reference*: Problems and possible improvements. *Arch Intern Med*. 1996;156(13):1375-1380. https://jamanetwork.com/journals/jamainternalmedicine/fullarticle/622098.

14. Medical Letter. Our mission and history. http://secure.medicalletter.org/mission. Accessed April 9, 2015.

15. Lasagna L. *The Doctors' Dilemma*. New York: Harper & Brothers; 1962:116-130.

16. Tobbell DA. *Pills, Power, and Policy: The Struggle for Drug Reform in Cold War America and Its Consequences*. Berkeley: University of California Press; 2012:168.

17. Tobbell DA. *Pills, Power, and Policy: The Struggle for Drug Reform in Cold War America and Its Consequences*. Berkeley: University of California Press; 2012:150,151.

18. Schwartz JL. Fifty years of expert advice: pharmaceutical legislation and legacy of the drug efficacy study. *N Engl J Med*. 2016;375:2015-2017. http://www.nejm.org/doi/full/10.1056/NEJMp1609763.

19. Tobbell DA. *Pills, Power, and Policy: The Struggle for Drug Reform in Cold War America and Its Consequences*. Berkeley: University of California Press; 2012:185.

20. Tobbell DA. *Pills, Power, and Policy: The Struggle for Drug Reform in Cold War America and Its Consequences*. Berkeley: University of California Press; 2012:122,123.

21. Healy D, Mangin D, Appelbaum K. The shipwreck of the singular. *Social Studies of Science*. June 11, 2014. http://sss.sagepub.com/content/ early/2014/06/11/0306312714536270.

22. Tobbell DA. *Pills, Power, and Policy: The Struggle for Drug Reform in Cold War America and Its Consequences*. Berkeley: University of California Press; 2012:176.

23. Hearings before the Subcommittee on Monopoly of the Select Committee on Small Business, U.S. Senate. On present status of competition in the pharmaceutical industry. http://archive.org/stream/competitiveprobl08unit/competitiveprobl08unit_djvu.txt.

24. Carpenter D, Tobbell DA. Bioequivalence: the regulatory career of a pharmaceutical concept. *Bull Hist Med.* 2011;85: 93-131. https://www.medscape.com/medline/abstract/21551918.

25. Skinner EF. Generic prescribing. *JAMA.* 1966;198(7):792-793. http://jama.jamanetwork.com/article.aspx?articleid=662245. Accessed January 26, 2015.

26. Tobbell DA. *Pills, Power, and Policy: The Struggle for Drug Reform in Cold War America and Its Consequences.* Berkeley: University of California Press; 2012:166,167.

27. Tobbell DA. *Pills, Power, and Policy: The Struggle for Drug Reform in Cold War America and Its Consequences.* Berkeley: University of California Press; 2012:167.

28. Tobbell DA. *Pills, Power, and Policy: The Struggle for Drug Reform in Cold War America and Its Consequences.* Berkeley: University of California Press; 2012:163.

29. Grabowski HG, Vernon JM. Effective patent time in pharmaceuticals. *Int J Technology Management.* 200;19(1-2):98-120. https://fds.duke.edu/db/attachment/182.

30. Fisher SH. The economic wisdom of regulating pharmaceutical "freebies." *Duke Law Journal.* 1991:206-239. http://scholarship.law.duke.edu/cgi/viewcontent.cgi?article=3141&context=dlj.

31. Tobbell DA. *Pills, Power, and Policy: The Struggle for Drug Reform in Cold War America and Its Consequences.* Berkeley: University of California Press; 2012:184-186.

32. Wright P. Louis Lasagna. *Lancet.* October 25, 2003;362. http://www.thelancet.com/pdfs/journals/lancet/PIIS0140-6736%2803%2914640-5.pdf.

33. Lou Lasagna Papers. University of Rochester. http://rbscp.lib.rochester.edu/3330.

34. CSDD history. Tufts Center for the Study of Drug Development. https://csdd.tufts.edu/.

35. Wallis WA. Law and medicine. In: Schwartz B, ed. *American Law: The Third Century.* South Hackensack, NJ: Fred B Rothman & Co.; 1976:351-363. Referenced in Nik-Khah E. Neoliberal pharmaceutical science and the Chicago School of Economics. *Social Studies of Science.* 2014. http://sss.sagepub.com/content/44/4/489.full.

36. Woodcock J, Junod S. PDUFA lays the foundation: launching into the era of user fee acts. Food and Drug Administration. http://www.fda.gov/AboutFDA/WhatWeDo/History/Overviews/ucm305697.htm.

37. Jauhar S. Why doctors are sick of their profession. *Wall Street Journal.* August 28, 2014. https://www.wsj.com/articles/the-u-s-s-ailing-medical-system-a-doctors-perspective-1409325361. Accessed January 26, 2015.

38. About Us: Corporations have their lobbyists in Washington, DC. The people need advocates too. Public Citizen. http://www.citizen.org/Page.aspx?pid=2306.

39. Fisher SH. The economic wisdom of regulating pharmaceutical "freebies." *Duke Law Journal.* 1991:206-239. http://scholarship.law.duke.edu/cgi/viewcontent.cgi?article=3141&context=dlj.

40. Tobbell DA. *Pills, Power, and Policy: The Struggle for Drug Reform in Cold War America and Its Consequences.* Berkeley: University of California Press; 2012:180.

41. S.1282(94th): Drug Utilization Improvement Act. https://www.govtrack.us/congress/bills/94/s1282.

42. Senator Edward Kennedy, Congressional Record 123, pt. 18. 1977:22262–22273. S. 2755: Drug Regulation Reform Act of 1978. Congressional Record 124, pt. 6. 1978:7205.

43. Peltzman, S. An evaluation of consumer protection legislation: the 1962 Drug Amendments. *J Political Economy.* 1973;81(5):1049-1091. http://www.jstor.org/discover/10.230 7/1830639?sid=21105156471131&uid=4&uid=3739576&uid=3739256&uid=2.

44. Newman E. *Pensions: The Broken Promise. NBC News.* September 12, 1972. http://archives.nbclearn.com/portal/site/k-12/flatview?cuecard=57200.

45. Pierron W, Fronstin P. ERISA pre-emption: implications for health reform and coverage. Employee Benefit Research Institute. February 2008. http://www.ebri.org/pdf/briefspdf/EBRI_IB_02a-20082.pdf.

46. 2 generic bills offered. *New York Times.* February 23, 1975:56 (NJ edition). Tobbell DA. *Pills, Power, and Policy: The Struggle for Drug Reform in Cold War America and Its Consequences.* Berkeley: University of California Press; 2012:189.

47. Tobbell DA. Eroding physicians' control of therapy. In: Greene JA, Watkins ES, eds. *Prescribed: Writing, Filling, Using, and Abusing Prescriptions in Modern America.* Baltimore, MD: Johns Hopkins University Press; 2012: Chapter 3. https://books.google.com/books?id=ArW-T3bPrOsC&pg=PT92&lpg=PT92&dq=NJ+1977+Generic+substitution+law&source=bl&ots=utU8dNRMXF&sig=RQ0_h3R_FZllEKRHvsdoYIbpb9Y&hl=en&sa=X&ei=uWjFVJTZD8TtgwTnhIKACA&ved=0CC0Q6AEwAg#v=onepage&q=NJ%201977%20Generic%20substitution%20law&f=false.

48. Grabowski HG, Vernon JM. Substitution laws and innovation in the pharmaceutical industry. *Law and Contemporary Problems.* 1979;43(1):43-66. http://scholarship.law.duke.edu/cgi/viewcontent.cgi?article=3569&context=lcp.

49. Wiesner JB. *Vannevar Bush: 1890–1974.* Washington, DC: National Academy of Sciences; 1979:99,100,101. http://www.nasonline.org/ publications/biographical-memoirs/memoir-pdfs/bush-vannevar.pdf.

50. Technology transfer: administration of the Bayh-Dole Act by research universities. May 1998. US Government Accounting Office. https://www.gao.gov/archive/1998/rc98126.pdf.

51. Markel H. Patents, profits and the American people: the Bayh-Dole Act. *N Engl J Med.* 2013;369:794-796. https://www.nejm.org/doi/full/10.1056/NEJMp1306553.

52. Allen J. The enactment of Bayh-Dole: an inside perspective. IP Watchdog. November 28, 2010. http://www.ipwatchdog.com/2010/11/28/the-enactment-of-bayh-dole-an-inside-perspective/id=13442/.

53. The Bayh-Dole Act: a guide to the law and implementing regulations. University of California Technology Transfer. Council on Government Relations. 1999. https://www.ucop.edu/research-policy-analysis-coordination/_files/cogr-guide.pdf.

54. Bayh-Dole Act. Association of University Technology Managers. https://www.autm.net/advocacy-topics/government-issues/bayh-dole-act/. https://www.autm.net/AUTMMain/media/Advocacy/Documents/BayhDoleTalkingPointsFINAL.pdf.

55. Loise V, Stevens AJ. The Bayh-Dole Act turns 30. *Science of Translational Medicine.* 2010; 2(52):52cm27. http://stm.sciencemag.org/content/2/52/52cm27.

56. Bayhing for blood or Doling out cash? *Economist*. December 2005. http://www.economist.com/node/5327661.

57. Office of Technology Assessment, *Patent Term Extension and the Pharmaceutical Industry*. Washington, DC: Government Printing Office; 1981. http://ota.fas.org/reports/8119.pdf.

58. Tobbell DA. *Pills, Power, and Policy: The Struggle for Drug Reform in Cold War America and Its Consequences*. Berkeley: University of California Press; 2012:195.

59. Weiswasser ES, Danzis SD. The Hatch-Waxman Act: history, structure and legacy. *Antitrust Law Journal*. 2003;71(2):585-603.

60. Boehm G, Yao L, Han L, Zheng Q. Development of the generic drug industry in the US after the Hatch-Waxman Act of 1984. *Acta Pharmaceutica Sinica B*. September 2013;3(5):297-311. http://www.sciencedirect.com/science/article/pii/S2211383513000762.

61. Generic drug facts. FDA. https://www.fda.gov/Drugs/ResourcesForYou/Consumers/BuyingUsingMedicineSafely/GenericDrugs/ucm167991.htm.

62. Spaulding R. Shkreli was right: everyone's hiking drug prices. Bloomberg News. February 2, 2016. https://www.bloomberg.com/news/articles/2016-02-02/shkreli-not-alone-in-drug-price-spikes-as-skin-gel-soars-1-860.

63. Cha AE. CEO Martin Shkreli: 4000 percent price hike is "altruistic," not "greedy." *Washington Post*. September 22, 2015. https://www.washingtonpost.com/news/to-your-health/wp/2015/09/22/turing-ceo-martin-shkreli-explains-that-4000-percent-drug-price-hike-is-altruistic-not-greedy/?utm_term=.a8e6ff8b83ef.

64. Martin A. Shkreli sentenced to seven years in prison for fraud. CNN. April 18, 2018. https://money.cnn.com/2018/03/09/news/martin-shkreli-sentencing/index.html.

65. McNeil DG. Selling cheap "generic" drugs, India's copycats irk industry. *New York Times*. December 1, 2000. http://www.nytimes.com/2000/12/01/world/selling-cheap-generic-drugs-india-s-copycats-irk-industry.html.

66. Clines FX. President is urged to press Japanese for freer trade. *New York Times*. December 18, 1983. http://www.nytimes.com/1983/01/18/business/president-is-urged-to-press-japanese-for-freer-trade.html.

67. Santoro MA, Paine LS. Pfizer: global protection of intellectual property. *Harvard Business Review*. 1995:9. https://hbr.org/product/Pfizer—Global-Protection/an/392073-PDF-ENG.

68. Drahos P, Braithwaite J. Who owns the knowledge economy? *Corner House Briefing*. September 30, 2004; 32. http://www.thecornerhouse.org.uk/resource/who-owns-knowledge-economy.

69. Beder S. Pfizer and intellectual property. *Business Managed Democracy*. 2009. http://www.herinst.org/BusinessManagedDemocracy/government/trade/Pfizer.html.

70. Gill K. What is the General Agreement on Tariffs and Trade (GATT)? ThoughtCo. March 16, 2018. http:// www.thoughtco.com/definition-of-gatt-3368065.

Chapter 10—Strange Bedfellows: Health Care, Politics, and the Christian Right

1. Glied SA, Frank RG. Care for the vulnerable vs. cash for the powerful—Trump's pick for HHS. *N Engl J Med*. January 1, 2017:103-105. http://www.nejm.org/doi/full/10.1056/NEJMp1615714.

2. AMA statement on the nomination of Rep. Tom Price to be HHS secretary. November 29, 2016. https://www.ama-assn.org/ama-statement-nomination-rep-tom-price-be-hhs-secretary.

3. Association of American Medical Colleges. AAMC commends president-elect Trump for nominating Rep. Price for HHS secretary. November 29, 2016. https://news.aamc.org/press-releases/article/price-hhs-nomination/.

4. Baker P, Thrush G, Haberman M. Health secretary Tom Price resigns after drawing ire for chartered flights. *New York Times*. September 29, 2017. https://www.nytimes.com/2017/09/29/us/politics/tom-price-trump-hhs.html.

5. Wallace G. IG: Tom Price's travel wasted $341,000. CNN Politics. July 14, 2018. https://www.cnn.com/2018/07/13/politics/tom-price-travel-review/index.html.

6. Editorial Board. An assault on efforts to prevent teenage pregnancy. *New York Times*. August 11, 2017. https://www.nytimes.com/2017/08/11/opinion/health-teenage-pregnancy-prevention.html.

7. Yoest Y. Transgender legal defense debates family research council. Fox News. November 13, 2006. https://www.youtube.com/watch?v=REZ4NuLmm-k&feature=youtube.

8. Belluck P. Programs that fight teenage pregnancy are at risk of being cut. *New York Times*. August 10, 2017. https://www.nytimes.com/2017/08/10/health/teen-pregnancy-prevention-trump-budget-cuts.html.

9. Tentler LW. *Catholics and Contraception: An American History*. Ithaca, NY: Cornell University Press; 2004:36,116.

10. Imbiorski WJ. *The Basic Cana Manual: Cana Conference of Chicago*. Chicago, IL: Delaney Publications; 1963:94-107.

11. Barry-Jester AM, Thomson-DeVeaux A. How Catholic bishops are shaping health care in rural America. FiveThirtyEight. July 25, 2018. https://fivethirtyeight.com/features/how-catholic-bishops-are-shaping-health-care-in-rural-america/?utm_source=STAT+Newsletters&utm_campaign=abe5154c2b-MR_COPY_09&utm_medium=email&utm_term=0_8cab1d7961-abe5154c2b-150335297.

12. Balmer R. The real origins of the religious right. *Politico*. May 27, 2014. http://www.politico.com/magazine/story/2014/05/religious-right-real-origins-107133.html#.VL7TOktggoM.

13. Paul Michael Weyrich. American National Biography Online. http://www.anb.org/articles/07/07-00849.html.

14. Hart-Smith A. "He'll do the right thing": a discussion of Jimmy Carter and Ronald Reagan's relationship with the evangelical community [dissertation]. University of Canterbury;

2013:12. http://ir.canterbury.ac.nz/bitstream/10092/8619/1/Hart-SmithAlexander480 FinalSubmission.pdf.

15. Navarro M. 2 decades on, Miami endorses gay rights. December 2, 1998. http://www .nytimes.com/1998/12/02/us/2-decades-on-miami-endorses-gay-rights.html.

16. Kelley K. Interview: Anita Bryant. *Playboy*. May 1978:73-96,232-250.

17. Clendinen D, Nagourney A. *Out for Good: The Struggle to Build a Gay Rights Movement in America*. New York: Simon and Schuster; 1990:291-311.

18. Holland J. When Southern Baptists were pro-choice. *Bill Moyers*. July 17, 2014. https:// billmoyers.com/2014/07/17/when-southern-baptists-were-pro-choice/.

19. Sizemore B. The Christian with four aces. *Virginian Pilot*. Spring 2008. http://www .vqronline.org/essay/christian-four-aces.

20. Robertson: Son conceived out of wedlock. *Pittsburgh Press*/UPI/*Washington Post*. October 8, 1987. http://news.google.com/newspapers?nid=1144&dat=19871008&id=Nt4cA AAAIBAJ&sjid=TGMEAAAAIBAJ&pg=2626,4526868.

21. Robertson P. Something's missing. From: *Shout It from the Housetops*. Newberry, FL: Bridge-Logos; 1972. http://www.patrobertson.com/SpiritualJourney/Something Missing.asp.

22. King W. Pat Robertson: a candidate of contradictions. *New York Times*. February 27, 1988. https://www.nytimes.com/1988/02/27/us/pat-robertson-a-candidate-of-contradictions .html.

23. Marley DJ. *Pat Robertson: An American Life*. Lanham, MD: Rowman and Littlefield; 2007:20,21.

24. About CBN. http://www1.cbn.com/about/cbn-partners-mission-statement.

25. Gerhardt MJ. How Jimmy Carter imperiled Roe v. Wade. Salon. March 30, 2013. http://www.salon.com/2013/03/30/how-jimmy-carter-imperiled-roe-v-wade/.

26. Le Beau BF. The political mobilization of the new Christian right. Creighton University. https://sites.google.com/site/apgovvocabwiki45/unit-4-terms/mobilization.

27. U.S. History. The Monkey Trial. http://www.ushistory.org/us/47b.asp.

28. History of BJU. https://www.bju.edu/about/history.php. News and Views: Bob Jones University apologizes for its racist past. *Journal of Blacks in Higher Education*. 2009. http:// www.jbhe.com/news_views/62_bobjones.html.

29. Bob Jones U. v. United States. May 24, 1983. Legal Information Institute. Cornell Law. https://www.law.cornell.edu/supremecourt/text/461/574.

30. Wertheimer L. Evangelical: religious right has distorted the faith—interview of Randall Balmer. NPR. June 23, 2006. http://www.npr.org/templates/story/story .php?storyId=5502785.

31. Koop CE. *The Right to Live, the Right to Die: Famous Pediatric Surgeon C. Everett Koop Speaks Out on Abortion and Mercy Killing*. Fort Collins, CO: Life Cycle Books; 1976.

32. Drake DC. Siamese twins: the surgery—an agonizing choice, parents, doctors, rabbis in dilemma. Originally printed in the *Philadelphia Inquirer*. October 16, 1977. *ASSAI*.

February 2001;4(1). http://www.daat.ac.il/daat/kitveyet/assia_english/drake-1.htm. Accessed February 10, 2015.

33. Koop CE, Schaeffer FA. *Whatever Happened to the Human Race?* Wheaton, IL: Crossway Books; 1978.

34. Hamilton MS. The dissatisfaction of Francis Schaeffer. *Christianity Today*. March 3, 1997. http://www.christianitytoday.com/ct/1997/march3/7t322a.html?start=1.

35. Specter M. Postscript: C. Everett Koop, 1916–2013. *New Yorker*. February 26, 2013. http://www.newyorker.com/news/news-desk/postscript-c-everett-koop-1916-2013.

36. Dr. Unqualified. *New York Times*. April 9, 1981. http://www.nytimes.com/1981/04/09/opinion/dr-unqualified.html.

37. Stobbe M. *Surgeon General's Warning: How Politics Crippled the Nation's Doctor*. Oakland: University of California Press:174.

38. Stobbe M. *Surgeon General's Warning: How Politics Crippled the Nation's Doctor*. Oakland: University of California Press:175,176.

39. Stobbe M. *Surgeon General's Warning: How Politics Crippled the Nation's Doctor*. Oakland: University of California Press:176.

40. Surgeon general biographies: C. Everett Koop (1982–1989). http://wayback.archive -it.org/3929/20171201191748/https://www.surgeongeneral.gov/about/previous/biokoop. html.

41. Weber B. Julius B. Richmond, who led Head Start and battled tobacco, dies at 91. *New York Times*. July 30, 2008. http://www.nytimes.com/2008/07/30/us/30richmond.html.

42. Reinhold R. Surgeon general report broadens list of cancers linked to smoking. *New York Times*. February 23, 1982. http://www.nytimes.com/1982/02/23/science/surgeon -general-report-broadens-list-of-cancers-linked-to-smoking.html. Accessed March 10, 2015.

43. Stobbe M. *Surgeon General's Warning: How Politics Crippled the Nation's Doctor*. Oakland: University of California Press:177.

44. Markel H. One man's rise from "Dr. Unqualified" to surgeon-in-chief. *PBS NewsHour*. November 15, 2013. http://www.pbs.org/newshour/rundown/one-mans-rise-from-dr -unqualified-to-a-household-name.

45. Arias DC. C. Everett Koop: the nation's health conscience. *AJPH*. October 10, 2011. http://ajph.aphapublications.org/doi/abs/10.2105/AJPH.2007.129114?journalCode =ajph.

46. Shilts R. *And the Band Played On: Politics, People, and the AIDS Epidemic*. New York: St. Martin's Press; 1987:68,69.

47. AIDS.gov. A timeline for AIDS. 1982. https://www.aids.gov/hiv-aids-basics/ hiv-aids-101/aids-timeline/.

48. Stobbe M. *Surgeon General's Warning: How Politics Crippled the Nation's Doctor*. Oakland: University of California Press:181,182.

49. Stobbe M. *Surgeon General's Warning: How Politics Crippled the Nation's Doctor*. Oakland: University of California Press:183.

50. The Age of AIDS. Interview with Margaret Heckler. PBS. January 11, 2006. http://www.pbs.org/wgbh/pages/frontline/aids/interviews/heckler.html.

51. Don't stop me now [editorial]. *Nature Immunology*. 2008;9:821. http://www.nature.com/ni/journal/v9/n8/full/ni0808-821.html.

52. Shilts R. *And the Band Played On: Politics, People, and the AIDS Epidemic*. New York: St. Martin's Press; 1987:456.

53. Shilts R. *And the Band Played On: Politics, People, and the AIDS Epidemic*. New York: St. Martin's Press; 1987:586.

54. Ocamb K. Ronald Reagan's real legacy: death, heartache, and silence over AIDS. February 7, 2011. Bilerico Project. http://www.bilerico.com/2011/02/ronald_reagans_real_legacy_death_heartache_and_sil.php http://harpercrusade.blogspot.com/2011/07/gary-bauers-focus-is-harper-governments.html.

55. Buckley WF. Crucial steps in combating the aids epidemic: identify all the carriers. *New York Times*. March 18, 1986. https://www.nytimes.com/books/00/07/16/specials/buckley-aids.html.

56. Berger J. Rock Hudson, screen idol, dies at 59. *New York Times*. October 3, 1985. http://www.nytimes.com/1985/10/03/arts/rock-hudson-screen-idol-dies-at-59.html.

57. Plante H. Reagan's legacy. San Francisco AIDS Foundation. http://www.sfaf.org/hiv-info/hot-topics/from-the-experts/2011-02-reagans-legacy.html.

58. Andriote JM. Doctor, not chaplain: how a deeply religious surgeon general taught the nation about HIV. *Atlantic*. March 4, 2013. http://www.theatlantic.com/health/archive/2013/03/doctor-not-chaplain-how-a-deeply-religious-surgeon-general-taught-a-nation-about-hiv/273665/.

59. Profiles in Science. National Library of Medicine. C. Everett Koop Papers. AIDS, the surgeon general, and the politics of public health. http://profiles.nlm.nih.gov/ps/retrieve/Narrative/QQ/p-nid/86.

60. Ryan White: 1971–1990. Ryan White: his story. http://ryanwhite.com/Ryans_Story.html.

61. Specter M. AIDs victim's right to attend public school tested in corn belt. *Washington Post*. September 3, 1985. https://www.washingtonpost.com/archive/politics/1985/09/03/aids-victims-right-to-attend-public-school-tested-in-corn-belt/8ffb6ac0-93cc-4c6f-88da-f3bb23664294/?utm_term=.aed27427cca3.

62. Crimp D. Before Occupy: how AIDS activists seized control of the FDA in 1988. *Atlantic*. December 6, 2011. https://www.theatlantic.com/health/archive/2011/12/before-occupy-how-aids-activists-seized-control-of-the-fda-in-1988/249302/.

63. Stobbe M. *Surgeon General's Warning: How Politics Crippled the Nation's Doctor*. Oakland: University of California Press; 2014:182-186. https://catalyst.library.jhu.edu/catalog/bib_7135916.

64. AZT's inhuman cost. *New York Times*. August 28, 1989. http://www.nytimes.com/1989/08/28/opinion/azt-s-inhuman-cost.html.

65. The Age of AIDS. Interview with Margaret Heckler. PBS. January 11, 2006. http://www.pbs.org/wgbh/pages/frontline/aids/interviews/heckler.html.

66. NIH Interview: Q and A with NIAID director Dr. Anthony S. Fauci. *Global Health Matters.* July-August 2011;10(4). https://www.fic.nih.gov/News/GlobalHealthMatters/August2011/Pages/niaid-tony-fauci.aspx.

67. Gonsalves G, Harrington M, Kessler DA. Don't weaken the F.D.A.'s approval process. *New York Times.* June 11, 2015. https://www.nytimes.com/2015/06/11/opinion/dont-weaken-the-fdas-drug-approval-process.html?_r=0.

68. FDA. Antiretroviral drugs used in the treatment of HIV infection. https://www.fda.gov/ForPatients/Illness/HIVAIDS/Treatment/ucm118915.htm.

69. Pear R. Faster approval of AIDS drugs is urged. *New York Times.* August 6, 1990. http://www.nytimes.com/1990/08/16/us/faster-approval-of-aids-drugs-is-urged.html.

70. Tobbell DA. *Pills, Power, and Policy: The Struggle for Drug Reform in Cold War America and Its Consequences.* Berkeley: University of California Press; 2012:121-162.

71. Lietzan E. FDA's reliance on user fees. *Yale Journal on Regulation Notice & Comment.* September 4, 2017. http://yalejreg.com/nc/fdas-reliance-on-user-fees/.

72. Woodcock J, Junod S. PDUFA lays the foundation: launching into the era of user fee acts. Food and Drug Administration. http://www.fda.gov/AboutFDA/WhatWeDo/History/Overviews/ucm305697.htm.

73. Effect of user fees on drug approval times, withdrawals, and other agency activities. September 2002. US Government Accountability Office. http://www.gao.gov/new.items/d02958.pdf. Accessed April 9, 2015.

74. Senator Edward M. Kennedy, 1932–2009. A lifetime of service. http://www.tedkennedy.org/service/item/health_care.html.

75. George Bush videos: acceptance speech—"Read my lips." August 18, 1988. History Channel. http://www.history.com/topics/us-presidents/george-bush/videos/read-my-lips.

76. Murugan V. Embryonic stem cell research: a decade of debate from Bush to Obama. *Yale J Biol Med.* September 2009;82(3):101-103. https://www.ncbi.nlm.nih.gov/pmc/articles/PMC2744932.

Chapter 11—Nigeria, CROs, and Research Biases

1. US Holocaust Memorial Museum. The doctors trial: the medical case of the subsequent Nuremberg Proceedings. https://www.ushmm.org/information/exhibitions/online-exhibitions/special-focus/doctors-trial#.

2. Miller MD. The informed-consent policy of the International Conference on Harmonization of Technical Requirements for Registration of Pharmaceuticals for Human Use: knowledge is the best medicine. *Cornell International Law Journal* 1997;30(1), article 5: 203-244. http://scholarship.law.cornell.edu/cgi/viewcontent.cgi?article=1398&context=cilj.

3. Beecher HK. Ethics and clinical research. *N Engl J Med.* June 16, 1966. https://www.nejm.org/doi/full/10.1056/NEJM196606162742405.

4. Michael DeBakey: inventor, surgeon, educator, doctor (1908–2008). Biography. https://www.biography.com/people/michael-debakey-9269009.

5. Kaplan S. Dr. Irwin Schatz, the first, lonely voice against infamous Tuskegee Study, dies at 83. *Washington Post*. April 20, 2014. https://www.washingtonpost.com/news/morning-mix/wp/2015/04/20/dr-irwin-schatz-the-first-lonely-voice-against-infamous-tuskegee-study-dies-at-83/?utm_term=.a361ba44bd10.

6. Beecher HK. Ethics and clinical research. *N Engl J Med*. June 16, 1966;274:1354-1360. http://www.nejm.org/doi/full/10.1056/NEJM196606162742405.

7. Hellert J. Syphilis victims in U.S. study went untreated for 40 years; syphilis victims got no therapy. *New York Times*. July 26, 1972. http://query.nytimes.com/gst/abstract.html?res=9B0CE7D71F3EE63BBC4E51DFB1668389669EDE.

8. "I Didn't Want to Believe It": Lessons from Tuskegee 40 years later. Planned Parenthood blog. November 15, 2012. http://blog.advocatesaz.org/2012/11/15/i-didnt-want-to-believe-it- lessons-from-tuskegee-40-years-later/.

9. Perkiss A. Public accountability and the Tuskegee syphilis experiments: a restorative justice approach. *Berkeley Journal of African-American Law and Policy*. 10(1), article 4:1-21. http://scholarship.law.berkeley.edu/cgi/viewcontent.cgi?article=1086&context=bjalp.

10. Remarks by the president in apology for the study done in Tuskegee. White House Office of the Press Secretary. May 16, 1997. http://clinton4.nara.gov/textonly/New/Remarks/Fri/19970516-898.html.

11. Carroll AE. Did famous Tuskeegee Study cause lasting mistrust of doctors among blacks? *New York Times*. June 17, 2016. https://www.nytimes.com/2016/06/18/upshot/long-term-mistrust-from-tuskegee-experiment-a-study-seems-to-overstate-the-case.html?_r=0.

12. LaMattina J. Pharma controls clinical trials of their drugs: is this hazardous to your health? *Forbes*. October 2, 2013. http://www.forbes.com/sites/johnlamattina/2013/10/02/pharma-controls-clinical-trials-of-their-drugs-is-this-hazardous-to-your-health/.

13. Bero L, Oostvogel F, Bacchetti P, Lee K. Factors associated with findings of published trials of drug—drug comparisons: why some statins appear more efficacious than others. *PLOS*. June 5, 2007. http://journals.plos.org/plosmedicine/article?id=10.1371/journal.pmed.0040184.

14. Magee M. Cholesterol: never having to say you're sorry. Health Commentary. November 20, 2013. http://www.healthcommentary.org/2013/11/20/cholesterol-never-having-to-say-youre-sorry-authors-reviewers-and-rwis/.

15. Bourgeois FT et al. Outcome reporting among drug trials registered in Clinical Trials .gov. *Annals of Internal Medicine*. 2010;153(3):18-66. http://www.annals.org/aim/article-abstract/745938/outcome-reporting-among-drug-trials-registered-clinicaltrials-gov.

16. Turner EH et al. Selective publication of antidepressant trials and its influence on apparent efficacy. *N Engl J Med*. 2008; 358:252-260. http://www.nejm.org/doi/full/10.1056/NEJMsa065779.

17. Goldacre B. *Bad Pharma: How Drug Companies Mislead Doctors and Harm Patients*. New York: Faber and Faber; 2013:111.

18. Le Carré J. *The Constant Gardener*. New York: Scribner; 2001.

19. Hutin Y, Luby S, Paquet C. A large cholera outbreak in Kano City, Nigeria. *Journal of Water and Health*. 2003;1:1. http://jwh.iwaponline.com/content/ppiwajwh/1/1/45.full.pdf.

20. Metz HC. Nigeria: a country study—civil war. Library of Congress Country Studies. 1991. http://countrystudies.us/nigeria/23.htm.

21. Nigeria becomes Africa's largest economy. *Al Jazeera*. April 6, 2014. http://www.aljazeera .com/news/africa/2014/04/nigeria-becomes-africa-largest-economy-20144618190520102 .html.

22. Mohammad I et al. A severe epidemic of meningococcal meningitis in Nigeria. 1996. *Trans R Soc Trop Med Hyg*. May-June 2000;94(3):265-270. http://www.ncbi.nlm.nih.gov/ pubmed/10974995.

23. Wallerstein R, Condit P, Kasper C, Brown J, Morrison F. Statewide study of chloramphenicol therapy and fatal aplastic anemia. *JAMA* 1969;208(11):2045-2050. http://jama .jamanetwork.com/article.aspx?articleid=346442.

24. Perlroth N. Pfizer's Nigerian nightmare. *Forbes*. November 20, 2008. http://www .forbes.com/forbes/2008/1208/066.html.

25. Goos H. Using Africans as "guinea pigs": Nigeria takes on Pfizer over controversial drug test. Spiegel Online. November 16, 2007. http://www.spiegel.de/international/ world/using-africans-as-guinea-pigs-nigeria-takes-on-pfizer-over-controversial-drug -test-a-517805.html.

26. French HW. Wide epidemic of meningitis fatal to 10,000 in West Africa. *New York Times*. May 8, 1996. http://www.nytimes.com/1996/05/08/world/wide-epidemic-of -meningitis-fatal-to-10000-in-west-africa.html.

27. Wise J. Pfizer accused of testing new drug without ethical approval. *BMJ*. January 27, 2001; 322(7280):194. http://www.ncbi.nlm.nih.gov/pmc/articles/PMC1119465/.

28. Pfizer Inc. summary Trovan, Kano State civil case—statement of defense. July 2007. http://www.pfizer.com/sites/default/files/news/trovan_statement_defense_ summary.pdf.

29. Stephens J. Pfizer to pay $75 million to settle Nigerian drug-testing suit. *Washington Post*. July 31, 2009. http://www.washingtonpost.com/wp-dyn/content/article/2009/07/30/ AR2009073001847.html.

30. Stephens J. Panel faults Pfizer in '96 clinical trial in Nigeria. *Washington Post*. May 7, 2006. http://www.washingtonpost.com/wp-dyn/content/article/2006/05/06/ AR2006050601338.html.

31. Boseley S. WikiLeaks cables: Pfizer "used dirty tricks to avoid clinical trial payout." *Guardian*. December 9, 2010. http://www.theguardian.com/business/2010/dec/09/ wikileaks-cables-pfizer-nigeria.

32. Umar A. Nigeria: Pfizer—victims' medical records missing. All Africa. October 5, 2009. http://allafrica.com/stories/200910050887.html.

33. Llamas M. Big pharma's role in clinical trials. Drug Watch. April 19, 2018. https:// www.drugwatch.com/featured/clinical-trials-and-hidden-data/.

34. Taylor N. FDA updates CRO and sponsor inspection guidance. OutsourcingPharma .com, March 22, 2011. https://www.outsourcing-pharma.com/Article/2011/03/22/FDA -updates-CRO-sponsor-inspection-guidance.

35. Walsh R. A history of: contract research organizations (CROs). PharmaPhorum, November 10, 2010. https://pharmaphorum.com/views-and-analysis/a_history_of_contract_research_organisations_cros/. Goldacre B. *Bad Pharma: How Drug Companies Mislead Doctors and Harm Patients.* New York: Faber and Faber; 2013:100-121.

36. Cohen LP. Lilly's "quick cash" to habitués of shelters vanishes quickly. *Wall Street Journal.* November 14, 1996. http://www.wsj.com/articles/SB847923261820633500.

37. Lustgarten A. Drug testing goes offshore. *Fortune.* August 8, 2005. http://archive.fortune.com/magazines/fortune/fortune_archive/2005/ 08/08/8267653/index.htm.

38. Piller CX, Bronshtein T. Faced with public pressure, research institutions up reporting of clinical trial results. STAT. January 9, 2018. https://www.statnews.com/2018/01/09/clinical-trials-reporting-nih/.

39. Top 10 global CROs in 2016. IGEA Hub. https://igeahub.com/2016/04/14/top-10-global-cros-in-2016.

40. Henry C. Top 10 clinical research organizations in the pharma and biotech industry. Pharma IQ. March 27, 2017. IQVia. https://www.pharma-iq.com/regulatorylegal/articles/top-10-clinical-research-organisations-in-the.

41. Goldacre B. *Bad Pharma: How Drug Companies Mislead Doctors and Harm Patients.* New York: Faber and Faber; 2013:1-99.

42. Goldacre B. *Bad Pharma: How Drug Companies Mislead Doctors and Harm Patients.* New York: Faber and Faber; 2013:41.

43. De Angelis C et al. Clinical trial registration: a statement from the Committee of International Medical Journal Editors. *N Engl J Med.* 2004; 351:1250-1251. https://www.nejm.org/doi/full/10.1056/NEJMe048225.

44. Mathieu S. et al. Comparison of registered and published primary outcomes in randomized controlled trials. *JAMA.* 2009;302(9): 977–984. https://www.researchgate.net/publication/26783446_Comparison_of_Registered_and_Published_Primary_Outcomes_in_Randomized_ Controlled_Trials.

45. Prayle AP et al. Compliance with mandatory reporting of clinical trial results on ClinicalTrials.gov: cross sectional study. *BMJ.* 2012;344:d7373. http://www.bmj.com/content/344/bmj.d7373.

46. Huser V, Cimino JJ. Linking ClinicalTrials.gov and PubMed to track results of interventional human clinical trials. *PLOS One.* July 9, 2013; 8(7):e68409. http://www.ncbi.nlm.nih.gov/pubmed/23874614.

47. Wislar JS, Flanagan A, Fontanarosa PB, DeAngelis CD. Honorary and ghost authorship in high impact biomedical journals: a cross-sectional survey. *BMJ.* October 25, 2011:343. doi: https://doi.org/10.1136/bmj.d6128.

Chapter 12—Viagra: "Everything That Rises Must Converge"

1. Jay E. Viagra and other drugs discovered by accident. BBC. January 20, 2010. http://news.bbc.co.uk/2/hi/health/8466118.stm.

2. Katzenstein L. *Viagra: The Remarkable Story of the Discovery and Launch.* New York: Medical Information Press; 2001:10.

3. Katzenstein L. *Viagra: The Remarkable Story of the Discovery and Launch*. New York: Medical Information Press; 2001:11.

4. Ignarro et al. Nitric oxide and cyclic GMP formation on electrical field stimulation cause relaxation of corpus cavernosum smooth muscle. *Biochem Biophys Res Commun*. 1990;170:843-850. https://www.sciencedirect.com/science/article/pii/0006291X9092168Y.

5. Rajfer J et al. Nitric oxide as a mediator of relaxation of the corpus cavernosum in response to noradrenergic, noncholinergic neurotransmission. *N Engl J Med*. 1992;326:90-94. https://www.nejm.org/doi/full/10.1056/NEJM199201093260203.

6. Altman L. Three Americans awarded Nobel for discoveries of how a gas affects the body. *New York Times*. October 13, 1998. http://www.nytimes.com/1998/10/13/us/three-americans-awarded-nobel-for-discoveries-of-how-a-gas-affects-the-body.html.

7. Katzenstein L. *Viagra: The Remarkable Story of the Discovery and Launch*. New York: Medical Information Press; 2001:15.

8. Tozzi J, Hopkins JS. The little blue pill: an oral history of Viagra. Bloomberg. December 11, 2017. https://www.bloomberg.com/news/features/2017-12-11/the-little-blue-pill-an-oral-history-of-viagra.

9. Katzenstein L. *Viagra: The Remarkable Story of the Discovery and Launch*. New York: Medical Information Press; 2001:33-37.

10. Feldman HA, et al. Impotence and its medical and psychological correlates: results of the Massachusetts Male Aging Study. *J Urol*. 1994; 151:54-61. https://www.researchgate.net/publication/14944126_Impotence_and_Its_Medical_and_Psychosocial_Correlates_Results_of_the_Massachusetts_Male_Aging_Study.

11. Katzenstein L. *Viagra: The Remarkable Story of the Discovery and Launch*. New York: Medical Information Press; 2001:38-41.

12. Katzenstein L. *Viagra: The Remarkable Story of the Discovery and Launch*. New York: Medical Information Press; 2001:34.

13. Katzenstein L. *Viagra: The Remarkable Story of the Discovery and Launch*. New York: Medical Information Press; 2001:15.

14. Osterloh IH. The discovery and development of Viagra (sildenafil citrate). In: Dunzendorfer U, ed. *Sildenafil: Milestones in Drug Therapy*. MDT. Birkhäuser, Basel; 2004. https://www.researchgate.net/publication /251403464.

15. Company overview. Robinson, Lerer, Montgomery. Bloomberg. https://www.bloomberg.com/research/stocks/private/snapshot.asp?privcapId=705713.

16. Burrough B, Helyar J. *Barbarians at the Gate: The Fall of RJR Nabisco*. New York: Harper Perennial; 1990.

17. Klein E. Here's to you, Mrs. Robinson. *Vanity Fair*. May 1990:122. http://edwardklein.com/pdfs/may_1990_VF_heres_to_you_mrs_robinson2.pdf.

18. McLeod E. *The Original Amos 'n' Andy: Freeman Gosden, Charles Correll and the 1928–1943 Radio Serial*. North Carolina: McFarland and Company, 2005.

19. Drahos P, Braithwaite J. Who owns the knowledge economy? *Corner House Briefing* 32, September 30, 2004. http://www.thecornerhouse.org.uk/resource/who-owns-knowledge-economy.

20. Beder S. Pfizer and intellectual property. Business Managed Democracy. 2009. http://www.herinst.org/BusinessManagedDemocracy/government/trade/Pfizer/html.

21. Chandler Chicco Agency. http://www.ccapr.com/about-us.

22. Yankelovich D. How public opinion really works. *Fortune*. October 5, 1992. http://archive.fortune.com/magazines/fortune/fortune_archive/1992/10/05/76926/index.htm.

23. Quinley H. Yankelovich Partners. a survey of the patient-physician relationship in America—executive summary. April 1998. http://www.healthcommentary.org/?page_id=7279.

24. Katzenstein L. *Viagra: The Remarkable Story of the Discovery and Launch*. New York: Medical Information Press; 2001:44-47.

25. Woolley S. Science and savvy. *Forbes*. January 11, 1999. http://www.forbes.com/forbes/1999/0111/6301122a.html.

26. Webb DJ et al. Sildenafil citrate and blood pressure lowering drugs: results of drug interaction studies with an organic nitrate and a calcium antagonist. *Am J Cardiol*. 1999;83:21C-28C. https://www.researchgate.net/publication/13211504_Sildenafil_citrate_and_blood-pressure lowering_drugs_Results_of_drug_interaction_studies_with_an_organic_nitrate_and_a_calcium_antagonist.

27. Big Pharma Report/ ED news you can use. ABC Viagra transcript. March 21, 1998. http://www.siliconinvestor.com/readmsgs.aspx?subjectid=5861&msgnum=629&batchsize=10&batchtype=Previous.

28. Werthmann MM. Timothy Johnson, long-time medical editor, to leave WCVB-TV. boston.com. December 6, 2012. http://www.boston.com/metrodesk/2012/12/06/timothy-johnson-long-time-medical-editor-leave-wcvb/QCHOv5UDGHDuhmfwz6bvbM/story.html.

29. Pear R. Gender gap persists in cost of health insurance. *New York Times*. March 3, 2012. https://www.nytimes.com/2012/03/19/health/policy/women-still-pay-more-for-health-insurance-data-shows.html.

30. Unintended pregnancies in the United States. Guttmacher Institute. July 2015. http://www.guttmacher.org/pubs/FB-Unintended-Pregnancy-US.html.

31. Katzenstein L. *Viagra: The Remarkable Story of the Discovery and Launch*. New York: Medical Information Press; 2001:47

32. Kolata G. U.S. approves the sale of impotence pill; huge market seen. *New York Times*. March 28, 1998. http://www.nytimes.com/1998/03/28/us/us-approves-sale-of-impotence-pill-huge-market-seen.html.

33. Katzenstein L. *Viagra: The Remarkable Story of the Discovery and Launch*. New York: Medical Information Press; 2001:49.

34. Langreth R. FDA approves Pfizer's impotence pill; firm's shares have risen nearly 10%. *Wall Street Journal*. March 30, 1998. http://www.wsj.com/articles/SB891017121342379500.

35. Comarow A. Viagra tale: how one man sought an impotence cure—and found one. *U.S. News & World Report*. May 4, 1998. http://backissues.com/issue/US-News-and-World-Report-May-04-1998.

36. Leckey A. Popular drugs give Pfizer health for years to come. *Chicago Tribune*. June–July 1998. http://articles.chicagotribune.com/1998-06-07/business/9806070478_1_pfizer-cholesterol-lowering-drug-lipitor-warner-lambert.

37. Katzenstein L. *Viagra: The Remarkable Story of the Discovery and Launch*. New York: Medical Information Press; 2001:47.

38. Magee M. Lessons learned from Viagra. Bell Labs Innovators Presentation. New Jersey. November 5, 1999. http://www.healthcommentary.org/?page_id=7298. Accessed August 7, 2015.

39. Press Release: Viagra label warnings strengthened due to deaths. Relias Media. February 1, 1999. https://www.reliasmedia.com/articles/60521-viagra-label-warnings-strengthened-due-to-deaths.

40. Goldstein I et al. Oral sildenafil in the treatment of erectile dysfunction. Sildenafil Study Group. *N Engl J Med*. 1998;338:1397-1404. http://www.nejm.org/doi/full/10.1056/NEJM199805143382001.

41. Hutchinson B. Impotence pill is OK with pope. *Daily News*. April 24, 1998. http://www.nydailynews.com/archives/news/impotence-pill-pope-article-1.792251.

42. PR Newswire. Viagra should be covered by insurance plans, Pfizer tells California managed care regulators. August 20, 1998. http://www.prnewswire.com/news-releases/viagra-should-be-covered-by-insurance-plans-pfizer-tells-california-managed-care-regulators-76273912.html. Accessed August 7, 2015.

43. Marquis J. Insurers should pay for Viagra, regulators told. *Los Angeles Times*. August 21, 1998. http://articles.latimes.com/1998/aug/21/news/mn-15253.

44. Feldman HA et al. Impotence and its medical and psychosocial correlates; results of the Massachusetts Male Aging Study. *J Urol*. 1994;151:54-61. http://www.ncbi.nlm.nih.gov/pubmed/8254833.

45. Personal communication.

46. Rundle R. Kaiser Permanente will raise rates to cover costs of providing Viagra. *Wall Street Journal*. January 4, 1999. https://www.wsj.com/articles/SB915183517344609000.

47. Keith A. The economics of Viagra. *Health Affairs*. March-April 2000:147-157. https://www.ncbi.nlm.nih.gov/pubmed/10718028.

48. Poll: insurers should pay for impotence treatment. *Orlando Sentinel*. October 27, 1998. http://articles.orlandosentinel.com/1998-10-27/news/9810270076_1_impotence-treatment-viagra-insurers.

49. Pfizer Government Relations organizational chart. 1999.

50. Olmos DR. Kaiser, citing cost, won't pay for Viagra. *Los Angeles Times*. June 20, 1998. http://articles.latimes.com/1998/jun/20/news/mn-61782.

51. U.S. orders Medicaid coverage of Viagra. *Los Angeles Times*. July 3, 1998. http://articles.latimes.com/1998/jul/03/news/mn-508.

52. Sisk R. VA won't provide Viagra, says it would bust budget. *New York Daily News*. July 24, 1998. http://www.nydailynews.com/archives/news/va-won-provide-viagra-bust-budget-article-1.811532.

53. Jim Harris, AP, July 23, 1998. From Magee M. Lessons learned from Viagra. Bell Labs Innovators Presentation. New Jersey. November 5, 1999. http://www.healthcommentary .org/?page_id=7298.

54. PR Newswire. IMS Health forecasts Viagra sales to reach $1 billion in first year; most successful product launch recorded. July 6, 1998. http://www.prnewswire.com/ news-releases/ims-health-forecasts-viagra-sales-to-reach-1-billion-in-first-year-most -successful-product-launch-recorded-75635267.html. Accessed August 7, 2015.

55. Berenson A. Sales of impotence drugs fall, defying expectations. *New York Times*. December 4, 2005. http://www.nytimes.com/2005/12/04/business/yourmoney/sales-of -impotence-drugs-fall-defying-expectations.html?_r=0.

56. *Larry King Live*. January 7, 2000. Bob and Elizabeth Dole discuss the state of American politics. CNN.com transcripts. http://www.cnn.com/TRANSCRIPTS/0001/07/ lkl.00.html.

57. Crouch I. Viagra returns to the Bob Dole approach. *New Yorker*. October 7, 2014. http://www.newyorker.com/business/currency/viagra-returns-bob-dole-approach.

58. Bob Dole Viagra commercials. *Rachel Maddow Show*. February 5, 2012. https://www .youtube.com/watch?v=nBdgpjnKInA.

59. Bob Dole "Courage" print ad. http://healthpopuli.com/wp-content/uploads/2012/08/ Bob-Dole-Viagra.jpg.

60. *National Men's Health Week* (Emmaus, PA). June 14, 1999. Quoted in Katzenstein L. *Viagra: The Remarkable Story of the Discovery and Launch*. New York: Medical Information Press; 2001:59.

61. Jacoby S. Great sex. What's age got to do with it? *Modern Maturity*. 1999. Quoted in Katzenstein L. *Viagra: The Remarkable Story of the Discovery and Launch*. New York: Medical Information Press; 2001:59.

62. Katzenstein L. *Viagra: The Remarkable Story of the Discovery and Launch*. New York: Medical Information Press; 2001:79.

63. Katzenstein L. *Viagra: The Remarkable Story of the Discovery and Launch*. New York: Medical Information Press; 2001:61.

64. Rosen RC et al. Development and evaluation of an abridged, 5-item version of the International Index of Erectile Dysfunction (IIEF-5) as a diagnostic tool for erectile dysfunction. *Int J Impot Res*. 1999;11:319-326. http://patientreportedoutcomes2.sites.olt .ubc.ca/files/2014/04/IIEF-5-Rosen-1999.pdf.

65. Katzenstein L. *Viagra: The Remarkable Story of the Discovery and Launch*. New York: Medical Information Press; 2001:62.

66. Carbone DJ et al. Incidence of previously undiagnosed urologic malignancies in a population presenting solely with the complaint of erectile dysfunction. *J Urol*. 1999;161:4. Abstract 695.

67. Pritzker MR. The penile stress test: a window to the hearts of man? Abstract presented at the American Heart Association National Meeting; November 10, 1999; Atlanta, GA.

68. Katzenstein L. *Viagra: The Remarkable Story of the Discovery and Launch*. New York: Medical Information Press; 2001:54,55.

69. Katzenstein L. *Viagra: The Remarkable Story of the Discovery and Launch*. New York: Medical Information Press; 2001:81.

70. Pfizer 2000 Annual Report, p. 20. http://www.pages.stern.nyu.edu/jbilders/Pdf/pfizer00ar.pdf.

71. Berke RL. Eye on 2000: Elizabeth Dole leaves Red Cross. *New York Times*. January 5, 1999. http://www.nytimes.com/1999/01/05/us/eye-on-2000-elizabeth-dole-leaves-red-cross.html.

72. White House 2000: Republicans. Elizabeth Dole. *New York Times*. January 5, 2000. http://partners.nytimes.com/library/politics/camp/whouse/gop-dole.html.

73. Viagra NASCAR commercial featuring Mark Martin. 2001. YouTube. https://www.youtube.com/watch?v=SP6rJZwPZ4Q.

74. Glasser DB, Pritchett J, Olson J. Nascar races: a targeted venue for health screening and identification of individuals at risk for cardiovascular disease. APHA. November 13, 2002. https://apha.confex.com/apha/130am/techprogram/paper_42416.htm.

75. Hospital closures: 1990–1999. Office of Inspector General. Atlanta, GA. December 2001. https://www.oig.hhs.gov/oei/reports/oei-04-02-00180.pdf.

76. United Healthcare Group: History. https://www.unitedhealthgroup.com/about/history.html.

77. Firozi P. Here's why rural independent pharmacies are closing their doors. *Washington Post*. August 23, 2018. https://www.washingtonpost.com/news/powerpost/paloma/the-health-202/2018/08/23/the-health-202-here-s-why-rural-independent-pharmacies-are-closing-their-doors/5b7da33e1b326b7234392b05/.

Chapter 13—New Rules

1. Emanuel EJ. The solution to drug prices. *New York Times*. September 9, 2015. https://www.nytimes.com/2015/09/09/opinion/the-solution-to-drug-prices.html?_r=0.

2. Simons J. The $10 billion pill: hold the fries, please. *Fortune*. January 20, 2003. http://archive.fortune.com/magazines/fortune/fortune_archive/2003/01/20/335643/index.htm.

3. O'Reilly B. The pills that saved Warner-Lambert led by the anti-cholesterol drug Lipitor: the company's shares have doubled in a year. *Fortune*. October 13, 1997. http://archive.fortune.com/magazines/fortune/ fortune_archive/1997/10/13/232535/index.htm.

4. CDC. MMWR. Achievements in public health, 1900–1999: decline in deaths from heart disease and stroke—United States, 1900–1999. https://www.webmd.com/heart-disease/guide/sudden-cardiac-death#1. Accessed August 7, 2015.

5. Williams O et al. Case 11—Merck (B): Zocor. University of Michigan Business. http://www-personal.umich.edu/~afuah/cases/case11.html.

6. Nawrocki JW. Reduction of LDL cholesterol by 25% to 60% in patients with primary hypercholesterolemia by atorvastatin, a new HMG-CoA reductase inhibitor.

Arteriosclerosis, Thrombosis, and Vascular Biology. 1995;15:678-682. http://atvb.ahajournals
.org/content/15/5/678.full.

7. Lipitor (atorvastatin calcium). CenterWatch. https://www.centerwatch.com/drug
-information/fda-approved-drugs/drug/1194/lipitor-atorvastatin-calcium.

8. Johnson LA. Against odds, Lipitor became world's top seller. *USA Today.* December 28,
2011. http://usatoday30.usatoday.com/news/health/medical/health/medical/treatments/
story/2011-12-28/Against-odds-Lipitor-became-worlds-top-seller/52250720/1.

9. Winslow R. Warner-Lambert, Pfizer win approval to market new drug. *Wall Street
Journal.* December 19, 1996. http://www.wsj.com/articles/SB850930655521266000.

10. Purvis L, Schondelmeyer SW. Rx price watch case study: efforts to reduce the impact
of generic competition for Lipitor. AARP Public Policy Institute. http://www.aarp.org/
content/dam/aarp/research/public_policy_institute/health/2013/lipitor-final-report
-AARP-ppi-health.pdf.

11. University of Michigan Case Study 25—Lipitor: at the heart of Warner-Lambert.
http://www-personal.umich.edu/afuah/cases/case25.html.

12. Langreth R, Harris G, Deogan N. Pfizer plans to tout new lineup of drugs, seeking
support for Warner-Lambert bid. *Wall Street Journal.* November 15, 1999. http://www
.wsj.com/articles/SB942431215148292128.

13. Lipin S, Langreth R, Harris G, Deogun N. In biggest hostile bid, Pfizer offers $80
billion for Warner-Lambert. *Wall Street Journal.* November 5, 1999. http://www.wsj.com/
articles/SB941761432116031917.

14. The history of American Home Products. HelpMe. http://www.123helpme.com/
view.asp?id=52267.

15. Langreth R, Lipin S. American Home Products discusses merger with Warner-
Lambert. *Wall Street Journal.* November 3, 1999. http://www.wsj.com/articles/
SB941602466851084149.

16. Warner criticizes Pfizer. CNN Money. November 9, 1999. http://money.cnn
.com/1999/11/09/news/warner/.

17. Langreth R. Warner-Lambert agrees to a deal with Pfizer worth $90 billion. *Wall
Street Journal.* February 7, 2000. http://www.wsj.com/articles/SB94988042510658
7767.

18. Petersen M. Pfizer gets its deal to buy Warner-Lambert. *New York Times.* February 8,
2000. http://www.nytimes.com/2000/02/08/business/pfizer-gets-its-deal-to-buy-warner
-lambert-for-90.2-billion.html.

19. Petersen M. Pfizer chief to retire, leaving successor hard act to follow. *New York Times.*
August 11, 2000. http://www.nytimes.com/2000/08/11/business/pfizer-chief-to-retire
-leaving-successor-hard-act-to-follow.html. Accessed August 9, 2015.

20. Pfizer Inc. (PFE). Historic prices. Yahoo Finance. http://finance.yahoo.com/q/hp?s=
PFE&a=01&b=1&c=2000&d=08&e=27&f=2010&g=d.

21. Elkind P, Reingold J. Inside Pfizer's palace coup. *Fortune.* July 28, 2011. http://fortune
.com/2011/07/28/inside-pfizers-palace-coup/.

22. Frank R, Hensley S. Pfizer to buy Pharmacia for $60 billion in stock. *Wall Street Journal*. July 15, 2002. http://www.wsj.com/articles/SB1026684057282753560. Accessed August 8, 2015.

23. Monsanto, Pfizer celebrate Celebrex. *St. Louis Business Journal*. July 20, 1999. http://www.bizjournals.com/stlouis/stories/1999/07/19/daily5.html.

24. Why COX-2 inhibitors such as Vioxx cause heart attacks and strokes. News/Medical and Life Sciences. December 2, 2006. https://www.news-medical.net/news/2006/12/02/21158.aspx.

25. FDA estimates Vioxx caused 27,785 deaths. Consumer Affairs. November 4, 2004. https://www.consumeraffairs.com/news04/vioxx_estimates.html.

26. Merck: A $5 billion settlement in Vioxx case. *Week*. November 15, 2007. http://theweek.com/articles/519390/merck-5-billion-settlement-vioxx-case.

27. Knox R. Merck pulls arthritis drug Vioxx from market. NPR. September 30, 2004. http://www.npr.org/templates/story/story.php?storyId=4054991.

28. Pfizer pulls plug on Bextra. PharmaTimes. April 8, 2005. http://www.pharmatimes.com/news/pfizer_pulls_plug_on_bextra_998436.

29. Tran L. Untangling the Vioxx-Celebrex controversy. Legal Electronic Document Archive, Harvard Law School. May 4, 2005. https://dash.harvard.edu/bitstream/handle/1/8889459/Tran05.html?sequence=2.

30. Berenson A. Pfizer to halt its advertising of Celebrex to consumers. *New York Times*. December 19, 2004. http://www.nytimes.com/2004/12/19/business/pfizer-to-halt-its-advertising-of-celebrex-to-consumers.html.

31. Berensen A. Celebrex ads are back, dire warnings and all. *New York Times*. April 29, 2006. http://www.nytimes.com/2006/04/29/business/media/29celebrex.html?gwh=2382767657FE5A9324F7488ACB35B9C8&gwt=pay.

32. 2006 Pfizer annual report: financial appendix. http://www.annualreports.com/HostedData/AnnualReportArchive/p/NYSE_PFE_2016.pdf.

33. Donohue JM, Cevasco M, Rosenthal MB. A decade of direct-to-consumer advertising of prescription drugs. *N Engl J Med*. 2007;357:673-681. http://www.nejm.org/doi/full/10.1056/NEJMsa070502.

34. Henderson DR, Hooper CL. Pfizer's $2.3 billion-dollar settlement. *Forbes*. September 9, 2009. https://www.forbes.com/2009/09/08/pfizer-bilion-dollar-settlement-fda-opinions-contributors-david-r-henderson-charles-l-hooper.html#70dccd235f9f.

35. PharmTech editorial. Pfizer exits Exubera and takes $2.8 billion charge. ePT. October 18, 2007. http://www.pharmtech.com/pfizer-exits-exubera-and-takes-28-billion-charge.

36. New FDA warning for anti-smoking drug Chantix. CBS News. March 10, 2015. https://www.cbsnews.com/news/new-fda-warning-for-anti-smoking-drug-chantix/.

37. Barter PJ, Caulfield M, et al. Effects of torcetrapib in patients at high risk for coronary events. *N Engl J Med*. November 22, 2007;357:2109-2122. http://www.nejm.org/doi/full/10.1056/NEJMoa0706628.

38. OpenSecrets.org. Pfizer Inc. Year 2000, Lobbyists. https://www.opensecrets.org/lobby/clientlbs.php?id=D000000138&year=2000.

39. Kerr P. Jersey Speaker sprints for governor's job. *New York Times*. March 17, 1989. https://www.nytimes.com/1989/03/17/nyregion/jersey-speaker-sprints-for-governor-s-job.html.

40. Nagourney A. The 2002 elections: the overview—the GOP retakes control of the Senate in a show of presidential influence; Pataki, Jeb Bush, and Lautenberg win. *New York Times*. November 6, 2002. http://www.nytimes.com/2002/11/06/us/2002-elections-overview-gop-retakes-control-senate-show-presidential-influence.html. Accessed 8/9/2015.

41. Federal elections 2002: election results for the U.S. Senate and the U.S. House of Representatives. http://www.fec.gov/pubrec/fe2002/cover.htm.

42. Weisman J. Prescription bill fuels lobbying blitz on hill: competition fierce for $400 billion pot. *Washington Post*. June 13, 2003. http://www.highbeam.com/doc/1P2-273987.html.

43. Drotleff EA. The Medicare Part D prescription drug benefit: who wins and who loses? *Marquette Elder's Advisor*. 2006;8:1, article 7. http://scholarship.law.marquette.edu/cgi/viewcontent.cgi?article=1065&context=elders.

44. Trends and analysis of Medicare Managed Care plan withdrawals in 2002. California Healthcare Foundation. October 2001. https://www.chcf.org/wp-content/uploads/2017/12/PDF-MedicareTrends1.pdf.

45. Merck & Co. completes Medco purchase. *New York Times* News Service. November 19, 1993. http://articles.baltimoresun.com/1993-11-19/business/1993323090_1_medco-merck-wygod.

46. Dewar H, Goldstein A. Medicare bill squeezes through House at dawn. *Washington Post*. November 23, 2003. http://www.highbeam.com/doc/1P2-310294.html.

47. Oliver TR, Lee PR, Lipton H. A political history of Medicare and prescription drug coverage. *Milbank Q*. June 2004;82(2):283-354. http://www.ncbi.nlm.nih.gov/pmc/articles/PMC2690175/.

48. White paper: Managed Medicare's rapid expansion. Managed Care. August 1997. http://www.managedcaremag.com/sites/default/files/imported/9708/9708.managedcare.pdf.

49. Freudenheim M. A windfall from shifts to Medicare. Market Place. *New York Times*. July 18, 2006. http://www.nytimes.com/2006/07/18/business/18place.html?pagewanted=all. Accessed August 9, 2015.

50. Pear R. Medicare debate focuses on merits of private plans. *New York Times*. June 9, 2003. https://www.nytimes.com/2003/06/09/us/medicare-debate-focuses-on-merits-of-private-plans.html.

51. Health Canada. Protecting Canadians from excessive drug prices. June 28, 2017. https://www.canada.ca/en/health-canada/programs/consultation-regulations-patented-medicine/document.html.

52. Iglehart JK. The new Medicare prescription-drug benefit: a pure power play. *N Engl J Med*. 2004;350:826-833. February 19, 2004. http://www.nejm.org/doi/full/10.1056/NEJMhpr045002 Accessed August 9, 2015.

53. Broder DS. AARP's tough selling job. *Washington Post*. February 18, 2004. http://www.democraticunderground.com/discuss/duboard.php?az=view_all&address=103x4045.

54. Blumenthal P. The legacy of Billy Tauzin: the White House–pharma deal. Sunlight Foundation. February 12, 2010. https://sunlightfoundation.com/2010/02/12/the-legacy-of-billy-tauzin-the-white-house-phrma-deal/.

55. Dionne EJ. Medicare monstrosity. *Washington Post.* November 18, 2003. https://www.washingtonpost.com/archive/opinions/2003/11/18/medicare-monstrosity/38c06221-f1a6-4141-aa43-c7429c2c6dfe/?utm_term=.65ecbedfb3c8.

56. Pear R, Toner R. Medicare plan covering drugs backed by AARP. *New York Times.* http://www.nytimes.com/2003/11/18/us/medicare-plan-covering-drugs-backed-by-aarp.html.

57. Porter Novelli. https://www.porternovelli.com/.

58. Connolly C. Democratic candidates rail at AARP on Medicare drugs. *Orlando Sentinel.* November 19, 2003. http://articles.orlandosentinel.com/2003-11-19/news/0311190156_1_aarp-new-hampshire-medicare.

59. Seelye KQ. A mini-mutiny at AARP over health care. *New York Times.* August 18/, 2009. https://prescriptions.blogs.nytimes.com/2009/08/18/a-mini-mutiny-at-aarp-over-health-care/.

60. Bush signs landmark Medicare bill into law. CNN.com. Politics: America Votes 2004. December 8, 2003. http://www.cnn.com/2003/ ALLPOLITICS/12/08/elec04.medicare/.

61. Feldman BS. Big pharmacies are dismantling the industry that keeps U.S. drug costs even sort of under control. Quartz. March 17, 2016. https://qz.com/636823/big-pharmacies-are-dismantling-the-industry-that-keeps-us-drug-costs-even-sort-of-under-control/.

62. De la Merced M, Abelson R. CVS to buy Aetna in a $69 billion deal that may reshape the health industry. *New York Times.* December 2, 2017. https://www.nytimes.com/2017/12/03/business/dealbook/cvs-is-said-to-agree-to-buy-aetna-reshaping-health-care-industry.html.

63. Merck—our history. https://www.merck.com/about/our-history/home.html.

64. Express Scripts Incorporated—company profile, information, business description, history, background. http://www.referenceforbusiness.com/history2/41/Express-Scripts-Incorporated.html.

65. Magee M. The basics of pharma kickbacks—opaque and complex. Health Commentary. March 7, 2018. http://www.healthcommentary.org/2018/03/07/basics-pharma-kickbacks-opaque-complex/; http://www.healthcommentary.org/2017/05/30/u-s-pharmaceutical-supply-chain-gray-black-market.

66. Schulman KA, Richman BD. The evolving pharmaceutical benefits market. *JAMA.* 2018:319(22):2269-2270. https://jamanetwork.com/journals/jama/fullarticle/2678286?utm_source=silverchair&utm_medium=email&utm_campaign=article_alert-jama&utm_content=etoc&utm_term=061218.

67. Allen TJ. Gray market drug. CorpWatch. January 22, 2012. http://www.corpwatch.org/article.php?id=15666.

68. Silverman E. Most emergency docs report shortages of critical medicines, and the problem is "getting worse." STAT. May 22, 2018. https://www.statnews.com/pharmalot/2018/05/22/emergency-doctors-shortages-opioids/.

69. FDA drug shortages, 2018. https://www.accessdata.fda.gov/scripts/drugshortages/default.cfm.

70. Fry E. Pfizer's drug supply problem. *Fortune.* May 22, 2018. http://fortune.com/longform/pfizer-drug-problem-fortune-500/.

71. Foley KE. Drug wholesalers shipped 9 million pain pills over two years to a single West Virginia pharmacy. December 19, 2016.

72. Mattioli D, Cimilluca D. Cigna agrees to buy Express Scripts for more than $50 billion. *Wall Street Journal.* March 8, 2018. https://www.wsj.com/articles/cigna-nears-deal-to-buy-express-scripts-1520482236?mod=djemalertNEWS.

73. Horowitz J, Wiener-Bronner D. CVS is buying Aetna in massive deal that could transform health care. CNN Money. December 3, 2017. https://money.cnn.com/2017/12/03/investing/cvs-health-aetna-merger/index.html.

74. Armour S, Overberg P. Nearly 600 Russia-linked accounts tweeted about the health law. *Wall Street Journal.* September 12, 2018. https://www.wsj.com/articles/nearly-600-russia-linked-accounts-tweeted-about-the-health-law-1536744638.

Chapter 14—Time to Deal

1. Berenson A. Long shot becomes Pfizer's chief executive. *New York Times.* July 29, 2006. http://www.nytimes.com/2006/07/29/business/29pfizer.html?pagewanted=all&_r=0.

2. Herper M. Drug drought. *Forbes.* October 29, 2007. http://www.forbes.com/part_forbes/2007/1029/044.html. Accessed August 9, 2015.

3. Elkind P, Reingold J. Inside Pfizer's palace coup. *Fortune.* July 28, 2011. http://fortune.com/2011/07/28/inside-pfizers-palace-coup/.

4. Pfizer's heart drug's trial failings detailed. Reuters/*Los Angeles Times.* March 27, 2007. http://articles.latimes.com/2007/mar/27/business/fi-pfizer27. Accessed August 9, 2015.

5. Tran L. Untangling the Vioxx-Celebrex controversy. Legal Electronic Document Archive. Harvard Law School. May 4, 2005. http://dash.harvard.edu/bitstream/handle/1/8889459/Tran05.html?sequence=2.

6. Berenson A. Pfizer to cut its U.S. sales force by 20%. *New York Times.* November 28, 2006. http://www.nytimes.com/2006/11/28/business/28cnd-pfizer.html.

7. LaMattina JL. The impact of mergers on pharmaceutical R&D. *Nature Reviews Drug Discovery.* August 2011;10:559-560. http://www.nature.com/nrd/journal/v10/n8/full/nrd3514.html.

8. Lenzer J. Doctors refuse exhibit space to group campaigning against drug company influence. *BMJ.* 2005; 331(7518): 653. Retrieved on September 13, 2018. https://www.bmj.com/content/suppl/2005/09/22/331.7518.653-a.DC1

9. Tyler D, Pickering K. Sales reps struggle to access doctors. ZS Associates/PM Group. September 30, 2014. http://www.pmlive.com/pharma_intelligence/sales_reps_struggle_to_access_doctors_601905.

10. Sorkin AR, Wilson D. Pfizer agrees to pay $68 billion for rival drug maker Wyeth. *New York Times.* January 25, 2009. http://www.nytimes.com/2009/01/26/business/26drug.html?pagewanted=all&_r=0.

11. Rost P. Pfizer CEO backs Hillary. CounterPunch. October 12, 2007. https://www
.counterpunch.org/2007/10/12/pfizer-ceo-backs-hillary/.

12. Pierce O. Medicare drug planners now lobbyists, with billions at stake. ProPublica.
October 20, 2009. http://www.propublica.org/article/ medicare-drug-planners-now
-lobbyists-with-billions-at-stake-1020.

13. Arnst C. Pfizer CEO: Wyeth takeover will be different. Bloomberg Business. January 26, 2009. https://www.bloomberg.com/news/ articles/2009-01-26/pfizer-ceo-wyeth
-takeover-will-be-different.

14. Abkowitz A. Will merger be Pfizer's miracle drug? *Fortune.* January 27, 2009. http://
money.cnn.com/2009/01/27/news/companies/pipeline.fortune/index.htm.

15. Woodruff B. Pfizer's political CEO: the pharma heavyweight who helped pass Obamacare. *National Review.* July 2, 2012. http://www.national review.com/article/304639/pfizers
-political-ceo-betsy-woodruff.

16. Blumenthal P. The legacy of Billy Tauzin: the White House–PhRMA deal. Sunlight
Foundation. February 12, 2010. https://sunlightfoundation.com/2010/02/12/the-legacy
-of-billy-tauzin-the-white-house-phrma-deal/.

17. Mangan D. Romney: Obamacare grew out of Romneycare. CNBC. October 23, 2015.
https://www.cnbc.com/2015/10/23/mitt-romney-admits-romneycare-had-to-precede
-obamacare.html.

18. Opinion: Big Pharma's ObamaCare big reward. *Wall Street Journal.* February 5, 2015.
http://www.wsj.com/articles/big-pharmas-obamacare-reward-1423180690.

19. Speights K. Is Obamacare a disaster waiting to happen for Big Pharma? *Motley Fool.*
March 23, 2013. http://www.fool.com/investing/general/2013/03/23/is-obamacare-a
-disaster-waiting-to-happen-for-big.aspx.

20. Herper M. Why pharma wants Obamacare. *Forbes.* August 20, 2009. http://www.forbes
.com/2009/08/19/pharmaceuticals-obamacare-reform-business-healthcare-washington
.html.

21. Open Secrets.org. Pharmaceutical Research and Manufacturers Association. 2009.
https://www.opensecrets.org/lobby/clientsum.php?id=D000000504&year=2009.

22. Physician Financial Transparency Reports (Sunshine Act). AMA. http://www.ama
-assn.org/ama/pub/advocacy/topics/sunshine-act-and-physician-financial-transparency
-reports.page?.

23. President Obama: address to Congress on health insurance reform. *New York Times.*
September 10, 2009. https://www.nytimes.com/2009/09/10/us/politics/10obama.text.html.

24. AMA, AARP back House health care bill. CNN. December 23, 2009. http://www.cnn
.com/2009/POLITICS/11/05/health.care/.

25. Clifton E. Exclusive: shady double-agent's Obamacare sabotage. *Salon.* April 8, 2014.
https://www.salon.com/2014/04/08/obamacares_shady_double_agent_how_phrma_
publicly_backed_the_bill_while_ quietly_funding_its_opposition/.

26. Singer EC. GOP attacked "secret" 2010 passage of ACA. They're now doing the same
with the AHCA. Mic. March 23, 2017. https://mic.com/articles/171935/gop-attacked
-secret-2010-passage-of-aca-they-re-now-doing-the-same-with-the-ahca#.h884QxFmp.

27. Kirkpatrick DD, Wilson D. One grand deal too many costs lobbyist his job. *New York Times*. February 12, 2010. http://www.nytimes.com/2010/02/13/health/policy/13pharm .html.

28. Wilson D. Pfizer's chairman and chief resigns unexpectedly. *New York Times*. December 5, 2010. http://www.nytimes.com/2010/12/06/business/06drug.html.

29. Teachout Z. "America's Bitter Pill," by Steven Brill [review]. *New York Times*. January 7, 2015. https://www.nytimes.com/2015/01/11/books/review/americas-bitter-pill-by -steven-brill.html?_r=0.

30. Lenzner R. ObamaCare enriches the health insurance giants and their share-holders. *Forbes*. October 1, 2013. https://www.forbes.com/sites/robertlenzner/ 2013/10/01/obamacare-enriches-only-the-health-insurance-giants-and-their -shareholders/#5fdbb21b3077.

31. Brill S. *America's Bitter Pill*. New York: Random House; 2015:108,119.

32. Brill S. *America's Bitter Pill*. New York: Random House; 2015:101-103.

33. Doctors and the cost of care. *New York Times*. June 13, 2009. http://www.nytimes .com/2009/06/14/opinion/14sun1.html.

34. Fox L, Lee MJ, Mattingly P, Barrett T. Senate rejects proposal to repeal and replace Obamacare. CNN Politics. July 26, 2017. https://www.cnn.com/2017/07/25/politics/ senate-health-care-vote/index.html.

35. *Economist*/YouGov poll. April 2, 2017. https://d25d2506sfb94s. cloudfront.net/ cumulus_uploads/document/divhts7l9t/econTabReport.pdf

Chapter 15—The MIC: "Tapeworm of American Economic Competitiveness"

1. Penn Medicine [news release]. FDA approves gene therapy for inherited blindness developed by the University of Pennsylvania and Children's Hospital of Philadelphia. December 19, 2017. https://www.pennmedicine.org/news/news-releases/2017/december /fda-approves-gene-therapy-for-inherited-blindness-developed-by-university-of -pennsylvania-and-chop.

2. Johnson CY. Gene therapy for inherited blindness sets precedent: $850,000 price tag. *Washington Post*. January 3, 2017. https://www.washingtonpost.com/news/wonk/ wp/2018/01/03/gene-therapy-for-inherited-blindness-sets-precedent-an-850000-price -tag/?utm_term=.2ac5e17a599d.

3. Bayer R, Galea S. Public health in the precision medicine era. *N Engl J Med*. 2015; 373:499-501. http://www.nejm.org/doi/full/10.1056/NEJMp1506241.

4. Kaiser J. Senate spending panel approves $2 billion raise for NIH in 2018. *Science*. September 6, 2017. http://www.sciencemag.org/news/2017/09/senate-spending-panel -approves-2-billion-raise-nih-2018.

5. Pear R. Medical research? Congress cheers. Medical care? Congress brawls. *New York Times*. January 6, 2018. https://www.nytimes.com/2018/01/06/us/politics/congress -medical-research-health-care.html.

6. Carroll AE, Frakt A. The best health care system in the world: which one would you pick? *New York Times*. September 18, 2017. https://www.nytimes.com/interactive/2017/09/18/upshot/best-health-care-system-country-bracket.html.

7. Cha AE. "An embarrassment": U.S. health care far from the top in global study. *Washington Post*. May 18, 2017. https://www.washingtonpost.com/news/to-your-health/wp/2017/05/18/an-embarrassment-u-s-health-care-far-from-the-top-in-global-study/?utm_term=.1185709b60d7.

8. Holm E. Buffett: Medical costs are the tapeworm of American competitiveness. *Wall Street Journal*. May 6, 2017. https://www.wsj.com/livecoverage /berkshire-hathaway-2017-annual-meeting-analysis/card/1494101158.

9. Sorkin AR. Forget taxes, Warren Buffett says. The real problem is health care. *New York Times*. May 8, 2017. https://www.nytimes.com/2017/05/08/business/dealbook/09dealbook-sorkin-warren-buffett.html?_r=0.

10. Morrissey J. Companies respond to an urgent health care need: transportation. *New York Times*. August 9, 2018. https://www.nytimes.com/2018/08/09/business/health-care-transportation.html?utm_source =STAT+Newsletters&utm_campaign=3aee612af2-MR_COPY_08&utm_medium=email&utm_term=0_8cab1d7961-3aee612af2-150335297.

11. Santhanam L. Millennnials rack up the most medical debt, and more frequently. PBS Health. July 26, 2018. https://www.pbs.org/newshour/health/millennials-rack-up-the-most-medical-debt-and-more-frequently.

12. Zumbrun J. Just four large countries have a higher debt burden than the U.S. *Wall Street Journal*/MSN. December 28, 2017. https://www.msn.com/en-us/finance/markets/just-four-large-countries-have-a-higher-debt-burden-than-the-us/ar-BBHuqrN.

13. Scott D. The Republican tax bill is a disaster for income inequality. Vox. December 20, 2017. https://www.vox.com/policy-and-politics/2017/12/20/16790606/gop-tax-vote-2017-income-inequality.

14. Marans D. Paul Ryan: secretary getting $1.50 more a week shows the effect of GOP tax cuts. Huffpost. February 3, 2018. https://www.huffingtonpost.com/entry/paul-ryan-tax-cut-weekly-pay-bump_us_5a76151de4b06ee97af318e8.

15. Jiwani A, Himmelstein D, Woolhandler S, Kahn JG. Billing and insurance-related administrative costs in United States health care: synthesis of micro-costing evidence. *BMC Health Services Research*. 2014; 14:556. https://bmchealthservres.biomedcentral.com/articles/10.1186/s12913-014-0556-7.

16. Hilton R. The collapse of the Soviet Union and Ronald Reagan. Stanford University Department of History. https://wais.stanford.edu/History/history_ussrandreagan.htm.

17. Watkins, T. The economic collapse of the Soviet Union. San Jose University Department of Economics. A forty year rise in Russia's mortality rate. Percentage change in the age-standardized, all-cause mortality rate, ages 25–64. https://www.bing.com/images/search?view=detailV2&ccid=gYpP% 2b7Bg&id=1E977759166871BFC260A71DDA4D85FBCED8DFD7 &thid=OIP.gYpP-7BgTcu50s7u6CCAMgEoDT&mediaurl=https%3a% 2f%2fepeak.info%2fwp-content%2fuploads%2f2017%2f06% 2f1498507011_625_white-americans-mortality-rates-are-rising- something-similar-happened-in-russia-from-1965-to-2005.png&exph =998&expw=1401&q=russian+male+mortality+rate+

rose+30%25+ between+1965+and+1985&simid=607988803566832879&selectedIndex =0&qpvt=russian+male+mortality+rate+rose+30%25+between+1965+and +1985&ajax-hist=0.

18. Shkolnikov VM, Meslé F. The Russian epidemiological crisis as mirrored by mortality trends. RAND CF-124. 1995. https://www.rand.org/pubs/conf_proceedings/CF124/cf124.chap4.html.

19. Donnelly G. Here's why life expectancy dropped in the U.S. again this year. *Fortune.* February 9, 2018. http://fortune.com/2018/02/09/us-life-expectancy-dropped-again/.

20. U.S. health in perspective: shorter lives, poorer health. National Research Council and Institute of Medicine. 2013. http://itsoureconomy.us/2013/01/institute-of-medicine -report-u-s-health-care-failing-as-americans-pay-more-have-shorter-lives-and-poorer -health/.

21. The opioid epidemic: from evidence to impact. Johns Hopkins Bloomberg School of Public Health. October 2017. https://www.jhsph.edu/events/2017/americas-opioid -epidemic/report/2017-JohnsHopkins-Opioid-digital.pdf.

22. Kolata G. Death rates rising for middle-aged white Americans, study finds. *New York Times.* November 2, 2015. https://www.nytimes.com/2015/11/03/health/death-rates -rising-for-middle-aged-white-americans-study-finds.html.

23. Ingraham C. CDC releases grim new opioid overdose figures: "We're talking about more than an exponential increase." *Washington Post.* December 21, 2017. https:// www.washingtonpost.com/news/wonk/wp/2017/12/21/cdc-releases-grim-new-opioid -overdose-figures-were-talking-about-more-than-an-exponential-increase/?utm_term= .fd90c09a9325.

24. The opioid epidemic and socioeconomic disadvantage. Institute for Research on Poverty. University of Wisconsin. Fast Focus Brief No. 32-2018. March 2018. https:// www.irp.wisc.edu/publications/fastfocus/pdfs/FF32-2018.pdf.

25. Cramer M, Cote J. A horrific injury. A heroic rescue effort. And a desperate plea: Please don't call the ambulance, it costs too much. *Boston Globe.* July 2, 2018. https://www .bostonglobe.com/metro/2018/07/02/woman-got-her-leg-caught-gap-orange-line-train -and-then-begged-for-ambulance-because-cost/q6gBPV8ujcfH0qLrQ6HjEJ/story.html.

26. Mangan D. Medical bills are the biggest cause of US bankruptcies: study. CNBC. June 25, 2013. https://www.cnbc.com/id/100840148.

27. Chappell B. U.S. births dip to 30-year low; fertility rate sinks further below replacement level. NPR. May 17, 2018. https://www.npr.org/sections/thetwo -way/2018/05/17/611898421/u-s-births-falls-to-30-year-low-sending-fertility-rate-to -a-record-low.

28. IOM and National Research Council. U.S. health in international perspective. January 1, 2013. http://itsoureconomy.us/2013/01/institute-of-medicine-report-u-s-health-care -failing-as-americans-pay-more-have-shorter-lives-and-poorer-health/.

29. LaVeist TA, Gaskin DJ, Richard P. The economic burden of health inequalities in the United States. Joint Center for Political and Economic Studies. 2003–2006. http:// jointcenter.org/sites/default/files/Economic%20Burden%20of%20Health%20 Inequalities%20Fact%20Sheet.pdf.

30. Fung B. How the U.S. health care system wastes $750 billion annually. *Atlantic.* September 7, 2012. https://www.theatlantic.com/health/archive/2012/09/how-the-us-health-care-system-wastes-750-billion-annually/262106/.

31. OECD data. Insurance spending. 2015. https://data.oecd.org/insurance /insurance-spending.htm. December 3, 2014. http://www.pewresearch.org/fact-tank/2014/12/03/health-affairs-among-11-nations-american-seniors-struggle-more-with-health-costs/.

32. Terhune C. Health care in America: an employment bonanza and a runaway-cost crisis. Kaiser Health News. April 14, 2017. https://khn.org/news/health-care-in-america-an-employment-bonanza-and-a-runaway-cost-crisis/.

33. Becker's Hospital CFO Report. Why U.S. hospital administrative costs are the highest in the world: 7 things to know. September 8, 2014. https://www.beckershospitalreview.com/finance/why-u-s-hospital-administrative-costs-are-among-the-highest-in-the-world-7-things-to-know.html.

34. Du L, Lu W. U.S. health-care system ranks as one of the least efficient. Bloomberg. September 28, 2016. https://www.bloomberg.com/news/articles/2016-09-29/u-s-health-care-system-ranks-as-one-of-the-least-efficient.

35. Modh N. The truth about physician pay. Huffington Post. September 24, 2016. https://www.huffingtonpost.ca/nadia-alam/ontario-doctors-pay_b_8180000.html.

36. 2017 Medscape physician compensation report: US. April 5, 2017. https://www.medscape.com/slideshow/compensation-2017-overview-6008547?src=wnl_physrep_170420_mscpmrk_comp2017&uac=268262SJ&impID=1331481&faf=1#2.

37. South EC et al. Effect of greening vacant land on mental health of community-dwelling adults. *JAMA.* 2018;1(3):e180298. https://jamanetwork.com/journals/jamanetworkopen/fullarticle/2688343.

38. Castele N. Meet the Republican governors who don't want to repeal Obamacare. NPR. January 23, 2017. https://www.npr.org/2017/01/23/510823789/meet-the-republican-governors-who-dont-want-to-repeal-all-of-obamacare.

39. Cambell D, Morris S, Marsh S. NHS faces "humanitarian crisis" as demand rises, British Red Cross warns. January 6, 2017. *Guardian.* https://www.theguardian.com/society/2017/jan/06/nhs-faces-humanitarian-crisis-rising-demand-british-red-cross.

40. Health and social care spending as a percentage of GDP. 2015. Commonwealth Fund. https://www.commonwealthfund.org/chart/2015/health-and-social-care-spending-percentage-gdp.

41. Squires D, Anderson C. U.S. health care from a global perspective. Commonwealth Fund. October 8, 2015. http://www.commonwealthfund.org/publications/issue-briefs/2015/oct/us-health-care-from-a-global-perspective.

42. Health Canada. Mission. https://www.canada.ca/en/health-canada/corporate/about-health-canada/activities-responsibilities/mission-values-activities.html.

43. Health care in Sweden. https://sweden.se/society/health-care-in-sweden.

44. Feldman BS. Big pharmacies are dismantling the industry that keeps U.S. drug costs even sort of under control. Quartz. March 17, 2016. https://qz.com/636823/big-pharmacies-are-dismantling-the-industry-that-keeps-us-drug-costs-even-sort-of-under-control/.

45. Swetlitz I. The Trump administration can't decide whether drug industry middlemen are the enemy—or part of the solution. STAT. August 22, 2018. https://www.statnews.com/2018/08/22/pbms-trump-enemy-solution/?utm_source=STAT+Newsletters&utm_campaign=49cff58daf-MR_COPY_12&utm_medium=email&utm_term=0_8cab1d7961-49cff58daf-150335297.

46. Weigel D. Medicare-for-all has broad support—but pollsters worry it hasn't been tested. *Washington Post.* March 19, 2018. https://www.washingtonpost.com/news/powerpost/wp/2018/03/19/medicare-for-all-enjoys-broad-support-but-pollsters-worry-that-it-hasnt-been-tested/?utm_term=.ac4f2c78a276.

47. Newport F. Majority in U.S. support idea of a federally funded healthcare system. Gallup Poll. March 16, 2016. https://news.gallup.com/poll/191504/majority-support-idea-fed-funded-healthcare-system.aspx.

48. Armour S, Overberg P. Nearly 600 Russia-linked accounts tweeted about the health law. *Wall Street Journal.* September 12, 2018. https://www.wsj.com/articles/nearly-600-russia-linked-accounts-tweeted-about-the-health-law-1536744638.

Afterword

1. Magee M. Qualities of enduring cross-sector partnerships. *Am J Surgery.* January 2003;185(1):26-29. https://www.americanjournalofsurgery.com/article/S0002-9610(02)01143-1/abstract.

Appendix: Time Line of Pfizer's Penalties and Transgressions

1. Mattera P. Pfizer: corporate rap sheet. Corporate Research Project. August 27, 2014. http://www.corp-research.org/pfizer.

2. Mooney RE. 6 concerns cited by the F.T.C. on fixing antibiotic prices; charges involve production of "broad spectrum" drugs attacking many diseases. All counts are denied. Agency sets Oct. 1 hearing here to seek order for companies to desist. 6 drug concerns accused by F.T.C. *New York Times.* August 3, 1958. http://query.nytimes.com/gst/abstract.html?res=9C03E5D8163EE43BBC4B53DFBE668383649EDE.

3. Ranzal E. 3 drug concerns indicted with officers in trust suit; price-fixing laid to 3 drug makers. *New York Times.* August 18, 1961. http://query.nytimes.com/gst/abstract.html?res=9F01E0D81239EE32A2575 BC1A96E9C946091D6CF.

4. 6 drug companies get pricing order; told by agency to reset fee on antibiotic independently. *New York Times.* January 7, 1964. http://query.nytimes.com/gst/abstract.html?res=9E06EEDA1338E13ABC4F53D FB766838F679EDE.

5. Cray DW. Drug makers get maximum fines; Bristol-Myers, Pfizer and Cyanamid must each pay $150,000 on charges. Three counts involved. Case centers on conspiracy to control production and sale of antibiotics. *New York Times.* February 29, 1968. http://query.nytimes.com/gst/abstract.html?res=950DEEDB1138E134BC4151DFB4668383679EDE.

6. Bird D. U.S. demands Pfizer clean waste—not dump it at sea. *New York Times.* October 10, 1971. http://query.nytimes.com/gst/abstract.html ?res=9F05E1DB1F3FE63ABC48 52DFB667838A669EDE.

7. Agreement backed in antitrust pact. *New York Times.* September 27, 1973. http://query .nytimes.com/gst/abstract.html?res=9B05EEDF1E30E63ABC4F51DFBF668388669EDE.

8. Stuart R. Kraftco, Pfizer report payments; disciplinary actions cited companies deny top aides knew of outlays. *New York Times.* March 20, 1976. http://query.nytimes.com/ gst/abstract.html?res=940DE0D9143BE334BC4851DFB566838D669EDE.

9. Rothschild M. Death by prescription. *Progressive.* June 1986;50:6. http://search. opinionarchives.com/Summary/TP/V50I6P18-1.htm.

10. Meier B. Pfizer unit to settle charges of lying about heart valve. *New York Times.* July 2, 1994. http://www.nytimes.com/1994/07/02/business/pfizer-unit-to-settle-charges-of -lying-about-heart-valve.html.

11. The media business: advertising; Pfizer's pact on Plax ads. *New York Times.* February 21, 1991. http://www.nytimes.com/1991/02/21/business/the-media-business-advertising -pfizer-s-pact-on-plax-ads.html.

12. Company news; Pfizer pays fine. *New York Times.* May 2, 1991. http://www.nytimes .com/1991/05/02/business/company-news-pfizer-pays-fine.html.

13. Davis liquid waste superfund. U.S. EPA. January 3, 2011. http://scorecard.goodguide .com/env-releases/land/npl-prp.tcl?epa_id=RID980523070.

14. Freudenheim M. Pfizer is told to end claims about antidepressant's uses. *New York Times.* August 8, 1996. http://www.nytimes.com/1996/08/08/business/pfizer-is-told-to -end-claims-about-antidepressant-s-uses.html.

15. Freudenheim M. Drug makers settle suit on price fixing. *New York Times.* February 10, 1996. http://www.nytimes.com/1996/02/10/business/drug-makers-settle-suit-on -price-fixing.html.

16. Pazniokas M. Pfizer to pay fine. The company has agreed to pay $625,000 for environmental violations, including spills in the Thames River. *Hartford Courant.* December 1, 1998. http://articles.courant.com/1998-12-01/news/9812010156_1_pfizer-spokeswoman -epa-s-new-england-discharges.

17. Status Report: Criminal Fines. March 28, 2001. Department of Justice. http://www .justice.gov/atr/public/speeches/8063.htm.

18. Adams C. FDA warns Pfizer, Pharmacia Celebrex ads are misleading. *Wall Street Journal.* December 12, 2000. http://www.wsj.com/articles/SB976576131675578398.

19. Pfizer to pay $49 million in fraud case. *New York Times.* October 29, 2002. https:// www.nytimes.com/2002/10/29/business/pfizer-to-pay-49-million-in-fraud-case.html.

20. Pear R. Investigators find repeated deception in ads for drugs. *New York Times.* December 4, 2002. http://www.nytimes.com/2002/12/04/us/investigators-find -repeated-deception-in-ads-for-drugs.html.

21. NJ DEP reaches settlement agreement with Pfizer for wastewater monitoring violations. NJ Department of Environmental Protection. August 7, 2002. http://www.nj.gov/ dep/newsrel/releases/02_0065.htm.

22. Shelby, Roden & Cartee announce Solutia, Monsanto and Pharmacia settle Anniston cases for $700 million. Business Wire. August 20, 2003. http://www.businesswire.com/ news/home/20030820005543/en/Shelby-Roden-Cartee-Announce-Solutia-Monsanto -Pharmacia#.VWY9X0umYoM.

23. Petersen M. Pfizer settles an inquiry into ads for an antibiotic. *New York Times*. January 7, 2003. http://www.nytimes.com/2003/01/07/business/pfizer-settles-an-inquiry-into-ads-for-an-antibiotic.html.

24. Warner-Lambert to pay $430 million to resolve criminal and civil health care liability relating to off-label promotion. Department of Justice. May 13, 2004. http://www.justice.gov/archive/opa/pr/2004/May/04_civ_322.htm.

25. $60 million deal in Pfizer suit. Business Day. *New York Times*. August 3, 2004. http://www.nytimes.com/2004/07/03/business/60-million-deal-in-pfizer-suit.html.

26. Pharmaceutical company agrees to pay $22,500 for failing to notify officials of explosion. EPA news release. January 18, 2004. http://www.greengovernmentnews.com/environment/Air/Pharmaceutical+Company+Agrees_to+Pay+%2422%2c500+for+Failing+to+Notify+Officials+of+Explosion.

27. Berenson A, Harris G. Pfizer says 1999 trials revealed risks with Celebrex. *New York Times*. February 1, 2005. http://www.nytimes.com/2005/02/01/business/01drug.html.

28. Saul S. Pfizer settles claims over Bextra and Celebrex. *New York Times*. October 17, 2008. http://www.nytimes.com/2008/10/18/business/18drug.html?_r=0.

29. EPA reaches agreement with Pharmacia and Upjohn. EPA news release. October 14, 2005. https://archive.epa.gov/epapages/newsroom_archive/newsreleases/ea0147c7b73cf7d6852570bc00711692.html.

30. Pfizer Inc. Pharmacia subsidiaries reach $34.7 million settlement with DOJ; resolve allegations of improper activities prior to acquisition by Pfizer. April 2, 2007. http://press.pfizer.com/press-release/pharmacia-subsidiaries-reach-347-million-settlement-doj-resolve-allegations-improper-a.

31. Update 1—Pfizer to pay $975,000 for clean air violations. Reuters. June 23, 2008. https://www.reuters.com/article/pfizer-fine/update-1-pfizer-to-pay-975000-for-clean-air-violations-idUSN2334031520080623.

32. Justice News. Associate Attorney General Tom Perrelli at Pfizer settlement press conference. Department of Justice. September 2, 2009. http://www.justice.gov/asg/speech/associate-attorney-general-tom-perrelli-pfizer-settlement-press-conference.

33. Wyeth. Financial report. 2007. http://library.corporate-ir.net/library/78/781/78193/items/283760/Wyeth_FR_07_lo.pdf.

34. Stephens J. Pfizer to pay $75 million to settle Nigerian Trovan drug-testing suit. *Washington Post*. July 31, 2009. http://www.washingtonpost.com/wp-dyn/content/article/2009/07/30/AR2009073001847.html.

35. Freeley J, Lawrence J. Pfizer to pay $142.1 million over Neurontin marketing. Bloomberg Business. January 28, 2011. http://www.bloomberg.com/news/articles/2011-01-28/pfizer-ordered-to-pay-142-1-million-in-damages-over-neurontin-marketing.

36. Pollack A, Wilson D. A Pfizer whistle-blower is awarded $1.4 million. *New York Times*. April 2, 2010. http://www.nytimes.com/2010/04/03/business/03pfizer.html.

37. Wilson D. Pfizer gives details on payments to doctors. *New York Times*. March 31, 2010. http://www.nytimes.com/2010/04/01/business/01payments.html.

38. Pfizer to pay $14.5 million for illegal marketing of drug Detrol. Department of

Justice. October 21, 2011. http://www.justice.gov/opa/pr/pfizer-pay-145-million-illegal -marketing-drug-detrol.

39. DHHS communication to Pfizer. August 29, 2011. In: McCutchin K. Social media: changing the way the industry interacts one click at a time. JDSUPRA. October 1, 2011. https://www.jdsupra.com/legalnews/social-media-changing-the-way-the-indus-15424/.

40. US Securities and Exchange Commission. August 7, 2012. SEC charges Pfizer with FCPA violations. http://www.sec.gov/News/PressRelease/Detail/PressRelease/1365171483696.

41. Pfizer consumer healthcare, CSPI resolve Centrum labeling issues [news release]. Center for Science in the Public Interest. July 5, 2012. http://www.cspinet.org/new/201207051 .html.

42. Pfizer Inc. Third quarter 2012 results, p. 21. http://www.sec.gov/Archives/edgar/ data/78003/000115752312005612/a50457010ex99.htm.

43. A.G. Schneiderman announces settlement with Pfizer to end deceptive advertising practices and off-label promotion of immunosuppressive drug Rapamune. August 6, 2014, http://www.ag.ny.gov/press-release/ag-schneiderman-announces-settlement-pfizer-end -deceptive-advertising-practices-and.

44. Bray C. Pfizer and Allergan call off merger after tax-rule changes. *New York Times*. April 7, 2016. https://www.nytimes.com/2016/04/07/business/dealbook/pfizer-allergan-merger.html. Retrieved April 7, 2016.

Index

Celgene, 295
Center for the Study of Drug Development
(CSDD)
"drug lag" and, 189–194, 219–222
founding of, 187–189
General Agreement on Tariff and Trade
and, 199
Lasagna's background, 184–187
as leading to MIC as equal parts politics and
science, 199–200
patent law changes and, 194–197
Centers for Disease Control and Prevention
ADHD and, 164, 173, 174
on AIDS, 212–213
on life expectancy, 306
on New England Compounding Center, 29
reform for, 320–321
WWII funding, 66
Centers for Medicare and Medicaid Services.
See also Medicaid; Medicare
AMA and billing by, 12
billing and coding, 116
Joint Commission on Accreditation of
Healthcare Organizations and, 99, 100
cGMP, 244–245
Chain, Ernst Boris, 63–64
Chandler, Bob, 250–251
Charter Med, 285
Chassin, Mark, 99, 103
Chemie Grünenthal, 43
Chicco, Gianfranco, 250–251
Children and Adults with Attention Deficit
Hyperactivity Disorder (CHADD), 165,
168
cholesterol drugs. *See* statins
Christian Broadcasting Network, 207–208
Christian Coalition, 208
Christian Herald, 157
Christian Medical Society, 205
Christian Right, 201–222
Bush (George H. W.) administration and,
216–217, 221
Bush (George W.) administration and, 221
Catholic Church and, 203–205
Evangelical Christians on health policy,
205–209
pharmaceutical industry and, 217–221
Reagan administration and, 209–216
religious orthodoxy vs. scientific fact, 201–202
Trump administration and, 202–203,
221–222

CIBA, 167
Cigna
Express Scripts and, 287–288
Medicare Advantage investigation, 121
profit margin of, 122
Circulation, 230
Citizens for the Treatment of High Blood
Pressure, 84
citric acid, early use of, 23
Civil Rights Act (1964), 140, 143
Clarke, A. Grant, 156
Clemente, Constantine "Lou"
at Pfizer, 247–248, 272, 277, 324
TRIPS and, 197–200
Cleveland, Clement, 78
ClinicalTrials.gov, 240–241, 316
Clinton, Bill
health care reform attempt, 108, 146–147,
294
on Medicare, 278, 279
pharmaceutical advertising and, 252
on Tuskegee Study, 229
Clinton, Hillary, 292
Clowes, George H. (Alec), 25–26
coding and billing system
data management by PBMs vs., 284–288,
313–314
hospital administration and, 96–97,
115–117, 122
Codman, Ernest, 100–101
Cohen, Wilbur, 144
Collier, Peter, 31
Collins, Chris, 91
Collins, Francis, 73
Columbia University/Columbia-Presbyterian
Medical Center, 103–105, 110
compensation
hospital CEOs, 104
physicians in United States vs. Canada, 309
physicians' wages during Great Depression,
105
compounding pharmacies, 29–31
Conant, James B., 56
Concerta (Johnson & Johnson), 170–171, 174
Congress. *See* government funding of medical
research; *individual legislation*
Conifer, 117
Conners, Keith, 166–171, 173–174
Connor, John T., 50, 67
Constant Gardener, The (film), 1, 231
Continus, 175